CW01371004

HISTORY OF
THE SECOND WORLD WAR

UNITED KINGDOM MEDICAL SERIES

Editor-in-Chief:

Sir Arthur S. MacNalty, k.c.b., m.d., f.r.c.p., f.r.c.s.

THE EMERGENCY MEDICAL SERVICES

BY
Lieut. Colonel C. L. DUNN,
C.I.E., I.M.S. (ret.)

VOLUME I
England and Wales

The Naval & Military Press Ltd

Published by

The Naval & Military Press Ltd
Unit 5 Riverside, Brambleside
Bellbrook Industrial Estate
Uckfield, East Sussex
TN22 1QQ England

Tel: +44 (0)1825 749494

www.naval-military-press.com
www.nmarchive.com

In reprinting in facsimile from the original, any imperfections are inevitably reproduced and the quality may fall short of modern type and cartographic standards.

FOREWORD
by the Editor-in-Chief

THE EMERGENCY MEDICAL SERVICES

THE two volumes on the work of the Emergency Medical Services, of which this is the first, have been prepared, written and edited by Lieut. Colonel C. L. Dunn, C.I.E., I.M.S. (ret.), who had practical experience of the Service as a Regional Hospital Officer in the first two years of the war.

In this responsible task Colonel Dunn has been aided by a number of collaborators with special experience of their individual subjects. Here thanks are particularly due to Dame Katherine Watt, Dr. Janet Vaughan, the late Sir Philip Panton, the late Dr. A. E. Barclay, Sir Robert Stanton Woods and Lieut. Colonel E. S. Goss, whose contributions appear in Vol. I. In Vol. II, Sir Andrew Davidson, Chief Medical Officer of the Department of Health for Scotland and Dr. A. K. Bowman are responsible for the history of the Emergency Medical Services in Scotland, Dr. J. Boyd and Mr. S. E. Taylor for the history of the Emergency Medical Services in Northern Ireland and the medical officers of health concerned for contributions on the air raids on industrial centres, 1940–1 and the 'Baedeker' raids, 1942.

Under the black clouds of threatening war, much work had to be devoted by the Ministry of Health to medical emergency services, hospital provision for air raid and military casualties, and arrangements for the evacuation from urban centres and reception in other areas of school children and others.

Up to June 1938, the provision of casualty clearing hospitals in the event of war had been the concern of local authorities as part of their air raid precautions schemes, while the cost of providing base hospitals was to be borne solely by the Exchequer. At the beginning of June 1938, the Ministry of Health assumed responsibility for the organisation of an emergency hospital scheme for the reception and treatment of large numbers of casualties in England and Wales. The Department of Health for Scotland and the Ministry of Home Affairs in Northern Ireland assumed similar responsibilities for their countries. This arrangement abolished the unworkable distinction between responsibility for casualty clearing hospitals and for base hospitals. By the provisions of the Civil Defence Act, 1939, the Minister of Health and the Secretary of State for Scotland were made responsible for securing that in the event of war, facilities would be available for the treatment of casualties occurring in Great Britain from hostile attack.

The Ministry of Health had now to set up a regional organisation and a central organisation in Whitehall for this new and onerous responsibility. In each Region a Hospital Officer or Officers appointed by the Ministry worked on the preparation of the scheme in co-operation with the local authorities and their medical officers of health. The problems on the medical side were so complex and various that a medical organisation was also planned in five regions of England by a redistribution of part of the Ministry of Health's central medical staff in Whitehall, at the head of which was a Principal Medical Officer. This Officer and the Hospital Officer formed part of the Departmental Staff at the Regional Commissioner's headquarters town and worked in close co-operation with him. Through the Principal Medical Officer and the Hospital Officer, headquarters at Whitehall was kept in close touch with the work of the local authorities and of the voluntary hospitals in preparing for air raid casualties and evacuation or reception of women and children. These officers were continually advising local authorities and local organisations on medical problems throughout the war.

Centrally, a special department of the Ministry of Health was set up to deal with air raid precautions. On the lay side there was a Principal Assistant Secretary with an Assistant Secretary, Principals and clerical staff. On the medical side, under the supervision of the Chief Medical Officer, Dr. J. H. Hebb, C.B., C.B.E. (afterwards Sir John Hebb), Director-General of Medical Services at the Ministry of Pensions, was seconded to the Ministry of Health and was appointed Director-General of Emergency Medical Services. Sir John Hebb's expert knowledge of hospitals and their administration proved of the utmost value. Working long hours and never sparing himself, his health failed and he was forced to retire in 1941. In the last few months of his life he prepared for this History an account of the initial planning and organisation of the Emergency Medical Service which has been utilised by Colonel Dunn in the first volume.

Sir John Hebb was succeeded as Director-General of the Emergency Medical Services by Sir Francis Fraser, M.D., F.R.C.P., under whose able direction the Service was maintained and developed during the remaining years of the war.

The Emergency Medical Services Department directed and organised the hospital services. The liaison with local authority hospitals was easily effected through the medical officers of health of counties and county boroughs. It was necessary, also, to organise the voluntary hospitals in each Region. This had never been done before, except in certain areas on a limited scale. The organisation was effected through the public spirit of the voluntary hospital authorities and their medical staffs in London and the provinces. The planning and the difficulties were enormous for, above all, the organisation had to be elastic and capable of providing for the casualties of an area or adjoining area in the event of destruction of hospitals by enemy bombing. It provided for military casualties as well as for the civilian population. In addition, there were the ancillary services to build up—the Civil Defence Services, the Ambulance Services, Medical Supplies, the Emergency Hospital Pathological Services, the Blood Transfusion Service which saved thousands of lives, Radiology, Physical Medicine, the provision of medical personnel and the Nursing Services.

It was inevitable in a task of this magnitude that errors would be made, that provision should be made for possible eventualities that did not arise and that the medical needs of the war would take a different course to initial anticipations. Reading the history of the Emergency Medical Services, one finds that it is a narrative in which the best medical and scientific knowledge, self-sacrifice, devotion to duty and the co-operation of all concerned played a worthy part.

Hitherto, the work of the Emergency Medical Services in England and Wales has been chiefly mentioned. The organisations in Scotland and Northern Ireland were planned on similar lines in co-operation with the English Authorities and are described fully in Colonel Dunn's second volume. Here also appear accounts of the air raids on industrial centres, 1940–1 and of the 'Baedeker' raids of 1942.

THE EMERGENCY MEDICAL SERVICES AND CIVIL DEFENCE IN THE WAR

The intensive stage of the Battle of Britain lasted from August 3 to October 31, 1940, during which the country was exposed to heavy daylight air raids and the Channel ports were evacuated of large numbers of sick persons and others. At the same time there were numerous air raid casualties. Thereafter the enemy resorted to night bombing and heavy attacks were made on London, Coventry, Birmingham, Hull, Plymouth, and other large cities. This phase lasted until about May 1941, and for the rest of the year the intensity of air raids on Great Britain greatly diminished. Throughout the period of intensive air raids the Emergency Hospital medical organisation was severely tested. It had been designed, principally, to deal with air raid casualties and to provide for an outflow of wounded from receiving hospitals in the dangerous areas to hospitals in the periphery and to others still more remote. In practice the method proved highly successful. As an example, in one heavy raid on London in the spring of 1941, all but a few of the patients had been operated upon, or otherwise treated, and removed to peripheral hospitals by the afternoon of the day after the attack. The emergency hospitals were also used to a large extent to accommodate chronic sick who were found in shelters and rest centres in the London area, and for people who needed to be evacuated from the coastal area in view of the possibility of invasion.

In 1942 came the 'Baedeker' raids on cathedral cities of England—Exeter, Bath, Norwich, York and Canterbury—acts of sheer vandalism with no military objective. In 1943 there was a comparative lull in the bombing of this country, but in the following year during the liberation of France came the flying bombs and the long-range rockets, (V1 and V2). The last rocket bomb fell on England in March 1945.

The Civil Defence organisation of this country stood up nobly to these repeated onslaughts. Much of its preliminary work had been devoted to arrangements for dealing with aerial gas attacks. Gas was not used, but the organisation and the distribution of gas masks to the civil population were probably an insurance against this inhuman type of warfare. Through the provision of shelters and the precautions taken for their healthy conditions, by the provision of rest centres, national fire service, first-aid centres and transport, the effects of the bombing raids were minimised as far as possible. The public health and medical work done by medical officers of health, doctors, nurses, sanitary inspectors, health visitors and others was beyond all praise. For example, the bombardment of water-mains and sewers involved great risk of outbreaks of enteric disease, yet owing to the precautions taken by the public health authorities, no cases of enteric fever occurred which could be assigned to this cause. The Women's Voluntary Service rendered great assistance. A high tribute must be paid to the efficiency of the ambulance service and to the courage, zeal and resourcefulness of the drivers, many of whom were young women. Countless epic stories are related of their heroism and exploits. Some died at the wheel; others carried on when wounded, thinking not of themselves but of the patients they were conveying to hospital. All were imbued with the spirit of patriotism and self-sacrifice.

This outline of the history of the organisation and part played by the Emergency Medical Services in the Second World War indicates the vast field which Colonel Dunn and his collaborators have covered in these two volumes of this History. It is a history of team work, where lay and medical administrators worked together for the prevention of disease, the saving of life and the alleviation of suffering under the unprecedented and deadly conditions of modern warfare. The failures of the Service were few, its successes conspicuous. Here stands the record, a plain tale of great achievement.

A. S. M.

EDITORIAL BOARD

Sir CYRIL FLOWER, C.B., F.S.A. (*Chairman*)

Sir WELDON DALRYMPLE-CHAMPNEYS, Bart., D.M., F.R.C.P.
Sir FRANCIS R. FRASER, M.D., F.R.C.P.
} *Ministry of Health*

Sir ANDREW DAVIDSON, M.D., F.R.C.P. Ed., F.R.C.S. Ed.
A. K. BOWMAN, M.B., Ch.B., F.R.F.P.S.
} *Department of Health for Scotland*

J. BOYD, M.D., F.R.C.P.I. — *Government of Northern Ireland*

SIR HAROLD HIMSWORTH, K.C.B., M.D., F.R.C.P.
JANET VAUGHAN, O.B.E., D.M., F.R.C.P.
} *Medical Research Council*

Surgeon Vice Admiral Sir C. E. GREESON, K.B.E., C.B., M.D., Ch.B., K.H.P.
} *Admiralty*

Lt. General Sir NEIL CANTLIE, K.B.E., C.B., M.C., M.B., F.R.C.S., K.H.S.
Brigadier H. T. FINDLAY, M.B., Ch.B.
} *War Office*

Air Marshal J. M. KILPATRICK, O.B.E., M.B., B.Ch., D.P.H., K.H.P.
} *Air Ministry*

Brigadier H. B. LATHAM
A. B. ACHESON, ESQ., C.M.G.
} *Cabinet Office*

Editor-in-Chief: Sir ARTHUR S. MACNALTY, K.C.B., M.D., F.R.C.P., F.R.C.S.

Secretary: W. FRANKLIN MELLOR

The following persons served on the Editorial Board for varying periods:

The Rt. Hon. R. A. Butler, P.C., M.A., F.R.G.S., M.P. (*Chairman*); Brigadier General Sir James E. Edmonds, C.B., C.M.G., D.Litt. (*Committee of Imperial Defence*); Surgeon Vice Admiral Sir Sheldon F. Dudley, K.C.B., O.B.E., M.D., F.R.C.P., F.R.C.S. Ed., F.R.S.; Surgeon Vice Admiral Sir Henry St. Clair Colson, K.C.B., C.B.E., F.R.C.P. (*Admiralty*); Lt. General Sir William P. MacArthur, K.C.B., D.S.O., O.B.E., M.D., B.Ch., D.Sc., F.R.C.P.; Lt. General Sir Alexander Hood, G.B.E., K.C.B., M.D., F.R.C.P., LL.D.; Major General H. M. J. Parry, C.B., O.B.E.; Brigadier L. T. Poole, C.B., D.S.O., M.C., M.B., Ch.B.; Brigadier J. S. K. Boyd, O.B.E., M.D., F.R.S. (*War Office*); Air Marshal Sir Harold E. Whittingham, K.C.B., K.B.E., M.B., Ch.B., F.R.C.P., F.R.C.S., LL.D.; Air Marshal Sir Andrew Grant, K.B.E., C.B., M.B., Ch.B., D.P.H.; Air Marshal Sir P. C. Livingston, K.B.E., C.B., A.F.C., F.R.C.S. (*Air Ministry*); Sir Edward Mellanby, K.C.B., M.D., F.R.C.P., F.R.S. (*Medical Research Council*); Professor J. M. Mackintosh, M.A., M.D., F.R.C.P. (*Department of Health for Scotland*); Lt. Colonel J. S. Yule, O.B.E., Philip Allen, Esq., G. Godfrey Phillips, Esq., M. T. Flett, Esq., A. M. R. Topham, Esq., D. F. Hubback, Esq. (*Cabinet Office*).

EDITORIAL COMMITTEE

Sir ARTHUR S. MACNALTY, K.C.B., M.D., F.R.C.P., F.R.C.S.
(*Chairman*)

Surgeon Commander J. L. S. COULTER, D.S.C., M.R.C.S., L.R.C.P. (Barrister at Law) } *Admiralty*

Professor F. A. E. CREW, D.Sc., M.D., F.R.C.P. Ed., F.R.S. } *War Office*

Squadron Leader S. C. REXFORD-WELCH, M.R.C.S., L.R.C.P. } *Air Ministry*

A. K. BOWMAN, M.B., Ch.B., F.R.F.P.S. { *Department of Health for Scotland*

J. BOYD, M.D., F.R.C.P.I. { *Government of Northern Ireland*

F. H. K. GREEN, C.B.E., M.D., F.R.C.P.   *Medical Research Council*

J. ALISON GLOVER, C.B.E., M.D., F.R.C.P.   *Ministry of Education*

A. SANDISON, O.B.E., M.D.   *Ministry of Pensions*

Lt. Colonel C. L. DUNN, C.I.E., I.M.S. (ret.)
V. ZACHARY COPE, M.D., M.S., F.R.C.S. } *Ministry of Health*

Secretary: W. FRANKLIN MELLOR

The following persons served on the Editorial Committee for varying periods:

Surgeon Commander J. J. KEEVIL, D.S.O., M.D.; Surgeon Lieutenant L. D. de LAUNAY, M.B., B.S.; Surgeon Lieutenant Commander N. M. MCARTHUR, M.D.; Surgeon Commander A. D. SINCLAIR, M.B., Ch.B. (*Admiralty*); Colonel S. LYLE CUMMINS, C.B., C.M.G., LL.D., M.D. (*War Office*); Wing Commander R. ODDIE, M.B., B.Ch.; Wing Commander E. B. DAVIES, M.B., B.Ch.; Squadron Leader R. MORTIMER, M.B., B.S.; Squadron Leader H. N. H. GENESE, M.R.C.S., L.R.C.P. (*Air Ministry*); Charles E. NEWMAN, M.D., F.R.C.P.; N. G. HORNER, M.D., F.R.C.P., F.R.C.S. (*Ministry of Health*).

PREFACE

IN order to present a readable account of the inception and growth of the Emergency Medical Services and the functions they fulfilled during the war, the story must of necessity be told more or less chronologically. It has been found, however, that certain features can be more conveniently dealt with in special chapters.

A full account of the widespread organisation, with so many diverse but nevertheless closely linked activities, which formed the Emergency Medical Services, would fill many volumes. This narrative does not attempt to do more than give a concise account of the work of these services, an object which could only be attained by a general description of the organisation and its functions, illustrated by selected examples of the activities of some of its more important component parts. The application of this principle was found to be specially necessary in compiling chapters 4–6 of Volume I, Part I, and Part III of Volume II.

Like the other volumes of the Official Medical History, those on the Emergency Medical Services are divided into three groups—Administrative, Campaigns and Clinical. Volume I, Part I, describes the administration, evolution and work of these services during the period of the war in England and Wales, while Part II contains special chapters on The Provision of Medical Personnel, The Ancillary Hospital Services, The Ambulance Services and The Civil Defence Casualty Services. Volume II is divided into three parts: Parts I and II dealing with the Emergency Medical Services in Scotland and Northern Ireland, while Part III, which may be compared with the Campaigns Group in the volumes dealing with the combatant services, describes the working of the Emergency Medical Services in London and other large industrial areas in the United Kingdom under the strain of intensive raids.

The clinical contributions will be found in the clinical volumes, it having been decided that the description of this aspect of the work of the Emergency Medical Services should be recorded together with that of the other Services, an arrangement which avoids a great deal of overlapping.

The chapters in Volume I, Part II, and Volume II, Part III have been contributed largely by those who were directly concerned with the events described, and a debt of gratitude is due to them for their great help and co-operation in connexion with the History. These contemporary contributions are obviously of far greater value than any accounts written at a later period.

London, December 1951. C. L. D.

CONTENTS

PART I: THE EVOLUTION AND OPERATION OF THE EMERGENCY MEDICAL SERVICES

	PAGE
INTRODUCTION: HISTORICAL REVIEW, 1923—MARCH 1935	3
CHAPTER 1: EARLY STEPS TO CREATE A CASUALTY ORGANISATION, MARCH 1935 TO SEPTEMBER 1938	7
CHAPTER 2: EXPANSION OF THE EMERGENCY MEDICAL SERVICES, OCTOBER 1938 TO SEPTEMBER 1939	29
CHAPTER 3: FURTHER EXPANSION AND ORGANISATION, SEPTEMBER 1939 TO APRIL 1940	61
CHAPTER 4: THE PERIOD OF ACTIVE OPERATIONS IN BRITAIN, MAY 1940 TO JUNE 1941	96
CHAPTER 5: PERIOD OF CONSOLIDATION AND IMPROVEMENT, JULY 1941 TO DECEMBER 1943	125
CHAPTER 6: PERIOD OF ACTIVE OPERATIONS JANUARY 1944 TO END OF HOSTILITIES	149

APPENDICES TO PART I

1. Official publications on Air Raid Precautions issued by the Home Office (Air Raid Precautions Department) . . . 206
2. Consultant Advisers at Headquarters and Special Centres . . . 207
3. Civilian Transferred Patients (Form E.M.S. 116), January 1, 1940, to December 31, 1945 (England and Wales) . . . 209
4. Classes of E.M.S. Patients (Form E.M.S. 227 revised) . . . 210
5. Extract from Memorandum 'Medical Arrangements in Region IV and Notes on the Action to be taken on Invasion or Severe Enemy Action from the Air'. (April 1942) . . . 212
6. Classes of E.M.S. Patients in Hospital . . . 216
7. Estimated number of Patients admitted to E.M.S. Hospitals for Disabilities not due to Enemy Action, 1943–5 . . . 217
8. Estimated number of Patients admitted to E.M.S. Hospitals for Disabilities due to Enemy Action, 1939–45 . . . 218

CONTENTS

PART II: THE ANCILLARY SERVICES

	PAGE
CHAPTER 7: THE CIVIL DEFENCE SERVICES	221
CHAPTER 8: THE AMBULANCE SERVICES	276
CHAPTER 9: MEDICAL SUPPLIES	309
CHAPTER 10: THE EMERGENCY HOSPITAL PATHOLOGICAL SERVICES	326
CHAPTER 11: THE CIVILIAN BLOOD TRANSFUSION SERVICE	334
CHAPTER 12: RADIOLOGY	356
CHAPTER 13: PHYSICAL MEDICINE	366
CHAPTER 14: THE PROVISION OF MEDICAL PERSONNEL	388
CHAPTER 15: THE CIVIL NURSING SERVICES IN WAR-TIME	438
INDEX	455

LIST OF PLATES

Plate *Following page*

I. Ward in Hutted Hospital
II. Searching for Radium, Marie Curie Hospital, Hampstead
III. Searching for Radium, Marie Curie Hospital, Hampstead
IV. Searching for Radium, Marie Curie Hospital, Hampstead
V. Casualties from Dunkirk
VI. Casualties from Dunkirk
VII. Guy's Hospital Underground Operating Theatre
VIII. Middlesex Hospital Underground Operating Theatre
IX. Underground Male Ward, City Corporation Hospital, Cheapside
X. Putney Dance Hall Incident, November 7, 1943
XI. Pilotless Plane Crash on Hospital, June 17, 1944
XII. Walking Patients being removed to Ambulances, June 17, 1944
XIII. Checking Bed Patients after Evacuation of Hospital hit July 6, 1944
XIV. Evacuation of Patients from a Damaged Hospital, July 6, 1944
XV. Patients entering Bus Ambulance after Evacuation of Hospital, July 8, 1944
XVI. Casualty being lowered from Damaged House after Pilotless Plane Strike, June 23, 1944

} 112

XVII. Man rescued after Pilotless Plane Strike, after Burial in Debris for 3½ hours, June 24, 1944
XVIII. Casualty being rescued from Debris after Pilotless Plane Strike
XIX. Members of Civil Defence Force attending Casualties after Pilotless Plane Strike in a London Road, July 11, 1944
XX. First Aid on the spot after Pilotless Plane Strike in London
XXI. Alsatian Dog searching for Casualties after Pilotless Plane Strike
XXII. Woman rescued from Roof of Public-house after Pilotless Plane Strike
XXIII. Casualty dug out from under Debris; he was buried for over an hour

} 208

xvi   LIST OF PLATES

Plate   *Following page*

XXIV. American Ambulance in Action after Convent and Block of Flats had been hit
XXV. Rescuers freeing Casualties from Debris in Farringdon Street after Long-Range Rocket Strike on March 8, 1945 .
XXVI. View of Damage caused by Long-Range Rocket in Islington .
XXVII. A Mobile Unit at Work in a Basement .
XXVIII. A Mobile Operating Theatre—Preston .
XXIX. L.M.S. Brake Van fitted for Stretcher Cases . } 208

XXX. Exterior of Casualty Evacuation Train—Southern Railway .
XXXI. L.M.S. Kitchen Compartment .
XXXII. L.M.S. Kitchen Compartment .
XXXIII. Stretcher Van fitted with Stretchers—Southern Railway .
XXXIV. Bus Ambulance being loaded—London Passenger Transport Board .
XXXV. Part of American Ambulance Fleet, Great Britain .
XXXVI. Redeveloping Thigh Muscles .
XXXVII. Infantile Paralysis in both Arms—Recovery of Muscles by using Loom .
XXXVIII. Knee Injuries—Restoring Strength of Thigh Muscles .
XXXIX. Restoring Strength of Calf Muscles .
XL. Daily Exercises carried out in Bed .
XLI. Watch Repairing . } 304

LIST OF FIGURES

		Page
1.	Layout of a Hutted Hospital .	36
2. 3.	}Plans of three of the Huts .	38
4.	Sketch Map of London Sectors .	45
5.	Plan of a Combined First-Aid Post and Cleansing Station .	224
6.	Blood Transfusion Standard Needle for Sternal Puncture .	339
7.	Standard Flask with Rubber Bung and Glass Tubing .	340
8.	Standard Bung replaced by Perforation Cap .	340
9.	Wire Gauze Filter .	342
10.	Gas Mantle Filter .	342
	Graph: Park Prewett Hospital Admissions and Operations D Day to D+96 .	167

PART I

The Evolution and Operation of the Emergency Medical Services

INTRODUCTION

HISTORICAL REVIEW: 1923 to March 1935

THE Emergency Medical Services may be said to have been born in June 1938, but no account of their growth through childhood and adolescence to maturity would be complete without some reference to the events which led to their conception and to the discussions on which the policy governing their evolution was based.

COMMITTEE OF IMPERIAL DEFENCE

Standing Sub-Committee on Air Raid Precautions. During the years succeeding the War of 1914–18, the policy of the Government was to promote disarmament by example and it was not considered desirable openly to discuss measures for defence; however, the need for studying the provisions which would have to be made in preparation for another war was not completely forgotten, although such an eventuality was then considered highly improbable. A sub-committee of the Committee of Imperial Defence was therefore constituted fully to examine the vulnerability of the British Isles to air attack from the Continent of Europe. In the report of this sub-committee the extreme danger to the country —and to London in particular—was emphasised, with the result that in January 1924, the Committee of Imperial Defence decided that a further sub-committee should be set up 'to inquire into the question of air raid precautions'. This was duly appointed and was composed of representatives of the three Defence Departments, the Ministry of Health, the Office of Works, the Treasury, the Post Office, the Board of Trade and the Ministry of Transport, with the Permanent Under Secretary of State (Home Office) as chairman. In the following year, this sub-committee produced its First Report containing a recommendation, which the Committee of Imperial Defence accepted, that it should be placed on a more permanent basis as a standing sub-committee, and as such it continued to function, with few changes in membership, until 1935.

The 'Brock' Committee, 1924. In the meantime, another sub-committee of the Committee of Imperial Defence, with Sir Laurence Brock as chairman had considered and reported in July 1924, among other matters, on the part to be played by the Ministry of Health in the distribution of medical personnel and in advising the Services as to suitable localities for hospitals, etc. This sub-committee endorsed the measures that had been approved as a result of war experience, and recommended that an organisation should be at the disposal of the Government to advise it, though without executive functions.

It proposed the re-appointment of the Central Medical War Committee of the British Medical Association to deal with questions of medical personnel, and the Committee of Reference of the Royal Colleges of Physicians and Surgeons to deal specifically with the staffing of the London hospitals.

The Ministry of Health's Preliminary Report—1925–6. In the same year the standing sub-committee requested the Ministry of Health to draw up a casualty scheme for the London area to provide for:

(*a*) The medical treatment of casualties, including the co-ordination of the existing ambulance services and their expansion if necessary;

(*b*) Hospital accommodation;

(*c*) The evacuation of wounded outside the area of bombardment.

The necessary inquiries had to be undertaken under a strict rule of secrecy; consequently information was obtained only with considerable difficulty and was limited in scope; but the sub-committee was able to issue a preliminary report in February 1926, containing the Ministry of Health's recommendations as to the most suitable method by which the ultimate object in view might be attained. The report showed that even at this time the Ministry of Health were aware of the kind of organisation which would be required, and also that a much more modest view was then held of the number of casualties to be provided for than in 1938. In 1923–6, the Royal Air Force considered that for each ton of bombs dropped the casualties would be about 17 killed and 33 wounded, and that about 100 tons of bombs would be dropped on the first day of the attack. This provided a figure of 3,300 wounded which was expected to decline to about half that number by the third day, remain at that level on each succeeding day for a month and thereafter gradually and continually to fall. It was also thought that the moral effect would be infinitely more serious than any material damage to be expected. At this time, it was estimated that during the first month there would be some 50,000 injured, of whom 36,000 would require admission to hospital. Assuming an average of thirty days' stay, 36,000 beds would be required.

The existing accommodation in the voluntary and local authority hospitals was then reviewed, but the question of any further accommodation was, for the time being, deferred. It was found that 8,245 beds in the voluntary hospitals in the London area were in use and that at the most, 4,000 beds in these hospitals could be made available for casualties if the necessary equipment could be supplied from store. In the local authority hospitals, it was expected that 11,000 to 12,000 beds might be made available, but only if most of the normal occupants of these hospitals could be accommodated elsewhere. It was also considered that 6,000 beds in the mental hospitals could be provided in a few hours; a most optimistic assumption. Thus, 21,000 beds were pictured as being quickly available for casualties. To meet the deficiency of 15,000 beds, it was suggested that schools might be adapted as hospitals.

There seems to have been no clear conception at this time of what the term 'evacuation of the wounded outside the area of bombardment' actually meant. It was realised, however, that if the intention was to keep the metropolis clear of wounded, a somewhat different scheme from that being explored would be required. Some evacuation would, in any case, be necessary to keep beds available at central hospitals and it was thought that this could most conveniently be done by motor ambulance convoys for a distance up to 40 or 50 miles.

The ambulances available were then reviewed. For duty in the London area it was found that 25 L.C.C. and 87 Metropolitan Asylums Board ambulances, and 5 ambulance steamers, with a carrying capacity of 160 cot cases, belonging to the latter body, might be regarded as available and that by drawing on the ambulances belonging to the Joint Council of the British Red Cross and the St. John Ambulance Brigade, a total of 150 vehicles could be mobilised in twenty-four hours. There were also 110 ambulances belonging to other local authorities which could be regarded as a reserve.

The lack of uniformity in design of these ambulances and stretchers, which would not be interchangeable, was criticised and the report suggested that steps to remedy this defect would be necessary. For the evacuation of casualties from the area of bombardment it was estimated that 225 ambulances each carrying 4 cot cases would be adequate, and among other suggestions for the provision of this fleet, the conversion of motor buses into ambulances was mooted.

An operational scheme consisting of a first-aid section, an ambulance section and an independent hospital section was set out in some detail, but the opinion was expressed that this organisation might be more efficiently administered on a military rather than on a civil basis.

The War Office, however, did not accept this view and it was finally agreed to set up an inter-departmental sub-committee under a chairman, Mr. H. W. S. Francis, C.B., appointed by the Ministry of Health, to work out a scheme for the medical services in London. This committee was known as the 'Francis' Sub-Committee (See Chapter 7: Civil Defence Casualty Services). It included representatives of the Ministry of Health, the War Office, the Home Office and the Ministry of Transport. It made its first report in July 1927, and also made a number of subsequent reports to the Organisations Sub-Committee of the Committee of Imperial Defence, until by 1934 it had worked out a comprehensive scheme for the first-aid treatment of casualties and their removal to hospital, which was subsequently found to be of considerable value.

No further action appears to have been taken at this time, but it is probable that, had these recommendations been actively followed up, particularly in view of the scheme ultimately adopted, an efficient organisation might have been ready years before the emergency for which it was contemplated did arise, and much of the hasty action which became necessary in 1938–9 would have been avoided. In the following few years, occasional mention was made, usually in the course of disarmament debates in the House of Commons, of the fact that precautionary measures for civil defence were being investigated; but few practical steps were taken to plan for the protection of the civilian population from air attack or for the succour of the injured.

THE WHITE PAPER, MARCH 1935

It was not until 1935 that publicity was given to any proposals for measures to safeguard the civil population against air attack. In that year, following on debates in the House of Commons, a White Paper was issued in which it was stated that provisions for defence, which had been allowed to fall to a level which was defeating the object in view, namely the maintenance of peace, could no longer be postponed. At the same time, the Government expressed confidence in the peaceful methods they were pursuing, a confidence not shared by their advisers, who for the past few years had been of opinion that Europe would be involved in another war within ten years and that the position was becoming one of increasing danger. Although a mass of information had been accumulated and certain schemes mooted, the policy of secrecy had militated against anything but the preliminary marshalling of ideas but, the Government having now decided on a restricted degree of publicity, real progress was made possible by enlisting the active co-operation of the local authorities, industrial undertakings and the general public.

REFERENCE

Statement Relating to Defence [Cmd. 4827], H.M.S.O., 1935.

CHAPTER 1
EARLY STEPS TO CREATE A CASUALTY ORGANISATION
March 1935 to September 1938

THE AIR RAID PRECAUTIONS DEPARTMENT OF THE HOME OFFICE
MAY 1935

THE first definite steps towards giving practical effect to air raid precautions were taken when it was decided to set up from May 1, 1935, a new department with executive powers—the Air Raid Precautions Department of the Home Office—to act on behalf of the various Government departments concerned.[1]

The accuracy of the information at the disposal of the Government at that time is suggested by the fact that the Committee of Imperial Defence asked that there should be an endeavour to complete defence preparations by 1939. In the light of subsequent events it is fortunate they did so. The narrative of the activities of this department from the medical point of view is adequately dealt with in Part II, Chapter 7 of this volume; but it is appropriate to mention here some of the more important matters regarding the growth of the casualty organisation during this period.

This new department was to be responsible for advising local authorities and the civil population generally in accordance with the approved policy of the Government and, in a memorandum,[2] local authorities were asked to make provision for the mobilisation and expansion of the medical and first-aid resources of each area so as to provide first-aid posts, casualty clearing stations and hospitals for more extended treatment, together with an adequate ambulance service; hospitals were as far as possible to be provided outside the areas of special danger. Facilities for the decontamination of gas casualties and their clothing were also to be provided. To aid local authorities, various handbooks on anti-gas precautions and first aid for air raid casualties, memoranda on the treatment of casualties, decontamination of personnel and the organisation of air raid casualty services were issued from time to time. In these instructions the type of organisation necessary was indicated in considerable detail and specimen plans for the layout of first-aid posts were included, but no mention of first-aid training for those who did not already belong to one of the peace-time organisations carrying out these duties was contained in any of these instructions until August 1938.[3] A list of the relevant handbooks will be found in Appendix I at the end of Part I of this volume.

In 1936 the Home Office, realising that medical men of the present generation could have little or no knowledge of gas warfare, appointed a number of medical officers to instruct members of the medical profession in the treatment of gas casualties. Two civilian anti-gas schools were opened—one at Falfield in Gloucestershire in 1936 and the other at Easingwold in Yorkshire in 1937—to which local authorities were invited to send representatives for courses of instruction in order that they in turn would be able to teach this subject to the casualty personnel in their own areas.

In general, the medical organisation for air raid precautions was being undertaken by the medical officers of health. As regards London, however, it was recognised that a special scheme would be required and the task of preparing a co-ordinated plan, which had been originally entrusted to the Ministry of Health, was taken over by the Air Raid Precautions Department. A medical officer was appointed to the staff of the department for this purpose, and arrangements were made for the Ministry of Health to hand over all the material which they had collected on the subject. Thus, with the exception of the special arrangements for London, the original policy was to entrust the medical and ancillary provisions for air raid casualties to local authorities, responsible to the Home Office as the co-ordinating central department.

The burden of the medical organisation of the Air Raid Precautions Department of the Home Office fell on the shoulders of Major H. S. Blackmore, O.B.E., R.A.M.C.(ret.). Major Blackmore was on the branch staff of the Chemical Warfare Research Station at Porton from 1923 to 1927 where he gained the extensive knowledge of that subject which qualified him for his later work. In March 1936, he was appointed Chief Medical Officer in the Air Raid Precautions Department of the Home Office, a post which he filled until his death on June 25, 1938. From the beginning Major Blackmore threw his heart and soul into his work and his keenness and anxiety for the success of the A.R.P. Department exhausted his energies and perhaps hastened his end. He laboured unremittingly to create a well-organised and efficient A.R.P. medical service, and in this task encountered many difficulties. That at the outbreak of war the country was to a large extent prepared medically to deal with gas warfare was largely due to Blackmore, and the thoroughness of his plans was possibly a potent insurance against this form of warfare.

THE AIR RAID PRECAUTIONS ACT, 1937

Legislative sanction and authority for the work of the Air Raid Precautions Department was given in December, when the Air Raid Precautions Act, 1937, was passed. The Act stated in general terms that it was the duty of all local authorities to assist each other where possible in making provision to protect persons and property from injury or damage in the event of hostile attack from the air. The responsibility for preparing air raid precautions schemes for their areas was laid upon county and county borough councils which were known as 'scheme-making authorities'. Local plans were to be subject to the approval of the Home Secretary. In the Schedule of Statutory Rules and Orders No. 251, issued under the Act on March 10, 1938, it was provided that 'arrangements for dealing with casualties including the organisation of first-aid parties, first-aid posts, casualty clearing stations and ambulance services' were to be made by local authorities.

THE 'GOODWIN' COMMITTEE

While the Air Raid Precautions Department were actively engaged in the organisation of these casualty services, the Government was giving consideration to certain other aspects of the medical problems involved, and the Minister for Co-ordination of Defence appointed a sub-committee of the Committee of Imperial Defence with Sir John Goodwin, K.C.B., D.S.O., formerly Director-General of the Army Medical Services, as chairman, to consider the co-ordination of medical arrangements in time of war. This was subsequently known as the 'Goodwin' Committee and included representatives of all Government departments with hospital interests.*

The committee met in November 1936, and in view of the wide field which the terms of reference covered it was agreed to deal with the question under the following headings:

(1) To consider the medical arrangements that would be required in a national emergency to deal with:

(a) the sick and wounded of the three Fighting Services at home or evacuated from overseas;

(b) war casualties among the civil population.

(2) To make recommendations regarding the co-ordination of these arrangements.

(3) To make recommendations regarding the sources and provision of the necessary personnel, accommodation, equipment and transport.

The military representatives considered that it was a matter of urgency to endorse the proposals of the War Office for additional military hospital accommodation, and, as these proposals envisaged little encroachment on the civil hospitals, an interim report agreeing with the proposals of the War Office was issued after the first meeting.

---

* See Army Medical Services, Volume I, Chapter 6.

The committee considered that, in addition to the Defence Service hospitals fully expanded, beds would be required on the following basis:

For	At once on Emergency	Increasing to:			
		2 weeks	3 weeks	4 weeks	2 months
Navy	900	2,700	2,700	3,900	3,900
Army	7,950	9,450	10,700	11,825	24,414*
Air Force	1,020	2,065	3,105	3,625	6,370
A.R.P. Dept. Home Office	76,800	124,800	148,800	184,800	268,800*
Total	86,670	139,015	165,305	204,150	303,484

The estimate of the number of civilian hospital beds in the United Kingdom, excluding the mental, special and infectious diseases hospitals, was given as 175,000. Of these it was considered that 50 per cent. could be cleared in forty-eight hours, and that the number of beds could be increased by 50 per cent. giving an immediate provision of 175,000 to meet emergency requirements. This was a remarkably accurate forecast of the beds which were actually made available on the outbreak of the war by these methods.

The committee also submitted that additional medical personnel would be required on and after mobilisation on the following estimates:

	1st Month	2nd Month
Royal Navy	125	—
Army	1,680†	250
Royal Air Force	131	60
Home Office, Air Raid Precautions Department	8,237‡	3,432

After holding seven meetings, the sub-committee in submitting its report on March 11, 1937 made the following recommendations:

(i) that the casualties from the Defence Services should, as far as practicable, be admitted to Service hospitals and remain under Service control;

(ii) that the necessary steps, such as the earmarking of land and buildings and the initiation of building and other contracts for the additional hospital accommodation required by the War Office, should be taken immediately;

(iii) that the Navy should make its own arrangements for the additional hospital accommodation and equipment required;

(iv) that since the wide disposition of Air Force units made it impracticable to establish special Air Force hospitals at home, provision for Air Force casualties be made as part of the general hospital arrangements;

(v) that, subject to review of the financial implications, a central

---

* See Army Medical Services, Volume I, Chapter 6.
† 377 part-time.
‡ 50 per cent. part-time.

authority consisting of representatives of the local authority and voluntary hospitals in England and Wales be established forthwith under the aegis of the Minister of Health with representatives of other Government departments concerned and professional representation, to direct and supervise the provision and organisation of the hospital accommodation required for civilian casualties and in particular to survey and earmark sufficient buildings or sites for hospitals;

(vi) that a similar organisation be established in Scotland;

(vii) that on the outbreak of war a controlling authority representing the central authorities already mentioned and the Service Departments concerned be established to allocate, as pressure in different directions may require, the available hospital accommodation and to determine to what hospitals the casualties should be sent;

(viii) that an emergency committee should be set up by the British Medical Association in peace-time to ascertain to what extent the services of medical men and women could be placed at the disposal of the Government on mobilisation and how these services could most readily be made available, and to report to the Ministry of Health (in Scotland, to the Department of Health for Scotland);

(ix) that large numbers of subordinate personnel, e.g. hospital orderlies, stretcher bearers, etc., should be trained for the requirements of the civil population;

(x) that the Ministry of Transport be requested to review the existing transport and its adequacy for emergency needs (including hospital transport needs) and to prepare any necessary scheme to organise and equip road transport and assign it to its several purposes;

(xi) that sub-committees of the central authorities be set up to deal respectively with (*a*) the provision and quantities of hospital equipment, and (*b*) medical and surgical stores likely to be required.

A reservation was made by the two Air Force members of the sub-committee to the effect that they did not feel able to agree that the administrative machine which was proposed, a complex of departments and authorities without central ministerial control, would prove capable of the manifold and far-reaching action which would be necessary, and submitted that the central controlling authority in peace and war should be constituted as part of an existing department, presumably the Ministry of Health and under its ministerial head. This was a most important reservation. Attention was drawn to the fact that the sub-committee had worked on the scale of attack which was given by the Air Ministry in June 1934 although it was advised that these figures were likely to be increased three or four times in the near future as a result of the re-calculation of the weight of bombs which might be expected to be dropped. This re-estimate when construed into terms of casualties indicated the provision of at least one million beds—a wholly impracticable task, as the administrative departments well knew.

Of these recommendations, the Committee of Imperial Defence accepted (i)–(iv) and (viii) and deferred consideration of the others pending the recommendations of a committee of Heads of Departments which, under the chairmanship of Sir Warren Fisher, was considering the question of hospital provision having regard to expected air attacks on a large scale, as it was becoming increasingly clear that, in order to meet estimated needs and avoid overlapping, this part of the scheme would have to be undertaken centrally. The policy recommended by the Goodwin Committee differed from the policy of the Home Office in advocating provisions being made for the treatment of R.A.F. casualties in the civil hospitals as well as civilian casualties, and in recommending that the Ministry of Health should be the controlling central authority instead of the Home Office, but with a new central authority to be brought into being at the outbreak of war to allocate hospitals to civilian or Service uses as indicated by the pressure of events.

THE 'MacNALTY' COMMITTEE

On May 13, 1937, the sub-committee on Air Raid Precautions Services of the Committee of Imperial Defence recommended that the sub-committee on the co-ordination of medical arrangements in time of war (The Goodwin Committee) should be reconstituted under the chairmanship of Sir Arthur MacNalty, K.C.B., M.D., Chief Medical Officer of the Ministry of Health, with the addition of a representative of the Treasury, to give further consideration to the measures necessary for the treatment of air raid casualties in 'base hospitals'. The Minister for Co-ordination of Defence approved and this reconstituted committee (subsequently known as the 'MacNalty' Committee) began its work in June and submitted its report in October 1937. The committee pointed out that the term 'base hospital' was not one normally applied to civilian uses. They understood it to mean a hospital not serving the needs of any comparatively small area, such as a borough or local government district, but one available for the reception of transferred patients requiring prolonged treatment. It was thus distinct from a casualty clearing hospital for the immediate reception of casualties, at that time to be provided by a local authority as part of its air raid precautions scheme. This interpretation was supported by the intimation the committee received to consider the matters referred to them 'on a national basis'.

They expressed doubt whether it was advisable to distinguish between base hospitals and casualty clearing hospitals (see (3) below), noting that in time of war the local and general needs of the situation may be such that the same institution may at one time be in use for local purposes, e.g. as a casualty clearing hospital, and at another for general purposes as a base hospital. This expression of opinion clarified a question on which much doubt existed. As a result the untenable distinction between base and casualty clearing hospitals disappeared in practice.

The estimate of the anticipated weight of attack and casualties previously obtained by the committee was such (600 tons a day and 200,000 casualties a week of which 66,000 would be killed) that it was obvious it would be an impossible task to make adequate provision for them in the time allowed. The chairman, therefore, suggested at the outset that the most feasible practical step was to ascertain the existing hospital provision in the country, and then expand and supplement it as far as was possible. This suggestion was adopted by the committee. It had the advantage of providing a working basis of facts upon which a hospital emergency scheme could be built.

The recommendations of the committee were as follows:

(1) that the Minister of Health and the Secretary of State for Scotland should be charged with the organisation of the base hospital scheme;

(2) that on the outbreak of war a controlling authority representing the Minister of Health, the Secretary of State for Scotland and the Departments concerned be established to allocate the available hospital accommodation as pressure in different directions might require, and determine to what uses hospitals should be put and to what hospitals casualties should be sent;

(3) that these Ministers and the Secretary of State for Home Affairs should consider further the distinction at present suggested between base hospitals and casualty clearing hospitals and, if this distinction were to be maintained, make arrangements to co-ordinate the demands for accommodation, supplies, material and personnel for the two types of hospitals;

(4) that the Minister of Health and the Secretary of State for Scotland should appoint, under suitable central control, Hospital Officers for the various Civil Commissioners' Divisions, charged with the preparation of base hospital schemes for their areas;

(5) that the areas primarily considered within the Civil Commissioners' Divisions should be those described in their report, the objective being to provide so far as the available financial resources allow a sufficiency of hospital beds to cover the reasonable accommodation of the whole region;

(6) that the Nursing Sub-Committee be re-appointed with the further direction suggested;

(7) that the Minister of Transport be requested to include in his plans the anticipated transport needs of the hospital scheme set out in this report.

In December the Committee of Imperial Defence accepted the whole of this sub-committee's recommendations. The Minister of Health therefore became the hospital authority for civilian purposes so far as base hospitals were concerned, although for the moment the organisation of the so-called casualty clearing hospitals still remained the function of the local authorities under the supervision of the Home Office.

The work of this reconstituted committee marked an important step forward in the national emergency medical preparations. A practical goal was in sight by making use of existing hospital provision in the country for war purposes with expansions and additions to this provision.

The war clouds were thickening and the time for preparing for war casualties was getting short. Fortunately, with a definite plan in view, the work of setting up a comprehensive emergency medical scheme now began to move rapidly.

THE HOSPITAL SERVICES

THE HOSPITAL SURVEY: JANUARY–MAY 1938

Consequent on the acceptance of the MacNalty Committee's recommendations, the Ministry of Health took early steps to appoint officers, both lay and medical, from the Ministry's staff to carry out a survey of all the voluntary and local authority hospitals in the whole country. It was fully expected that a survey would reveal a shortage of beds and also the direction in which expansion would be possible; but it was clear that the provision of 1,000,000 casualty beds, which the Air Ministry had estimated would be required in the whole country, would be a complete impossibility. Moreover, as the base hospitals must be as far removed from the danger of attack as possible, there would be areas where the distinction between base and casualty clearing hospitals could not be applied to the existing hospitals. This was primarily the position in London.

It was, however, becoming increasingly evident by February 1938, that the Home Office was coming round to the view of the Committee of Imperial Defence that the organisation of base and casualty clearing hospitals was inseparable, and in March the Home Office informed local authorities that it would not be possible for them to consider in detail the measures which might be necessary in planning casualty clearing hospitals until the survey of hospitals being carried out by the Ministry of Health had been completed. Eventually, the Home Secretary on June 1 announced[4] that it had been agreed that the Ministry of Health would be the Department responsible for the administration of the Emergency Hospital Service (as it was then called) as a whole and not only of the base hospitals. In the meantime officers of the Ministry of Health were actively engaged in carrying out the hospital survey, the necessary information concerning each and every hospital in the country being collected on a form known as B.H.1—which had been carefully designed to bring out as much co-ordinated information as possible—and such rapid progress was made that the survey was completed before the end of May 1938. The report was a comprehensive one and the information which it gave was very valuable.

So many points, however, subsequently arose, leading to revision of some of the principles on which the report was framed, that reference here will be limited to the main conclusions. For the purpose of the survey institutions were graded into three classes:

Grade A. General hospitals capable of full medical and surgical services.

Grade B. Reasonably good hospitals without facilities for major surgical work, e.g. isolation hospitals and public assistance institutions with reasonably good wards.

Grade C. All institutions capable of taking patients not included under A or B and suitable for chronic sick, convalescent patients from Grades A and B hospitals and the more able-bodied patients.

It was found that the number of beds of all grades existing in the whole country was about 403,000 of which about 103,000 were usually vacant. Of these, 189,000 were Grade A beds in 1,205 hospitals, 134,000 Grade B beds in 1,071 hospitals, and 80,000 Grade C beds in 852 hospitals. By accelerating discharges and transferring patients to lower grade accommodation and using spare beds and equipment, the 103,000 vacant beds could be expected to be capable of an increase on the outbreak of war or within seven days to 233,000. By crowding and converting ancillary rooms it was considered that this figure could be further increased by 205,000, bringing the total that could be made available for casualties up to 438,000. The use of 42,000 beds in mental hospitals and 2,000 beds in the Ministry of Pensions hospitals would bring the total up to 482,000. The further addition of 145,000 beds was thought to be possible by the utilisation of buildings adjacent to existing institutions, giving a grand total of 627,000 beds available of which 364,000 would be in Grade A. Included in the total of beds in existing institutions were 7,000 which had been earmarked by the War Office as Territorial Army General Hospitals, but these were expected to be temporarily available for civilian use on the outbreak of an emergency. The report went on to state that if further provision were required, it would have to be made by the conversion of suitable buildings not in the immediate neighbourhood of existing hospitals or by providing new accommodation in temporary buildings.

It was noted that 424 hospitals in Grades A and B when fully expanded would each only hold 60 patients and that in 254 the limit would be 30 patients, these hospitals being small cottage hospitals mostly situated in rural areas. Attention was also drawn to the fact that the wisdom of increasing or even using the available supply of hospital beds in or near the centres of densely populated areas was questionable.

TERRITORIAL ARMY GENERAL HOSPITALS

In consequence of the acceptance of the recommendation of the Goodwin Committee that Army casualties should, as far as possible, be admitted to hospitals under Army control, discussions with a view to providing accommodation for Army casualties by allocating hospitals for this purpose and providing *ad hoc* hospitals in addition had been going on for some time. (See Army Medical Services, Volume I, Chapter 2.)

It was at first proposed to provide for 29 Territorial Army general hospitals of 600 beds each, capable of expansion to 2,000 beds, and for convalescent hospitals of 2,000 beds in each of the Commands. In August 1938, it was agreed to establish hospitals as follows:

5 in mental hospitals in Scotland, 4 in England and Wales;
3 in sanatoria;
3 in good general hospitals.

The remainder would be located in non-medical buildings or on open sites. It was realised, however, that if this number of hospitals were taken over solely for military purposes, the difficulty of supplying hospital accommodation for the displaced civilian sick and the large number of civilian casualties to be expected would be greatly increased. In addition, the calling up of large numbers of civilian medical practitioners to staff these hospitals, in addition to those required for the Field Armies, would further seriously deplete the available medical personnel.

In September 1938, the Minister of Health and the Secretary of State for Scotland took action which was eventually to have far-reaching effect. In a memorandum to the Secretary of State for War they urged that mobilisation, when it occurred, should not extend to medical units, and that all schemes to this end should be worked out by the three Departments concerned. It was clear that any plans for the treatment of casualties based on previous experience would have to be reconsidered in view of the type of warfare and number of casualties to be expected. The War Office agreed to relinquish their call on 25 of the 29 Territorial Army General Hospitals on the understanding that the Ministry of Health would hand over to the Army authorities such accommodation as might be required from time to time on forty-eight hours' notice. (See Chapter 2 and Army Medical Services, Volume I, Chapters 2 and 6.)

ADMINISTRATIVE RESPONSIBILITY, JUNE 1938

The Ministry of Health having been made responsible for the organisation of the whole of the Emergency Hospital system in England and Wales from June 1, it was found necessary to create an Administrative Division and Medical Section in the Ministry, with a Principal Assistant Secretary in charge, an Assistant Secretary, Principals and an Executive and Clerical Establishment. Dr. (afterwards Sir) John H. Hebb, C.B., C.B.E., Director-General of the Medical Services of the

Ministry of Pensions, who had been seconded for this purpose, was appointed Principal Medical Officer of the Emergency Medical Services, with a medical officer, Dr. W. A. Lethem, seconded from another branch of the Ministry, as his deputy. This new medical section, like the other medical branches was under the general direction of the Chief Medical Officer of the Ministry.

The Regional Hospital Organisation was also planned and brought into being, Regional Hospital Officers being appointed to the Defence Commissioners' Regions, with the exception of the London Region, which was administered from headquarters.

The Ministry at this stage had still no responsibility for the Civil Defence Services, including first-aid posts, local ambulance services, etc., for which the local authorities were responsible under the provisions of the Air Raid Precautions Act. These were still under the Home Secretary; but at this time responsibility for inter-hospital ambulances was handed over to the Ministry of Health. The primary purpose of the Ministry was to erect a stable framework within which the whole hospital treatment of casualties could be built on plans appropriate to the new type of warfare which was expected.

ADMINISTRATIVE POLICY

The previously conceived cut-and-dried medical arrangements for the home front for the War of 1914–18 would obviously not suffice for a war in which large numbers of civil and Service casualties might have to be dealt with in many areas of the country. Elasticity in all schemes was therefore essential so that the functions of most of the hospitals could be varied at will to meet changing conditions. It was therefore necessary, in view of the urgency of the matter, for the Ministry to expedite in every way the evolution of a workable scheme once the main principles had been decided, omitting the usual course of inviting and encouraging the criticism of the many conflicting interests concerned. The expert advice of persons of acknowledged repute was, however, always sought when necessary. It was also necessary to keep in view the possibility of having to bring into being a 'short-term' scheme at any stage of the evolution of a 'long-term' scheme.

THE 'SHORT-TERM' POLICY: PROVINCES

As the result of this policy the Ministry was able in August 1938, to issue to all scheme-making authorities a circular[5] in which were laid down the general principles on which Emergency Hospital Schemes in the provinces were to be based, namely, that the distinction hitherto drawn between base hospitals and casualty clearing hospitals was untenable; that all suitable accommodation in hospitals, voluntary or local authority, might in the event of a serious emergency be required to play some part; that every hospital must be prepared to receive casualties arising from a local air raid; that in addition every hospital, except those situated in areas which might be expected to be peculiarly subject to attack and hospitals where special medical considerations arise, must be prepared to receive, for such further treatment as might be required, both casualties and ordinary patients whom it might be necessary to transfer from the more dangerous areas. These authorities were further required to furnish the Regional Hospital Officers, who were actively engaged in considering what casualty organisation would be best suited to their respective areas, with all the assistance in their power.

THE REGIONAL HOSPITAL SCHEMES

In the meantime, the reports of the Hospital Officers on their Emergency Hospital Schemes were being received and examined. The aggregate results of these inquiries into the number and grade of suitable beds which could be made available are given in the following table:

Grade of beds	By clearing (24 hours)			Spare beds in store		
	A	B	C	A	B	C
London Region (6 counties) .	32,455	14,957	4,683	3,097	1,242	246
Rest of country . . .	54,620	39,022	22,976	4,044	3,719	1,700
Totals	87,075	53,979	27,659	7,141	4,961	1,946
Grand Totals	168,713			14,048		

From these figures it appeared that the hospital survey figures of potentially available beds were much too optimistic and that in the interests of a short-term scheme to meet any sudden emergency, as well as for a long-term scheme, it was of primary importance to get down to bedrock on the question of suitable hospital accommodation in order to be able to give a definite opinion on the additional accommodation required, the appropriate use to which beds should be put and the additional equipment required, etc. Forms were therefore issued in the middle of August to the Hospital Officers requesting the following information:

(*a*) The position of the hospital in relation to the centre of the town or district in which it is situated.

(*b*) Particulars of beds normally available.

(*c*) An estimate of the patients who could be sent home or decanted into other specific accommodation in twenty-four hours.

The information would show how the hospitals could best be utilised without any extra equipment, also the number of ambulances which would be required to effect decanting and the number of beds of different grades available at once in the event of a sudden emergency. By the middle of September the completed returns had been received.

They provided a definite practical basis on which to found a long-term policy of expansion by ' crowding ', by using additional accommodation and by equipping with surgical facilities or 'upgrading' hospitals not fitted to undertake surgical work. The Hospital Officers had also been requested to draw up operational orders for the partial evacuation of hospitals and the decanting of patients to other suitable hospitals in consultation with the medical officers of health of the scheme-making authorities in their area, and to complete the calculation of the number of patients to be moved by ambulance transport and the arrangements for the transfers with the hospitals from and to which they would be made. These arrangements were understood to be purely precautionary and were to be replaced in due course by more complete schemes.

LONDON REGION

The 'Wilson' Committee, May–July 1938. This committee, of which Sir Charles Wilson, M.C., M.D., F.R.C.P. (Afterwards Lord Moran), was chairman, was appointed in May 1938, to consider how best to plan an organised Casualty Hospital Scheme for the London area. Because of the urgency of putting such a scheme into operation with the least possible delay the committee issued an interim report in July. It made a number of definite recommendations and some provisional ones which it thought would require further consideration.

Estimates before the committee of the number of casualties to be expected daily on the outbreak of hostilities gave a figure of 30,000. This estimate referred to the whole of the country, but the committee appear to have based their recommendations on the assumption that such a figure might apply to the London area only. On this basis and an estimate of an average stay of two days in casualty clearing hospitals and fourteen days in base hospitals, the committee considered that 60,000 casualty clearing hospital beds, and 420,000 base hospital beds would be required. The committee made a complete survey of bed accommodation in the counties of London, Middlesex, Kent, Surrey, Essex and Hertfordshire and concluded that by moving patients, sending some to their homes and crowding others (excepting maternity hospitals and those for chronic sick) some 50,000 beds could be made available for the inner zone. To make up the number of beds available to 60,000 it was recommended that buildings such as hotels should be adapted and equipped as emergency hospitals.

As regards the outer zone, the committee suggested dividing the London area into five triangular sections with apices based on the larger London leading hospitals in order that patients in the inner portion of each segment could be directed to the corresponding hospitals in the outer portion. Of the estimated number of 420,000 beds required, only about 80,000 could be made available in existing hospitals. To meet the deficiency the committee recommended that schools and country houses should be earmarked for the purpose, and that hutted or tented hospitals should be constructed and equipped.

The recommendations and suggestions of the 'Wilson' Committee were brought to the notice of the local authority and voluntary hospitals in the London Region preparatory to working out a definite scheme for each hospital.

Short-term Arrangements for the London Area. The evolution of a casualty scheme for London, owing to the intricacy of the problem in an area which was expected to be the main target for attack from the air, was tending to lag behind the arrangements which were being brought into effect in the rest of the country. The L.C.C., however, at the request of the Ministry had seconded one of their medical staff, Dr. J. Nairn Dobbie, to act as Hospital Officer for the London Region and a further officer, Dr. J. G. Johnstone, to act as his part-time assistant. They had also placed at the Ministry's disposal their Chief Ambulance Officer to become Ambulance Officer for the London Region in the event of war. Arrangements were being made for the clearance of the voluntary hospitals in the inner zone of London to the outer zone and plans were on foot to fit up Green Line coaches as ambulances to carry 10 stretchers each to evacuate the patients. Arrangements had also been made for 10 L.C.C. fever hospitals to be used as casualty hospitals in addition to the existing voluntary and county council hospitals, and the L.C.C. had been authorised to spend £400 for each of these hospitals to enable it to undertake surgical work.

HOSPITAL EQUIPMENT

The Government had constituted a Supply Committee, on which the Ministry of Health was represented, to co-ordinate the requisition of drugs and other medical supplies by the various Government departments, and the Ministry of Health had already had under consideration the amount and types of equipment which would need to be supplied.

Attention at this time, owing to increased tension in the European situation, was chiefly devoted to ward equipment, e.g. bedsteads, blankets, mattresses and surgical equipment. The London County Council had been authorised to purchase 20,000 blankets at once. Proposals were made to utilise blankets belonging to the Ministry of Pensions as a reserve. As regards bedsteads, although the rigid three-piece type would be the best for hospitals the problem of storage at short notice was found to be insuperable. It was therefore decided that the bedsteads would have to be of the one-piece folding variety. The Office of Works devised a suitable bedstead of this type and an initial order for 50,000 was placed on September 9. A type of coir mattress was also decided upon and 50,000 of these were ordered on September 14. Because of the difficulties of storage the manufacturers were asked in the meantime to store the bedsteads, and the big local authorities the mattresses.

The Home Office in the meantime also had been considering the question of the best type of stretcher which would be durable and interchangeable, and a stretcher, eventually found to be suitable in every way, was devised. This stretcher was of light tubular metal with a wire bed clipped on to the frame treated with a cellulose finish; this permitted easy and rapid decontamination when necessary. These stretchers were designed to be used by the first-aid parties, in the first-aid posts, in ambulances and in ambulance trains instead of cots; they therefore eliminated the moving of the patient from one stretcher to another at all stages until he reached the hospital. The Home Office had placed an initial order for 100,000 of these.

THE PROVISION OF MEDICAL, NURSING AND TECHNICAL PERSONNEL

MEDICAL PERSONNEL

The Committee of Reference. The question of medical personnel for the Services and for the expansion of the civil hospitals had been under urgent consideration for some time and the Committee of Reference of the Royal Colleges of Physicians and Surgeons, constituted during the War of 1914–18 to advise on the needs of the medical schools and hospitals in London and to indicate the teachers and specialists to be retained in the interests of medical education and the hospital services, was revived in the summer of 1937. It was then decided that its functions should be expanded and that this committee should advise on the specialist staffing of hospitals generally, whether voluntary or local authority, and that in view of the large interests vested in the L.C.C., a representative of that body should be co-opted to the committee.

The Central Medical Emergency Committee. The Central Medical Emergency Committee was also reconstituted as the Central Emergency Committee of the British Medical Association in 1937 and it became again the Central Medical War Committee at the outbreak of hostilities. This committee had begun to compile a register eventually covering over 90 per cent. of the medical profession and proposed to set up Local Emergency Committees in each of the British Medical Association's divisions to assist the central body in preparing to meet the demands of the Defence and Civil Services. This register was completed in August 1938, in respect of about 44,000 medical practitioners and it was agreed later that the Central Medical War Committee would be the recruiting agency for the supply of medical personnel to the Services and the civil hospitals and would also be the authority for fixing the establishments of the latter. A full report of the evolution and activities of this body is recorded in Part II, Chapter 14.

NURSING PERSONNEL

The Central Nursing Emergency Committee. The shortage of trained nurses in peace-time had already given rise to anxiety and in 1937 the Inter-Departmental Committee on Nursing Services (known as the 'Athlone' Committee) had been appointed to advise how recruitment could be improved.[6] The question of providing reserves of nurses for the Defence Services in time of war had already been considered by a sub-committee of the Committee of Imperial Defence in 1927 and again by a sub-committee in 1936. The Nursing Sub-Committee was reconstituted under the chairmanship of Sir Arthur S. MacNalty, Chief Medical Officer of the Ministry of Health, in October 1937, with the following terms of reference:

(a) To attempt to secure for the trained nurses the establishment of an Emergency Committee to work on lines parallel to those of the Emergency Committee of the British Medical Association.

(b) To concert with the Order of St. John and the British Red Cross Society (who already had certain commitments for the provision of staff in an emergency) and other suitable organisations, arrangements for the supply of auxiliary and unqualified nursing staff.

This committee reported in September 1938, that in March of that year there were 89,254 trained nurses on the register but that there was no information available as to how many unregistered trained nurses there were in existence and that it was a vital necessity to appoint a co-ordinating body for the nursing profession. They advised that the College of Nursing should be asked to compile a register of all nurses and assistant nurses, that the British Red Cross Society and the Order of St. John be asked to compile one for auxiliary nurses prepared to offer their services and that the W.V.S. should deal with all hospital auxiliaries other than nurses. They therefore recommended that a Central Emergency Committee for the nursing profession similar to that of the Central Medical War Committee for the medical profession should be set up. The Central Emergency Nursing Committee was duly constituted in December 1938, to carry out the duties contained in these recommendations. The activities of the Central Nursing Committee are given in detail in Chapter 15.

THE CENTRAL DENTAL, OPTICAL AND PHARMACEUTICAL COMMITTEES

Although their Emergency and War Committees were not all appointed within the period with which this chapter mainly deals, it may be convenient here to refer also to the arrangements made for recruiting dentists, opticians and pharmacists.

Central Dental Emergency and War Committees. Arrangements for the recruitment of dentists began with the appointment towards the end of 1938 of a Central Emergency Committee and of District Committees, which were superseded on the outbreak of war by Central and District Dental War Committees. On the Central Committee were represented not only the various dental organisations, the Teaching Schools and the British Medical Association, but also the Service Departments, the Ministries of Health and Education, the Northern Ireland Ministry of Home Affairs and, for liaison between this and the Scottish Dental War Committee, the Department of Health for Scotland.

The procedure followed by the Central Dental War Committee was similar to that of the Central Medical War Committee, but it had a simpler task because of its narrower professional field. Although there was not the same variety in classes of employment in the dental as in the medical profession, the Central and District Dental Committee nevertheless carried out a difficult duty of considerable national importance in meeting the demands of the Services and at the same time ensuring under war conditions an adequate dental service for the community, including schools, hospitals and clinics.

The Central Committee was notified by the Service Departments of their requirements and, working mainly through its Commissions Sub-Committee, called upon District Committees for their quotas. It was the practice to nominate newly qualified dentists for commissions forthwith. Representations regarding local selections could be made to the District Committees, both by the dentists concerned and by other interested parties, and dentists also had the usual right of appeal to the Hardship Committees set up by the Ministry of Labour and National Service to deal with deferment of calling up on grounds of personal hardship. Appeals against the decisions of the District Committees were heard by the Commissions Sub-Committee, which appointed a further sub-committee of its members to consider questions affecting the calling up of dental mechanics and the employment of female mechanics, receptionists, nurses and secretaries. Two representatives of the Trades Union Congress were appointed to this sub-committee with the right to attend meetings and take part in the deliberations of the Central Committee when questions concerning dental mechanics were under consideration.

Marked absence of criticism indicated that the difficult work of the Central and District Dental War Committees was done with fairness and efficiency.

Central Emergency Committee for Opticians (England and Wales). This committee was set up early in 1939 for the purpose of compiling a special register of opticians who were prepared to offer their professional services in an emergency and to advise the Minister of Health on questions relating to the employment of optical personnel in the event of war. It consisted of all members of the Ophthalmic Benefit Approved Committee already established for National Health Insurance purposes, and included representatives of the Joint Council of Qualified Opticians (5), the National Association of Opticians (1), the Institute of Chemist-Opticians (1), Ophthalmic Supplies Ltd., (1) the Association of Dispensing Opticians Ltd. (1), the Association of Wholesale and Manufacturing Opticians (2) and Unattached Opticians (1), with representatives of the three Service Departments, the Ministry of Health and the Department of Health for Scotland attached to the committee as observers.

When the Ministry of Labour and National Service introduced the system of progressive de-reservation of men of military age in 'reserved occupations' the committee was called upon to advise the Minister on the deferment or recruitment of de-reserved opticians and later of their ancillary workers. It also dealt with the retention in or release from optical employment of Opticians' Women Technical Assistants of whom a register was set up in 1943. Scotland had a separate Central Emergency Committee for Opticians, which functioned on similar lines.

Central Pharmaceutical Emergency and War Committee. At the request of the Ministry of Health early in 1939, the Pharmaceutical Society of Great Britain set up a Central Pharmaceutical Emergency Committee to compile and maintain a register of all pharmacists and dispensers who were prepared to serve in an emergency. The register was to cover the whole of Great Britain, with a copy of the Scottish part lodged in Edinburgh. Local Emergency Committees, based on District Pharmaceutical Committees constituted for National Health Insurance purposes, were formed to advise the Central Committee from the local aspect. These Central and Local Emergency Committees were reconstituted respectively as the Central Pharmaceutical War Committee and District Pharmaceutical War Committees.

The Central Pharmaceutical War Committee consisted of representatives of the following bodies:

Pharmaceutical Society of Great Britain	6 members
North British Executive of Pharmaceutical Society of Great Britain	1 member
National Pharmaceutical Union	2 members
Guild of Public Pharmacists	1 member
Co-operative Societies	1 member
Wholesale Drug Trade Association	1 member
Society of Apothecaries	1 member
Company Chemists' Association	2 members
Pharmaceutical Standing Committee for Scotland	1 member
National Association of Insurance Committees	1 member
Scottish Branch of Pharmaceutical Society	1 member

The Ministry of Health had two observers, the Department of Health for Scotland one observer and the three Service Departments one observer each attached to the committee. Two representatives of the Trades Union Congress were added during the course of the war.

In 1942, the original register was brought to a close, and a complete census was taken of all pharmaceutical undertakings under the Pharmacy Undertakings Order, 1942. This provided detailed information as to the staffing and work carried out by retail pharmacies, hospital dispensaries and wholesale establishments, and was used for considering the recruitment or deferment of individual pharmacists and dispensers.

In the same year, the Central Pharmaceutical War Committee became an Approved Agency, under the Control of Engagement Order, for the control of the movements of women pharmacists and women dispensers. District Committees also were called upon to advise local offices of the Ministry of Labour and National Service on questions relating to the withdrawal of women dispensers under the National Service Acts and the Registration for Employment Order.

THE PERIOD OF ACUTE CRISIS LEADING UP TO MUNICH AGREEMENT

While this preliminary work to evolve a short-term scheme was going on, work on the long-term scheme had been more or less suspended. Meanwhile the political situation had gone from bad to worse and by the end of the second week in September 1938, it was considered necessary to proceed on the basis that an emergency might arise during the next week or two.

There ensued, therefore, a period of intense activity at the Ministry of Health in order to bring the Department in touch with as many as possible of the individuals and bodies who would be most intimately concerned in establishing a casualty organisation based on existing resources, with such improvisation as could be introduced in a matter of days. Daily contact was maintained with the L.C.C. and discussions were held from September 14 onwards with the medical officers of health throughout the country.

As regards London it was decided to decant a number of patients, who could not be sent to their homes, from thirty-four of London's principal hospitals to eight towns outside London. Brighton was to take 1,000; Eastbourne, 330; Hastings, 400; Oxford, 350; Reading, 450; Bedford, 500; Cambridge, 450 and Windsor, 100; a total of 3,580 patients. With the exception of those going to Windsor who would travel by road, all were to be transferred by rail and arrangements were made with the railway companies for 21 ambulance trains to be improvised for the purpose. At the same time the London Passenger Transport Board were converting a number of their Green Line coaches to carry 10 stretchers each, fittings being prepared in advance so that 320 of these coaches could be transformed into ambulances at from twelve to twenty-four hours' notice. These fittings were completed and stored in the garages by September 20. By September 22 it was possible to inform the Minister that plans for the evacuation scheme were complete, with the one exception, that there were no stretchers available. This defect was met by obtaining 4,000 G.S. stretchers and pillows on loan from the Army depot at Didcot. These all reached the Ministry by September 24 and the appropriate quota was delivered to each of the 34 hospitals on Sunday, September 25.

In the meantime the medical officers of health of the eight towns were summoned to a meeting in London and the decanting scheme was explained; the scheme entailed some very hard work by the medical officers of health in order to perfect arrangements, but whole-hearted co-operation was assured from the first. Similar arrangements were made for certain large provincial towns, from only one of which, however, was subsequent evacuation actually carried out. It was made clear to the medical officers of health concerned that during the emergency they would be acting in their own areas as agents of the Hospital Officer, which would bring them directly into relationship with the voluntary hospitals. On September 16, Hospital Officers were warned[7] that they might be required to take preparatory action without putting into force the whole scheme for evacuating hospitals: this preparatory action included a request to all hospitals to keep a daily record of patients who could if necessary be sent home and, in Grade A hospitals in the larger towns, a record of those fit to be decanted. Hospital Officers were also requested to arrange with local transport officers for suitable ambulances for this purpose. It was expected that on the average 30 per cent. to 50 per cent. of patients would be found fit for transfer, except in hospitals maintained for chronic sick. Hospitals were asked to make their own arrangements for stretcher bearers by using their own staff and medical students and to send blankets with the patients. Hospitals were also given advice on blacking-out rooms which it would be essential to use at night, on structural precautions, on protection against gas and the keeping of records. The above is merely a summary of the more important operational moves which were put in hand. Many other matters had to be provided for.

While the Ministry of Health were making these improvised arrangements, the Home Office authorities were endeavouring to improvise first-aid arrangements and, although these would have been admittedly inadequate had very heavy attacks from the air occurred, arrangements were made with all hospitals to use their out-patient departments, and with local authorities to use all their clinics where medical assistance could be supplied.

The Munich Agreement which was reached on September 29 had relieved the tension, although not sufficiently to warrant general relaxation of the emergency arrangements. But the Minister instructed the hospitals all over the country that there should be as little interference as possible with the treatment of peace-time sick and that the arrangements which had been in force for the limitation of admission and the keeping vacant of the beds of those discharged, might now be relaxed.

Subsequent reports from the Hospital Officers recounting their experiences during the crisis and the extent to which they were individually able to develop their preparations show that while the great efforts made produced tangible results, had the emergency come, not a few difficulties would have arisen. In the provinces the provision of transport for sending patients home and transferring others from one hospital to another had caused great anxiety from the uncertainty attached to requisition and improvisation.

The hospital authorities, both voluntary and municipal, almost without exception did their utmost to assist in preparing to implement the hospital scheme, and there is no doubt that in the time at their disposal the Hospital Officers and all those associated with them had done excellent work.

THE EMERGENCY HOSPITAL SERVICE IN SEPTEMBER 1938

If the emergency had occurred the state of affairs in the emergency services would have been as follows:

(i) About 170,000 beds in all grades of hospitals with a reserve of about 15,000 beds would have been available.

(ii) A skeleton administrative medical staff had been appointed.

(iii) Regional Hospital Officers had had several months' experience of the hospitals in their Regions.

(iv) The medical officers of health of Scheme-Making Authorities had been designated to carry out the Ministry's short-term scheme in their capacity of Agents to the Hospital Officers.

(v) Ambulance Officers had been appointed by all the Local Authorities and improvised arrangements had been made for the supply of ambulances, stretchers, stretcher bearers, etc.

(vi) A Central Nursing Committee had been appointed to organise the supply of extra nurses to the hospitals.

(vii) Improvised ambulance trains had been arranged for, to carry out the evacuation of patients from the hospitals in vulnerable areas.

(viii) The Home Office had made arrangements to improvise first-aid posts in the out-patient departments of general hospitals, in clinics and in other suitable buildings.

(ix) Improvised structural precautions for vulnerable portions of the hospitals had been arranged and instructions had been issued for the improvisation of black-out in portions of the hospitals.

Reflecting on what actually happened after the outbreak of war in 1939 there is no doubt, even if an enemy attack had been made by air on the scale experienced in the autumn of 1940, that these improvised arrangements would have been, more or less, adequate for most of the casualties; on the other hand if the scale of attack had been that forecast by the Air Force, it is obvious that they would have been totally inadequate, as indeed would the organisation brought into being after hostilities had been in progress for nearly a year. Probably rapid emergency improvisation would have combated the partial chaos that would have resulted.

REFERENCES

[1] *Parliamentary Debates, Official Report, House of Commons*, Sixth Vol. of Session 1934–5, Col. 1670. (300 H.C. Deb., Col. 1670).
[2] Home Office A.R.P. Dept. Circular 700,216/14, July 9, 1935.
[3] Home Office A.R.P. Dept. Circular 703,189/19, August 26, 1938.
[4] *Parliamentary Debates, Official Report, House of Commons*, Ninth Vol. of Session 1937–8, Col. 2091. (336 H.C. Deb., 2091).
[5] Min. of Health Circular 1732, August 12, 1938.
[6] *Interim Report of Inter-departmental Committee on Nursing Services*, December 20, 1938. H.M.S.O.
[7] Emergency Medical Services Instruction No. 6, September 16, 1938.

CHAPTER 2
EXPANSION OF THE EMERGENCY MEDICAL SERVICES
October 1938 to September 1939

THE crisis had awakened the country to its danger, and although the acute tension of September was relaxed, little confidence was felt that the clouds of war had been finally dispersed. The nation was therefore moved to look to its defences, which were now realised to be woefully inadequate. Since it was believed that war—so narrowly averted—would probably claim its first victims among the civilian population, the apathy which had previously impeded progress in civil defence was fortunately replaced by a widespread sense of reality and of the urgent need for advance provisions for dealing with casualties, thus stimulating action and giving the machine an impetus which it might otherwise have taken a long time to gain.

THE HOSPITAL SERVICES: THE LONG-TERM POLICY

HOSPITAL ACCOMMODATION

One of the first essentials was to accelerate and complete the inquiries in progress to ascertain the exact amount of hospital accommodation and equipment which could be made available for the treatment of casualties within a few days of the outbreak of war. Much had already been done, and the Ministry of Health forthwith resumed the activities which had been interrupted by the crisis. These resulted in the completion of approved registers for all the Regions, of hospitals suitable for inclusion in the Emergency Hospital Scheme. These contained reliable information verified by Regional Hospital Officers, regarding the grade, accommodation, facilities, equipment and potentiality of every hospital. These registers formed the basis for the Emergency Hospital Scheme until their revision in the autumn of 1941.

A considerable number of hospitals, however, were now excluded from the Emergency Hospital Scheme. Infectious diseases and maternity hospitals, which would be required for children and expectant mothers to be evacuated from large towns, were excluded and, as the demand on beds in sanatoria was considered likely to increase during war, as it did in 1914–18, the use of sanatoria for emergency hospitals was considerably modified.

RECLASSIFICATION OF HOSPITALS

As a result of the exact information now available the hospitals were reclassified in three groups instead of the previous

Grades A, B and C (see Chapter 1) and the following bed figures emerged:

		Beds to be available in 24 hours	Later
Group IA.	(Hospitals with full medical and surgical services)	136,425	48,505
Group IB.	(Small hospitals—usually less than 50 beds—with limited surgical facilities)	7,460	1,465
Group II.	(Hospitals with medical facilities only)	54,135	51,920
	Totals	198,020	101,890

Group III. Infectious diseases hospitals were not now included, but particulars of these, with a potentiality of some 48,000 casualty beds, were recorded for future use if necessary.

Note: The beds being arranged for in the mental hospitals—estimated at 40,000—are not included in the above figures.

MENTAL HOSPITALS

Plan for Surrender of Accommodation to the Emergency Medical Services. During the early months of 1938, the Board of Control undertook, at the request of the Ministry of Health, a survey of the accommodation in mental hospitals and mental deficiency institutions in England and Wales with a view to estimating the number of beds which could be made available for civilian casualties in the event of war. The proposals submitted by the Board as a result of the survey contemplated the evacuation and surrender to the Emergency Medical Services of 16 of the 101 county and borough mental institutions and 10 out of the 89 certified institutions for mental defectives administered by local authorities or joint boards.

The scheme involved the evacuation of rather more than 25,000 beds and it was estimated that by installing additional beds, a total of about 40,000 beds for casualties could be provided in the accommodation surrendered.

Good progress was made in working out the details of the scheme, which would in all probability have been brought into operation if the international crisis of September 1938, had culminated in war. During the latter part of the year, however, conferences between representatives of the Ministry of Health and the Board led to a fundamental change of plan. It was felt that a scheme based upon the complete evacuation of a comparatively small number of selected institutions might result in an excessive number of casualty beds in some areas and a shortage in others. To meet this objection the Board proposed and the Ministry accepted an alternative scheme under which the necessary beds would be found by the partial evacuation of most of the mental hospitals and the larger mental deficiency institutions found to be suitable for the object in view. Certain hospitals which were already overcrowded were omitted from the scheme and the general rule was adopted that in no hospital should more than 25 per cent. of the authorised accommodation be given up.

The administrative arrangements were that the medical superintendent remained in administrative charge of the whole hospital, including the portion allotted to the Emergency Medical Services. As regards the medical staffing of the E.M.S. wards, the usual arrangement was that medical officers of the E.M.S. should be specially appointed for this work, but in some hospitals it was found more convenient for members of the hospital staff to undertake the care of the E.M.S. patients in addition to their normal duties. A surgeon or physician of high professional status was, in all the larger E.M.S. units, appointed as the medical or surgical director and was in clinical charge of the unit.

The Visiting Committees were asked to undertake the responsibility (subject, of course, to financial reimbursement) for the supply of food and such common services as washing, heating and lighting, while the E.M.S. provided such extra theatre and ward equipment and ancillary services as might be required for the work of a casualty hospital. This scheme provided also for the complete or almost complete evacuation of a few selected mental hospitals and mental deficiency institutions.

Operation and Development of the Plan. When the time came to put this plan into operation it worked with such smoothness and rapidity that the necessary transfers of accommodation were completed within little more than twenty-four hours. The hospitals completely evacuated were Park Prewett Mental Hospital, Basingstoke; Horton Mental Hospital, Epsom; Hill End Mental Hospital, St. Albans; Westwood Mental Deficiency Colony, Leeds; and Shotley Bridge Mental Deficiency Colony, Newcastle. In the remaining mental hospitals, except for those in which further overcrowding was thought to be too dangerous, and in the larger mental institutions, space was released by transferring patients to other wards or institutions. Altogether sufficient accommodation was released to provide space for about 36,000 casualty beds in 43 mental hospitals and 18 mental deficiency institutions. This does not mean that this number of mental hospital and mental deficiency beds was lost. Mental hospitals and institutions, unlike general hospitals in which practically all the patients are in bed, have to provide considerable day space as well as night space, and the accommodation released was estimated to provide casualty bed space for approximately double the number of beds surrendered. In the mental hospitals 17,204 beds out of a total of 132,890 were released in 1939 and by the end of 1941 the total beds surrendered had increased to 24,078. In the mental deficiency institutions 5,926 beds out of 34,746 were surrendered in 1939 and a small additional number of beds was given up later on.

The original scheme, however, only took into consideration bed space for civilian casualties, for whom day room was not considered essential as most ambulatory patients could be discharged to their homes. But when the Ministry of Health undertook the responsibility of providing hospital accommodation for the great majority of Service sick and casualties from both home stations and overseas, this condition did not apply, Service casualties having to remain in hospital until fit for transfer to convalescent establishments; dining rooms and recreational facilities were therefore essential. It was also necessary to convert a proportion of the ward accommodation in the larger institutions handed over into additional operating suites, X-ray rooms, pathological laboratories, etc., in order to bring these institutions up to the standard of first-class general hospitals fully equipped to deal with large numbers of surgical cases at one time, coming in convoys from overseas.

When these alterations had been carried out the casualty bed space in these hospitals was materially reduced and was replaced, and where necessary increased, by the construction of hutted annexes.

The demands of the Emergency Medical Services were not the only ones which the Board of Control was called upon to meet. The Ministry of Health did not include in their hospital scheme any provision for the treatment of Service mental cases, as these by arrangement were to be dealt with by the Services themselves. For this purpose the Navy took over sections of two mental hospitals and one whole mental hospital for general purposes; the Army required one whole mental hospital and one mental deficiency institution and sections in ten other mental hospitals; while the R.A.F. took over one whole mental hospital for general purposes. In these institutions the patients remained under military discipline and could receive treatment for their mental disabilities without certification, which would otherwise have been necessary. This was done by giving temporary commissions in the R.A.M.C. to the superintendent and his deputy, and to other physicians with special qualifications in psychological medicine detailed for duties in these units.

THE INCREASE OF HOSPITAL ACCOMMODATION

The Basis of the Estimates of Requirements. In making plans for the hospital organisation the stage had been reached at which the fullest use had been made of existing hospital accommodation by introducing additional beds and by upgrading. By these expedients approximately 200,000 beds could be found in the first twenty-four hours and another 100,000 at the end of a week. These figures, however, included some 80,000 beds in large towns which it would probably prove impracticable to use except for 'clearing hospital' purposes, leaving 220,000 available for patients requiring a longer stay in hospital. Before an estimate of the number of additional beds which would be required could be arrived at it was necessary to get an appreciation of what the requirements of the civilian sick as well as those of the civilian casualties would be. In a future war, owing to altered conditions of warfare entailing the evacuation of civilians from the larger towns, etc., it was not expected that the civilian sick rate would be appreciably diminished as it was in the last war; consequently, beds vacated at the beginning of an emergency were expected gradually to be filled again by a flow into hospital of civilian patients. Therefore the 87,075 beds which it had been estimated could be made available by sending people home could only be considered as being temporarily available (see Table, page 18). In addition it had been estimated that some 50,000 beds would be required to accommodate the sick transferred from the larger towns, especially London. It followed that in round numbers an additional 140,000 beds would be required outside the large towns.

It appeared, therefore, that not more than 80,000 beds would be available for casualties outside the large towns and another 80,000 in these towns which could only be put to limited use. Estimates of the number of casualties to be expected from aerial attack had been very largely increased since the figures supplied to the Ministry in 1924. The figures given in 1938 estimated that the provision of at least 1,000,000 beds in hospitals was necessary; such a number was so fantastic as to be entirely beyond the capacity of the medical and nursing personnel which could be found to staff them. Air raid casualties on such a scale with the concurrent loss of personnel (which excluded provision for civilian sick, Service sick and casualties) and which were based on a stay in hospital of only sixteen days—a serious underestimate—could only have reduced some of the larger centres of population to a shambles.

The above figures had been arrived at by multiplying the casualties caused by a ton of bombs in recent warfare by the number of tons of bombs it was expected would be dropped in aerial attacks on this country, an estimate which might well be misleading. It therefore seemed desirable to the Minister that confirmation of these figures should be obtained from higher authority before finally submitting any estimates of beds required. In February, therefore, the Minister communicated with Lord Chatfield, Minister for Co-ordination of Defence on the subject and his reply was to the effect that the accepted proportion of wounded to killed would be two to one, that the Air Raid Precautions Department of the Home Office, on the advice of the Air Ministry, were working on an estimate of 24 deaths for every ton of bombs dropped and that 700 tons of bombs might be expected to be dropped daily on objectives in this country during the first fortnight of a war breaking out in 1939; but as the estimated bomb lift of the Luftwaffe was 2,500 tons this figure might be considerably exceeded. The estimate of wounded in one day was now 35,000 as compared with 3,300 in 1925 and 30,000 in 1935 and it was recognised that the whole of this number might conceivably occur in the London area.

In order to apply these figures to the problem with which the Ministry was confronted it was necessary to estimate what percentage of the wounded would be lightly wounded and not require in-patient treatment in hospital. The last war provided no guide, as then all wounded were admitted to hospital. A completely different type of warfare had now to be provided for. In Spain, however, the slightly wounded averaged 19 per cent. of all wounded, so it was considered that 20 per cent. would be a reasonable estimate on which to base figures. Eventually the following table based partly on the Air Ministry's figures, partly on figures from Spain and partly on conjecture, was put forward as a possible basis on which to arrive at some conclusion:

Next War		Spain	
33% killed per day	17,500	17% killed	7,000
66% wounded	35,000	83% wounded	35,000
Of these latter		Of these latter	
20% slightly wounded	7,000	19% slightly wounded	6,750
16% die within 48 hours	5,600	39% died within 48 hours	13,800
64% for further treatment	22,400	42% for further treatment	14,450

The estimate of 16 per cent. dying in hospital within forty-eight hours is just over double the percentage dying in hospital in this period in the last war, but this low figure was certainly due to the inevitable delay in getting casualties into hospital in that type of warfare and also to the fact that lightly wounded were included in admissions. In Spain the deaths in hospital within forty-eight hours seemed too high to serve as a basis for this country. The number of beds required was therefore based on the following estimates:

(i) 80 per cent. of the wounded would require in-patient treatment;

(ii) 16 per cent. of these would die within forty-eight hours and thus release beds;

(iii) the daily number of 35,000 wounded would continue for a fortnight but would fall by 25 per cent. in the third week and by a further 25 per cent. in the fourth week;

(iv) after the first fortnight 25 per cent. of the in-patients could be discharged or become out-patients.

The Deficiency of Beds. These assumptions showed that 322,000 beds would be required by the end of the second week and 433,000 by the end of the fourth week, or more than five times the number of beds which could be relied on as available for casualties in existing hospitals after the war had been in progress for four weeks. The deficiency was therefore estimated to be 353,000 beds. Inherent in the difficulty of meeting this deficiency was the problem of providing medical and nursing staff commensurate with the number of beds. On the War Office scale of 17 doctors to a base hospital of 600 beds, 24,225 would be required for the civilian hospital services alone out of 45,000 doctors available in the country, out of which the expanded needs of the Services, the staffing of the first-aid posts, the public health services and the medical needs of the outside hospitals would also have to be met. It was obvious that it would be quite impossible to meet these demands. A similar state of affairs would arise in the nursing profession and between 300,000 and 400,000 nursing auxiliaries would have to be recruited and given adequate hospital training.

In the above figures the demands of the Services for hospital accommodation for casualties from overseas had not been considered. It was therefore suggested in the interests of economy of personnel and uniformity of administration that the additional hospital accommodation required should be under one central authority which would permit of fully equipped units being handed over, if and when required, to the Services. This proposal had the merit of keeping medical and nursing personnel employed to the best advantage and avoided their immobilisation in Service institutions, where they might not be immediately required, at a time when the civilian hospitals were expected to be subjected to their severest strain. A further advantage would be that a considerable economy would be effected in the use of consultant advisers who otherwise would be appointed separately for each service.

The Proposals for New Construction. It will be observed that in these calculations no provision could be made for concentrated enemy attacks on a limited number of places as this would mean a further considerable increase in the demands for bed accommodation. It was therefore decided to recommend as a short-term policy the provision of 40,000 beds in huts at the earliest possible date and a provisional allotment to each Region was drawn up. This allotment provided hospital accommodation where it was normally most required, in non-vulnerable areas so that local authorities could use the beds pending the outbreak of an emergency, on terms to be agreed. Thus some return for the capital expenditure might be obtained.

When these works were well under way it was proposed to provide another 40,000 beds in new hospital units, also in places where there was need for additional beds. This would bring the number of beds on which continued reliance could be placed to 160,000. As a result of these proposals financial sanction was obtained to proceed with the immediate construction of huts to accommodate 20,000 beds on lands adjoining hospitals primarily to serve London, Birmingham and Tyneside. On receipt of this sanction the Minister of Health and the Secretary of State for Scotland submitted a memorandum to the Cabinet briefly outlining the position to date and suggesting:

(a) that approval be given to the principle of unified control of Emergency Hospital accommodation whether for civilian or Service requirements in this country;

(b) that a committee of Ministers be set up to consider the extent to which additional accommodation might be provided.

This was followed by a more comprehensive memorandum early in April asking for decisions on the following two points:

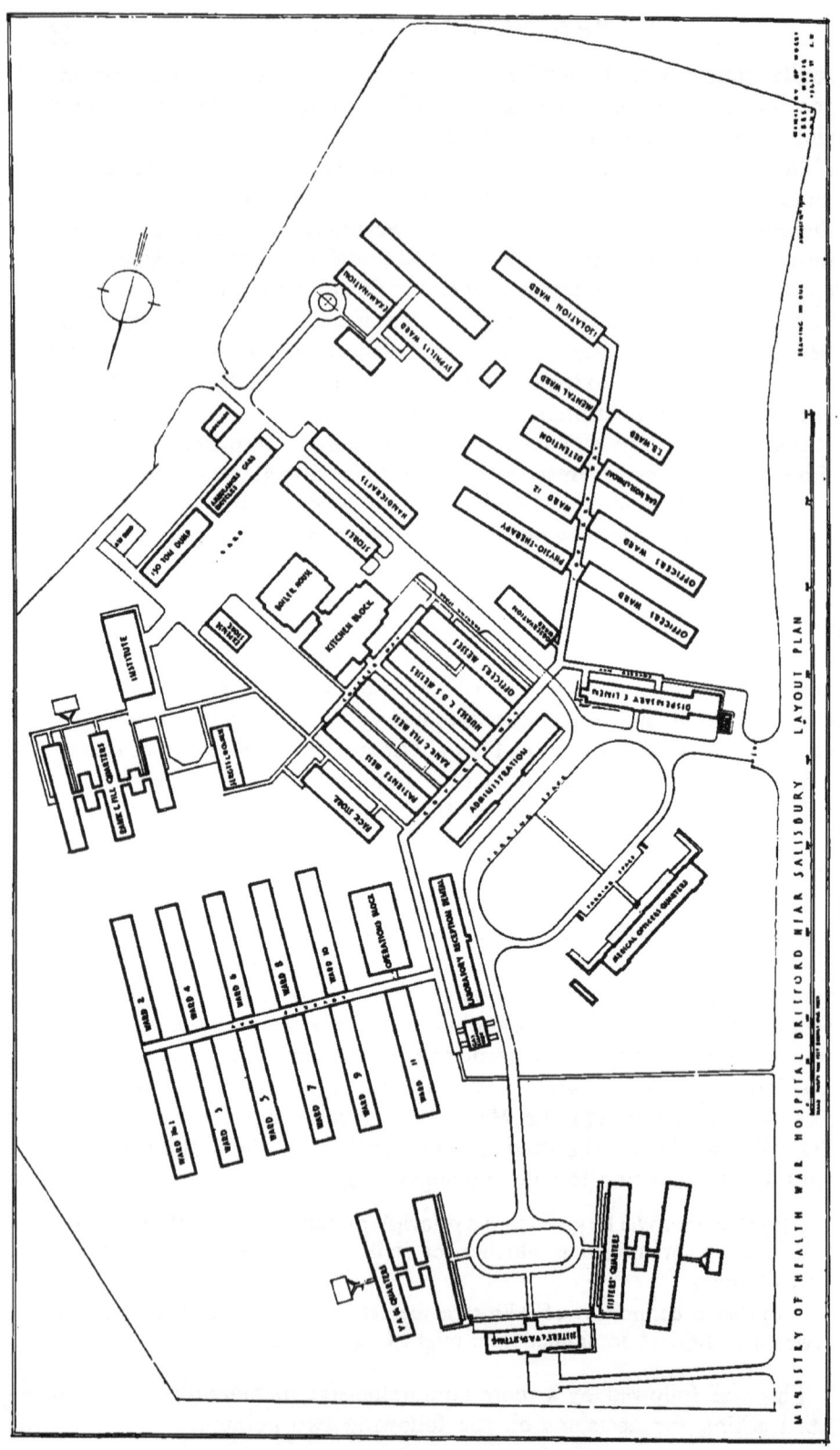

FIG. 1. Layout of a hutted hospital

(i) The extent to which additional accommodation should be provided. It was suggested that not less than 90,000 new beds should be aimed at.

(ii) It was suggested that the execution of this programme should be in stages:

> *Block A.* 26,000 beds as a first instalment already begun and estimated to cost £2,080,000.
> *Block B.* 26,000 further beds attached as far as possible to existing hospitals to be ordered at once at a cost of £2,560,000.
> *Block C.* 46,000 beds in new hospital units at a cost of £7,360,000 to be ordered after a further review of the position.

The figures above include in each case a quota of 6,000 beds for Scotland.

It was pointed out in making these suggestions that the provision for casualties had been scaled down from some 430,000 to roughly 300,000 but that the Ministers would not take the responsibility of adopting this lower figure without bringing the matter to the knowledge of their colleagues. The result was that the Cabinet Committee of Ministers on Emergency Hospital Organisation, appointed in accordance with recommendation (*b*) above, agreed on April 17 that the number of casualties to be provided for should be roughly 300,000 and that subject to the approval of the Chancellor of the Exchequer a further 20,000 beds for England and Wales in huts (Block B) should be ordered forthwith and that the decision regarding the further provision (Block C) be deferred until it had become possible to report progress on Blocks A and B.

This target of 300,000 beds for casualties, in addition to full provision for the normal requirements of the civil population, was made up as follows:

	Beds Approximate numbers
(*a*) Already provided in existing hospitals by crowding and upgrading	160,000
(*b*) To be provided by new construction	90,000
(*c*) To be provided in mental hospitals	36,000
	286,000
In addition to casualty beds provided by the E.M.S., considerable numbers of beds were provided by the Ministry of Pensions and the Armed Forces. These amounted to about 30,000 in June 1941. On average about half were constantly vacant, say	14,000
	300,000

220,000 of these were to be available for normal periods of hospitalisation and 80,000 in casualty clearing hospitals. These numbers could at any time be increased by 90,000 beds for short periods by restricting normal admission.

As regards hutted accommodation plans and specifications for the type of huts were agreed on, the Office of Works' layouts approved, land

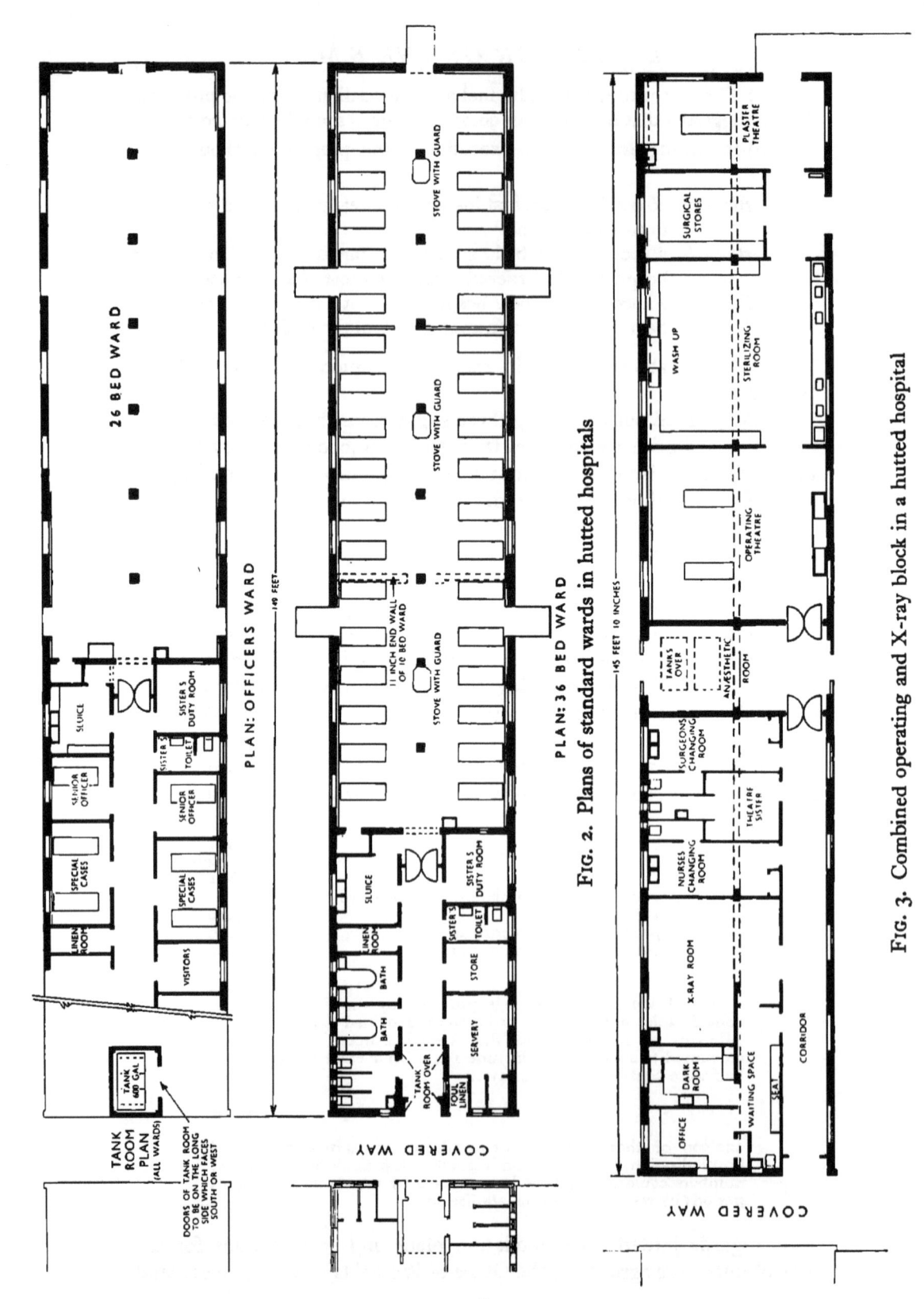

FIG. 2. Plans of standard wards in hutted hospitals

FIG. 3. Combined operating and X-ray block in a hutted hospital

acquired and contracts placed and eventually construction on Block A commenced, dates for the completion of the contracts being fixed in each case. The layout of a typical hutted hospital, and the plans of three of the huts are illustrated in Figs. 1-3. Plans were modified when necessary to meet local requirements. Plate I illustrates a typical ward.

In order that the new accommodation would be ready to be brought into use as soon as the buildings were completed, it was arranged that the Office of Works should deliver the necessary equipment of each unit as it was completed, rather than this should be done under the general arrangements for supply. Orders were, therefore, placed for surgical equipment, operating theatre and ward equipment for the 70,000 beds which it was proposed to 'crowd' into hospitals and institutions which were being upgraded, etc. The position in May, therefore, was that 150,000 bedsteads together with the necessary number of mattresses, sheets, blankets, etc., had been ordered. The Home Office had also increased the number of stretchers on order to 226,000 of which over 50 per cent. had already been distributed. Drugs and dressings estimated to provide for 250,000 casualty beds, 3,000 first-aid posts and 2,000 first-aid points had already been ordered. It was expected that these would be distributed by the end of June.

The Cabinet Committee also considered that agreement on the unified control of emergency hospital accommodation should be reached by inter-departmental discussion without further reference to the Cabinet. (See Army Medical Services, Volume I, Chapter 2.) Discussions with the War Department followed which resulted in May in an agreement that the medical officers required for the four Territorial General Hospitals for home service, eleven general hospitals and four casualty clearing stations, eventually to proceed overseas—which were the War Office's requirements for hospitals in Great Britain in the event of war (see Chapter 1)—would, after call-up, be temporarily released to civil duties, a nucleus of three medical officers only being retained to start the establishment of each hospital. As regards nurses, the calling up of four-fifths of the establishment for each hospital would be postponed until their services were actually required.

Upgrading. The various hospital authorities having submitted proposals for upgrading certain of their hospitals to Class I and for adaptations in both Class I and Class II, these proposals were now reviewed, and medical officers and engineers of the Ministry, in consultation with hospital authorities, considered what adaptations should be carried out. In order to save time, wherever possible the work was authorised and put in hand immediately, with the result that during the first two months of the year 156 hospitals and institutions were in the process of being upgraded.

Equipment and Storage. Orders for equipment had been placed on a large scale. Of 150,000 bedsteads and mattresses, 300,000 blankets and 200,000 pillows which had been ordered by May 1939, considerable quantities had already been delivered and stored. In addition, 400,000 blankets had been obtained by the Home Office for distribution to first-aid posts. An arrangement was made with the Chief Officer of Supplies whereby he acted as agent for the Ministry of Health, as well as for the Home Office and Department of Health for Scotland in purchasing reserves of drugs, dressings, etc., for hospitals and first-aid posts. This proved to be of the greatest value.

Centres for Special Treatment and the Appointment of Consultant Advisers. The general hospital arrangements were now well on their way and the Ministry took up the important question of providing specially equipped hospitals for the treatment of special types of disabilities. Although it was the policy of the Ministry to interfere as little as possible with the internal working of the hospitals and to leave to them the responsibility for actual clinical work, it was realised that the organisation of special treatment hospitals on a scale commensurate with the enormously increased demand for such facilities in time of war must involve a certain amount of central control. To provide for these special centres, suitable hospitals or other buildings which could be adapted to the particular object in view had to be chosen and arrangements made for the assembly of the necessary specialised personnel and special equipment. For this purpose it was decided in November 1938, to appoint forthwith Consultant Advisers for each of the types of disability for which special arrangements would have to be made as well as for general medicine and surgery, and the Advisory Committee of the Royal Colleges of Physicians and Surgeons was asked to make suitable nominations. The Minister desired to obtain advice from the consultants on the schemes to be worked out and, when an emergency arose, they would advise on the general administration and supervise the working of the scheme. In the first instance consultant advisers were appointed for psychiatry, neurology and surgery (general, head, orthopædic, chest, and maxillo-facial). These were followed by appointments in general medicine, physical medicine, and radiology, and in ear, nose and throat, ophthalmic and dental surgery. Later, consultant advisers in neurosurgery, gynæcology, anæsthetics, peripheral nerve injuries, and rehabilitation and in the organisation of casualty services were added. Subsequently consultant advisers were also appointed for the Regions. (See Chapter 4, and Appendix II.)

After the appointment of the first group of consultant advisers, plans for setting up centres for the treatment of special cases were taken up. Since it was expected that at the opening of hostilities every available bed would be required, definitely to earmark and equip certain institutions for special cases would be to sterilise accommodation which might be urgently required for general purposes. It therefore appeared that all hospitals must in the first instance be prepared, equipped and staffed to admit any type of casualty, and that special centres should be planned to form an integral part of the larger general hospitals. The main reason for this was that each special centre would require particular apparatus which in most cases already existed in the larger general hospitals and that specialists in such hospitals were usually already available. The number of beds both primarily and ultimately to be devoted to special work could be left indeterminate and so be regulated by the current demand as it arose. The scheme was therefore developed on these lines, and, as time went on, arrangements were made to transfer all special cases to the hospitals containing the appropriate facilities.

Neurosis Centres. As a departure from the general policy, exceptional arrangements were made for dealing with neurosis. Reports from countries recently at war indicated that an appreciable amount of hysteria and other neuroses must be expected to follow intensive bombing of the civilian population. It was obviously necessary to prepare a scheme which would effectively deal with the contingency if and when it arose and ensure the utilisation of the available specialist medical personnel to the greatest advantage. In October 1938, the Ministry sought the advice of specialists, whose general opinion was that psycho-neurotic casualties among the civil population were not only inevitable but would occur in large numbers. After many discussions it was decided to locate three intermediate hospitals for the treatment of neurosis, namely : at Mill Hill School, the Sutton Training Centre, and Isleworth Public Assistance Institution; Cox Heath in Kent was subsequently chosen as a fourth.

Peripheral base hospitals for London were also designated. Accommodation for neurosis cases was arranged for at the Park Prewett Hospital, Hampshire, the Horton Mental Hospital, Surrey, and the Bedford County Mental Hospital, providing potential accommodation for 6,000 cases should the need arise and other circumstances permit. Provincial Hospital Officers were asked to organise a similar scheme with the advice of the consultant advisers to serve large centres of population in their Regions. Of the special schemes, the neurosis centres were the first to take shape; this was, in a large measure, due to the unremitting energy of the two consultant advisers, Dr. Gordon Holmes and Dr. Bernard Hart.

Events subsequently disproved the estimates of civilian cases of neurosis; they were found to be only an infinitesimal percentage of the total war casualties. But, as the war went on, these neurosis centres served an increasing need and their provision was amply justified.

Numerous instructions were issued on the organisation and location of the centres for special treatment and in June 1941 these were consolidated in a booklet entitled *Medical Treatment and Special Centres*, issued by the Ministry of Health, to which supplements and amendments were added from time to time. The names of the consultant advisers and numbers of the special centres will be found in Appendix II.

THE PROVISION OF ANCILLARY SERVICES FOR THE HOSPITALS; RADIOLOGY, PATHOLOGY AND BLOOD TRANSFUSION

With the expansion of the hospitals and re-distribution of the medical staffs, especially in London, and the allotment to each hospital of its rôle in the Emergency Hospital Scheme, the question of efficient ancillary services for the hospitals had to be taken up. It was obvious that the peace-time provisions for services such as radiology, pathology, blood transfusion, the supply of anti-tetanic serum, etc., would have to be expanded and co-ordinated.

After full discussion on each subject it was agreed that the Medical Research Council would organise pathological and blood transfusion services for the London area, and that they would largely increase the output of anti-tetanic serum and issue an adequate supply of anti-gas gangrene serum. At the suggestion of the Medical Research Council the Hospital Officers of the provincial Regions were asked to nominate senior pathologists who would act as their advisers on the provision of the pathological services, and later were instructed to organise blood transfusion services in accordance with a scheme laid down by the Ministry for their Regions (see Chapter 4). They were also instructed to arrange for a suitable number of storage depots for sera supplied by the Medical Research Council for distribution, when required, to the hospitals and first-aid posts. The story of these organisations will be found in the special chapters on these subjects (Chapters 10–11) contributed by those chiefly concerned in bringing them into being, so that only a passing reference is necessary here. A chapter on the organisation of the radiological services is also included in this volume (Chapter 12).

REGIONAL BOUNDARIES AND RE-NUMBERING OF REGIONS

In February 1939, the various Regions into which the country had been divided were re-numbered as follows:

Old Number	New Number		Area Covered
No. 1	No. 1	Northern Region	Northumberland, Durham, Yorkshire (North Riding)
No. 2	No. 2	North-Eastern Region	Yorkshire (West and East Ridings, and York County Borough)
No. 4	No. 3	North-Midland Region	Derbyshire (less the High Peak District, in Region 10), Leicestershire, Lincs., Northampton, Nottinghamshire, Rutland, Soke of Peterborough

Old Number	New Number		Area Covered
No. 6	No. 4	Eastern Region	Beds, Cambs, Hunts, Norfolk, Suffolk, Isle of Ely, Essex (less the portion in No. 5 Region), Herts (less the portion in No. 5)
No. 9	No. 5	London Region	Metropolitan Police District
No. 7	No. 6	Southern Region	Berks, Bucks, Dorset (parts of), Hampshire, Oxfordshire, Isle of Wight, Surrey (less the portion in No. 5 Region)
No. 8	No. 7	South-Western Region	Cornwall, Devon, Gloucester, Somerset, Wiltshire, Dorset (less portions in No. 6 Region)
No. 10	No. 8	Wales Region	Wales and Monmouth
No. 5	No. 9	Midland Region	Herefordshire, Shropshire, Staffs, Warwick, Worcester
No. 3	No. 10	North-Western Region	Cheshire, High Peak District in Derbyshire, Cumberland, Lancashire, Westmorland
	No. 12	South-Eastern Region	Kent (less portion in No. 5 Region), Sussex and Surrey (less portion in No. 5 Region)

PROTECTION OF BUILDINGS

Emergency Medical Service Memorandum 1. The Home Office in conjunction with the Ministry of Health drew up a memorandum on structural precautions which was eventually issued to local authorities and hospitals as Memorandum 1 of the Emergency Medical Services.[1] This contained recommendations for protection against air raid risks which had necessarily to be taken at hospitals, as obviously patients could not be transported wholesale into bomb-proof shelters each time an air raid warning was given. No uniform scale of protection could be laid down as each case would have to be dealt with on its merits. The general recommendations were as follows:

(1) Protection of upper floors against incendiary bombs by providing boarding and asbestos sheeting over rafters under pitched roofs and spraying the wood-work with fire resisting paint.
(2) Protection of operating theatres by sand-bagging or otherwise protecting windows—if this were found impracticable provision should be made to set up emergency theatres on the ground floors or in basements.
(3) Prevention of injury from flying glass by providing wire or other screens for windows.
(4) Protection of ground floors by sand-bagging against the effects of blast and splinters.
(5) Provision of shelters for the staff off duty and ambulant patients by strengthening basements or providing trenches or steel shelters in the hospital grounds.

Owing to deterioration of sand-bags from the effects of the weather, brick walls, constructed according to special specifications which were found to be effective from experience, were later substituted for sand-bagging and similar forms of protection.

PUBLICATION OF THE MINISTRY'S HOSPITAL SCHEME

Emergency Medical Service Memorandum 2. In March 1939, it was decided to publish the Ministry's schemes for dealing with that part of the casualty service which was concerned with hospital organisation, thereby enabling the various hospitals to obtain a clear idea of what would be expected of them and of the division of responsibility. Regions and Sectors were supplied with detailed information about each of their areas and Emergency Medical Service Memorandum No. 2 was issued.[2] This memorandum explained in general terms the main lines on which a comprehensive scheme for war-time hospital organisation was being worked out, that the scheme would be liable to modification in the light of further experience and to that extent it was to be regarded as provisional. In addition, it was explained how it was intended to make beds available for casualties, and in an appendix details were given of the way the admission and discharge of casualties should be carried out and recorded, together with specimen forms for the purpose. One of the main sections in the memorandum was that on the affiliation of hospitals, since this introduced a system of co-operation foreign to the practice of the voluntary hospitals in peace-time when the aim of most of these was to preserve their identity inviolate. Hospital authorities having thus been made aware of the general principles of the Emergency Hospital Scheme, individual hospitals were approached as to the part that each would be expected to play; the functions of the Group Officers in the London Sectors and of the Regional Hospital Officers in the provinces were explained.

LONDON CASUALTY HOSPITAL SCHEME

The Sectors. Since October 1938, the Ministry had been endeavouring to arrive at an amicable agreement with the London voluntary hospitals in order to bring into being a scheme partly based on a recommendation of the 'Wilson' Committee, which aimed at dividing the London area into Sectors with inner and outer zones, each Sector to be based on one or more of the large teaching hospitals, with hospitals in outer zones affiliated to them—but the attitude of the governing bodies of the hospitals appeared to be suspicious of any Government scheme, which they feared might limit their independence or interfere with their traditional policy. This attitude hindered rapid progress. One thorny question was the medical administration of each Sector; the Minister considered that in the best interests of all parties the Medical Directors should be men who would be assured of the full co-operation of the voluntary hospitals as well as of the local authority hospitals, and who also had a full knowledge of their internal administration and their potentialities.

In the middle of January 1939, however, the Deans of the teaching hospitals became anxious about the delays and called a meeting the

FIG. 4

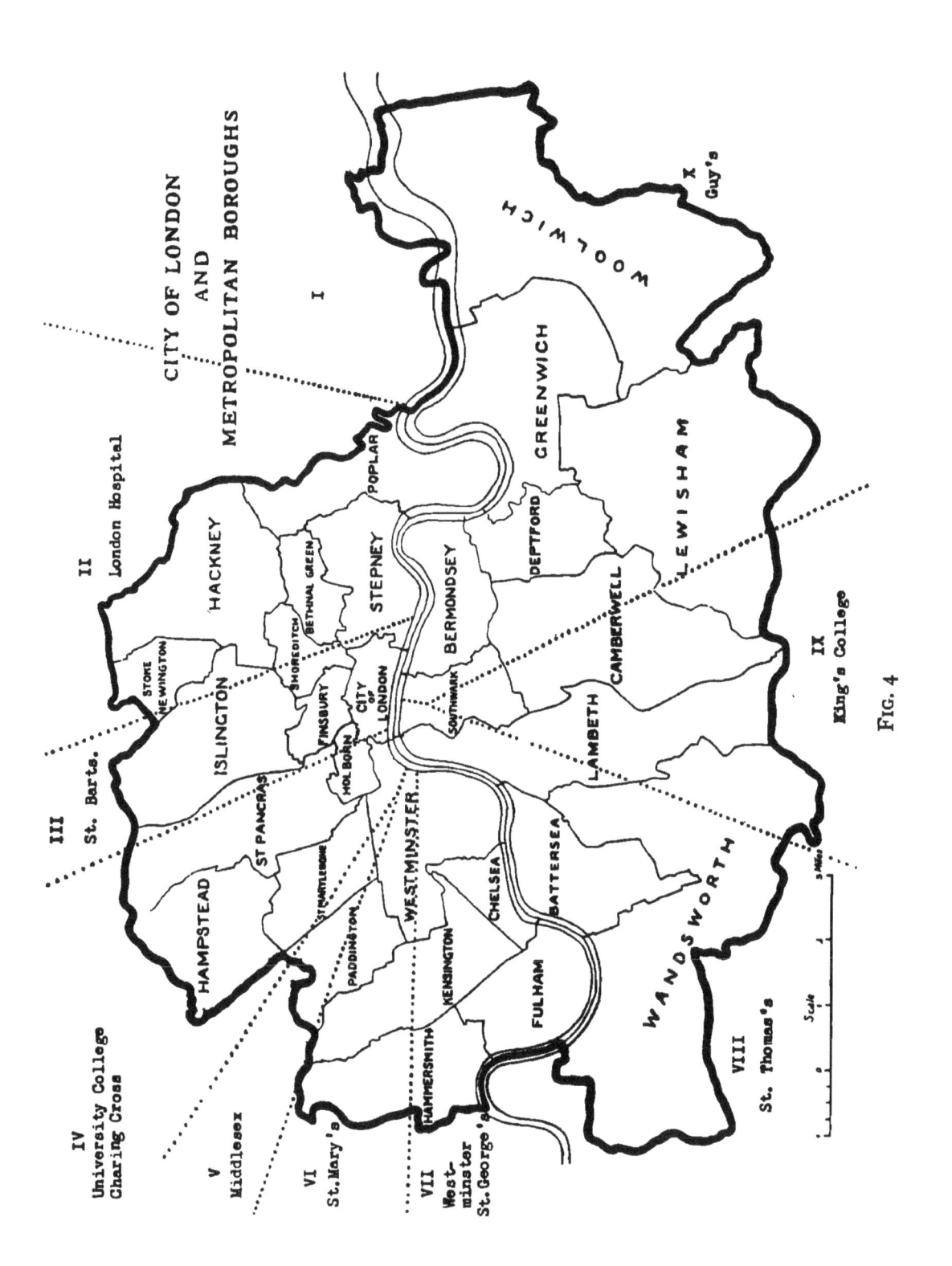

outcome of which was that Sir Girling Ball, the Dean of St. Bartholomew's Hospital was authorised to suggest to the Ministry that the Deans' Committee should be the body appointed to put into effect the London Zoning Scheme. In view of some of the difficulties already apparent this offer was both opportune and attractive. Before any definite decision was reached, it was considered desirable that the main details of the Ministry's scheme should be explained to the Deans' Committee; accordingly, at a meeting held in February the salient features of the scheme were discussed. It was explained that there had been a general recognition of the fact that the hospital organisation for London and its environs presented problems of its own owing to the heavy concentration of population, the wide area over which the movement of patients would have to be arranged and the number and diversity of hospital authorities.

Accordingly the London Region had been divided into ten Sectors each of which radiated from an apex in the centre out into the Home Counties (see map, Fig. 4). The hospitals whose representatives it was proposed should direct each of the Sectors were as follows:

Sectors I and II	London Hospital
Sector III	St. Bartholomew's Hospital
Sector IV	University College Hospital
Sector V	Middlesex Hospital
Sector VI	St. Mary's Hospital
Sector VII	St. George's Hospital
Sector VIII	St. Thomas's Hospital
Sector IX	King's College Hospital
Sector X	Guy's Hospital

In Sectors III, IV and VII, the Royal Free Hospital, Charing Cross Hospital and Westminster Hospital respectively, were to be asked to co-operate in the scheme.

The wide ends of the Sectors extended into the counties of Essex, Hertfordshire, Buckinghamshire, Surrey and Kent. In peace-time the functions of the Medical Director of a Sector would be to work out the organisation, to arrange, on the general plan laid down by the Ministry, the precise use to which each hospital was to be put, the distribution of the medical personnel between the inner and outer zone hospitals, and generally to act on behalf of the hospitals in the Sectors but also as agent of the Ministry in carrying out the Goverment's policy on hospital organisation. Since the L.C.C. and other municipal authorities' institutions would come within the scope of the scheme it would be necessary to work in co-operation with the representatives of the local authorities. The general scheme visualised:

(a) Central hospitals for the immediate admission of cases which would be evacuated as soon as conditions permitted.

(b) Hospitals about four miles from the centre of London to receive sick and casualties arising locally.
(c) A limited number of hospitals designated 'advance base hospitals' to which the more serious cases could be evacuated from the central hospitals. These hospitals would require to have a full range of surgical facilities.
(d) Base hospitals varying in distance from fifteen to fifty miles.
(e) Special hospitals or wards to be set aside for special types of cases.

The aim would be to maintain as few beds in the inner zone as was consistent with the immediate needs of the sick and for the first reception of casualties, and to make increasing provision in the outer areas by the expansion of existing institutions, by utilising the mental hospitals and, if necessary, by constructing additional hutted hospitals.

Team work was considered an integral part of any scheme, the advance base hospitals being considered the appropriate place for establishing mobile teams in order to reinforce the central or other hospitals which might require assistance. These mobile teams would not carry special equipment as this would be available at the hospitals where their services were required, but there should be at least one equipped mobile surgical unit in each sector available to proceed to any unit not in possession of the surgical facilities to meet any special contingency. It would be the duty of the head of each Sector to arrange for the dispersal of therapeutic equipment which would not be required in the central area; he would also be concerned with the recommendations for adaptations, which might be necessary in institutions suitable for the purpose, which he had in mind. Further, he would be responsible for schemes to obtain the dispersal and location of nursing and other technical staff. A list of the hospitals allocated to each sector had been prepared showing their grading and the functions which it was proposed each should assume during an emergency, in some cases the number of beds being increased and in others reduced, according to the situation of the hospital. The head of the Sector in war-time would assume responsibility for directing the movement of casualties and personnel within his sector, and the Hospital Officer of the Region would co-ordinate such movements for the whole Region. During the discussions which took place the representatives of the teaching hospitals unanimously expressed their wholehearted desire to give all the help in their power to make the scheme a workable one. The offer of their services was readily accepted.

The Sector Group Officers. The representatives of the London teaching hospitals were then appointed to be the first Sector Group Officers.

Functions of the Sector Group Officers and Consultant Advisers. With the appointment of Consultant Advisers and Sector Group Officers uncertainty arose as to their respective functions, in consequence of which a note was issued to clarify the position. Sector Group Officers were likened to Deputy Directors of Medical Services in the Army who in peace-time are purely organisers but who in war-time are in complete control, being responsible for all medical movements within their Sectors. Consultant advisers, on the other hand, were responsible for seeing that the special units were established on a proper scale and in the appropriate locations to meet the needs of the Sectors. It was also their function to recommend to Sector Group Officers the most suitable people to place in charge of the work of particular units; thereafter their duty would be generally to supervise their side of the work in the country as a whole, and to advise the Principal Medical Officer at the Ministry of further requirements which they thought necessary.

THE ORGANISATION IN THE REGIONS

London Region. At the end of June 1939, there was some anxiety about the state of preparedness of the London hospitals, and the Minister agreed to meet a deputation from the London teaching hospitals. To this deputation the Minister outlined the general scheme by which it was proposed to meet the needs of the casualty service for extra accommodation in hospitals. After discussion it was agreed that the chairmen of the boards of the hospitals should draw up a detailed memorandum of the points on which they would like guidance and decisions. At a later meeting this memorandum was discussed and answers were supplied whenever the development of the scheme made it possible. One of the chief points raised was that the lay organisations were incomplete. The Minister intimated that since in and around London the local authorities controlled a very large number of hospital beds, the solution would be to institute a system of regular weekly meetings of the representatives of both local authority and voluntary hospitals and officers of the Ministry, thus instituting systematised machinery for dealing with difficulties as they arose. At the first of these meetings proposals were put forward for the composition of the personnel of the Sector offices in order that all interests might be represented. Subsequently the Ministry drafted a formula setting out the decisions arrived at and the responsibilities of those concerned in war-time, including those of the Hospital Officers, as follows:

1. *Hospital Officers.* In peace-time the Regional Hospital Officers will become the constituted authority for the whole Emergency Hospital Service in their Regions either directly or through one of their deputies. A number of Regional Medical Officers of the Ministry will be seconded to act as deputies to the Hospital Officers. They will become also the ultimate ambulance authority whether for casualty or inter-hospital work. In London the Hospital Officers will be located at the headquarters of the Ministry together with the Chief Ambulance Officer and the Chief Casualty Officer for London.

(This latter arrangement did not take effect as the London Regional Hospital Officers and their staff were located at the offices of the London Civil Defence Region.)

2. *Officers in the Sectors.* In each Sector the Ministry will establish an office as the headquarters of the Group Officer. The Group Officer will have ultimate authority over his staff and will be responsible to the Hospital Officers.

3. The Group Officer's staff will fall into two main parts:
   (1) Representing the voluntary hospitals, there will be:
      (*a*) a medical officer who will be the Group Officer's deputy for dealing with the voluntary hospitals on matters of medical administration.
      (*b*) the Sector Matron who will similarly act as the channel of communication with the voluntary hospitals on nursing matters.
      (*c*) the Lay Sector Officer who will deal with transport, lay personnel such as domestic staff, etc., equipment and general supplies. He will be the channel of communication with the voluntary hospitals of the Sector on matters of administration and finance.
   (2) Representing the L.C.C. and other local authorities having hospitals in the Sector, there will be a medical officer, a matron and a lay officer recommended by the L.C.C., who will carry out in relation to the local authority hospitals, functions similar to those of the representatives of the voluntary hospitals.

Provincial Regions

Hospital Officers. The Hospital Officers were informed of their responsibilities for the whole of the Emergency Hospital Services in their Regions and for the ambulance services, both inter-hospital and local.

Group Officers. They were also advised that they should form groups of hospitals similar to the London Sectors based on large provincial cities with central inner zone hospitals and affiliated outer zone hospitals. They were instructed to arrange conferences with the representatives of the large voluntary hospitals in the cities selected as bases for groups, and to obtain recommendations from them for the appointment of suitable men of high professional standing as Group Officers. Recommendations were also required for the appointment of Sector Matrons and lay Sector Officers in these approved groups.

Eventually twenty-nine Group Officers were appointed for the approved groups of hospitals in the provinces and took up their appointments at the outbreak of hostilities.

Local conditions in the provinces, however, required considerable departures from the London plan. In certain cities there were well-founded objections to evacuating the inner zone hospitals to the same extent as in London and to the honorary and whole-time medical staffs being split up between the inner zone hospitals and the affiliated outer zone hospitals. There were also objections to affiliating the outer zone hospitals to these inner zone hospitals and to handing over their administration to the parent hospital. In most groups, therefore, their administration was carried out by the owning authority. As in London, the Group Officers were responsible for ensuring the proper equipment of the hospitals in the groups and for their staffing. They were also generally responsible to the Ministry for obtaining an adequate standard of professional efficiency in all the hospitals in the group.

THE TEACHING OF MEDICAL STUDENTS

The Chairman of the University Grants Committee had drawn attention to the question of the continued teaching of medical students during war and had stressed the importance of medical training not being interrupted. In London the problem presented considerable difficulties owing to the intention largely to reduce the numbers of beds in inner zone hospitals and transfer many of the teaching staff to affiliated peripheral hospitals, as the result of which it had been suggested that London students should be dispersed among other universities. At a meeting at the Ministry attended by the Vice-Chancellors of the London, Cambridge and Manchester Universities decided views were expressed that medical education could not be carried on in ordinary casualty hospitals and the Vice-Chancellor of London University considered that it could not be carried on in London at all. It was their definite opinion that teaching could only be carried out in units isolated from any casualty scheme and which dealt almost exclusively with disabilities common to peace-time. As they were of opinion that on a war-time footing one bed should be earmarked for each student, this meant segregating at least 6,000 beds for this purpose alone. If it was decided that clinical students from London might be distributed to provincial universities it was estimated that about 3,000 additional students could be taken into ten of the other universities in England and Wales provided that their respective teaching hospitals could be used for this purpose. Obviously some of these universities were situated in towns which would prove to be targets and whatever they planned might be frustrated by the course of events. The question continued to be discussed and it became clear that the Deans of the London teaching hospitals were increasingly opposed to the proposals for the dispersal of students. In the latter part of March a further meeting of Vice-Chancellors and Deans was held at the Ministry but no decision was arrived at. Eventually, the Deans of the London hospitals made their own arrangements for clinical teaching by their own teaching staffs, partly in the inner zone hospitals and partly in the affiliated hospitals, and the scheme thus brought into being functioned with considerable success.

In the provinces each teaching hospital carried on as it had been doing, and in spite of heavy attacks on Liverpool and Manchester, etc., clinical work went on with little or no serious interruption.

THE CASUALTY BUREAUX

The Ministry issued particulars about setting up casualty bureaux, in the Regions as well as in the Sectors; the procedure to be adopted in carrying out the evacuation of patients and the recording of bed-states and statistical returns, and the addresses of all Service record offices to which Service casualties were to be notified by the bureaux. Local authorities were also notified of the need for setting up casualty bureaux and the manner in which the casualties were to be notified. Information was also issued to the medical officers of health and hospitals dealing with the procedure for the admission, transfer, discharge or death of casualties and describing the records which should be kept by the hospitals at each stage. This information was included in Emergency Medical Services Memorandum No. 3 issued in October 1939, and revised in April 1940.[3]

In the Regions, casualty bureaux were set up by each scheme-making authority, i.e. county council or county borough council, but in places where the headquarters of the county council and county borough council were in the same town, their casualty bureaux were often combined. In the Sectors, as stated in the paragraphs on the London Hospital Organisation, there was only one casualty bureau for each Sector.

THE CIVIL DEFENCE CASUALTY SERVICES

FIRST-AID POSTS AND POINTS

Since the September crisis uneasiness had been voiced not only in Parliament but elsewhere at the casualty services being administered by two different departments and on November 30, 1938, it was announced in the House of Commons[4] that the responsibility for the first-aid posts would be transferred from the Home Office to the Ministry of Health. After discussions with the Home Office it was agreed that personnel for the first-aid posts would be recruited, as before, by the Home Office through the local authorities and that the Home Office would still be in charge of the arrangements for their initial training in first aid, etc. The Ministry of Health decided that the plans already worked out by the Home Office for the first-aid posts and points should be generally adhered to, although some modification might be advisable. It was considered that first-aid posts were likely to become more akin to dressing stations and that one or more doctors, according to the size of the post, would have to be appointed in charge.

These medical officers would be recommended by the Local Emergency Committees and appointed by the local authorities. A trained nurse also was considered necessary in each first-aid post.

First-aid parties, together with all other air raid precautions personnel, were still to be the responsibility of the Home Office. The first-aid parties being the first to give medical aid to casualties at incidents either under the supervision of a doctor, as eventually happened in most places on the appointment of 'incident doctors', or without such supervision, it would seem that they should have been made responsible to the Ministry of Health, as were the personnel of the first-aid posts of which they really formed an integral part, but with external duties (see also Chapter 7).

The decision was no doubt influenced by the close co-operation desirable between first-aid parties and rescue parties which were clearly the responsibility of the Home Office.

Emergency Medical Services, Memorandum 4 was issued by the Ministry for the guidance of medical officers and other first-aid personnel in the first-aid treatment of casualties.[5]

MOBILE FIRST-AID UNITS

It was felt that there was too much rigidity in the spacing of first-aid posts and that in less densely populated areas the number of fixed posts could be cut down. In order, however, that first-aid facilities should be available even to the more remote portions of a district, local authorities were asked to give consideration to supplementing fixed posts by 'mobile units' which could proceed to the area required and set up a post, the personnel and equipment being conveyed in a motor van or bus the fitting-up of which was to be undertaken in peace-time. Plans for these 'mobile units' were being worked out and were to be distributed as soon as possible. The size and layout of posts were to be left to the discretion of local authorities.

DECONTAMINATION UNITS

Decontamination arrangements were also being organised by the Home Office and the Ministry of Health; the Home Office were responsible for large cleansing units for contaminated but unwounded members of the public, and the Ministry of Health for wounded and contaminated casualties at first-aid posts and hospitals, separate decontamination arrangements being made at hospitals for stretcher cases.

AMBULANCES

The responsibility for local authority ambulances, the personnel of which also did external duties, having been handed over to the Ministry of Health, discussions with the Ministry of Transport had been taking place and general agreement had been reached on the procedure to be followed. The local ambulances were to be provided by the local authorities in the numbers considered necessary in each place, after approval by the Regional Hospital Officers. Suitable fitments for these ambulances, which would permit the efficient transport of casualties on the Ministry's standard type of stretcher were also agreed upon. The instructions of the Ministry on this subject were sent to the local authorities and amending instructions were issued from time to time in the light of experience; suitable fleets of ambulances came into being with adequate garage accommodation and arrangements for their maintenance. The efficient state of affairs eventually attained naturally took many months during which defects in adaptation and organisation were gradually eliminated. Details of the evolution of the first-aid and ambulance services will be found in the special chapter on the Casualty Services, as this section of the Emergency Medical Services Organisation eventually became known (Chapter 7).

CIVIL DEFENCE ACT, 1939

On July 13, the Civil Defence Act was passed with a view to giving legislative authority for the schemes already in hand. It included powers for the Minister of Health to make arrangements for the treatment in hospital of casualties occurring in Great Britain, the training of nurses, the provision of services controlling the spread of infectious diseases and the removal of sick persons and persons of unsound mind from one locality to another when necessary. The Minister was given power to acquire land, to erect buildings, to obtain and hold medical stores and equipment, to provide for storage and transport and to enter into agreement with local authorities and voluntary hospitals for effecting these ends in providing for the treatment of casualties. The duties of local authorities were defined and councils were required to place any officer temporarily at the disposal of the Minister. The basis of the respective financial responsibilities of the Government and the local authorities was also laid down.

MEDICAL PERSONNEL*

HEADQUARTERS STAFF

From the appointment of Dr. Hebb as Principal Medical Officer of the Emergency Medical Services on July 13, 1938, the whole-time medical staff at headquarters of the Service consisted at first only of Dr. Hebb and his deputy, Dr. Lethem.

In December 1938, Dr. Murchie and Dr. Charles Seeley were seconded by the Ministry of Pensions to Dr. Hebb's staff—Dr. F. Murchie as Director of the Emergency Medical Services for London and the Home Counties and Dr. Seeley in charge of the administration of the

---

* See also Chapter 14.

first-aid posts—and Dr. Johnstone, who had been lent to the Ministry by the L.C.C. to assist the Hospital Officer for London, was absorbed into the headquarters staff—at first on a part-time basis and afterwards whole-time—as advisory officer on medical equipment. In July 1939, Lt. Col. E. T. Potts, C.M.G., D.S.O., R.A.M.C. (ret.) was recruited by a selection board to act as Deputy Director-General for personnel, Col. T. J. Scott, D.S.O., M.C., R.A.M.C. (ret.) was recruited to act as liaison officer with the Services, and Dr. P. D. Oakley was appointed medical officer in charge of civil evacuation trains. From time to time, as the work expanded, other officers were recruited to the headquarters staff such as Col. L. W. Proger as blood transfusion liaison officer, Dr. (afterwards Sir) Philip N. Panton in charge of the pathological services, Dr. S. Cochrane Shanks in charge of the radiological services, etc. A principal matron, Miss K. C. Watt, R.R.C. (afterwards Dame Katherine Watt) was also appointed to control the nursing arrangements. Mr. A. H. Mahoney, Senior Dental Officer of the Ministry was put in charge of the dental arrangements.

In June, the Lord Privy Seal and the Minister of Health decided that a greater degree of co-ordination was required between the Air Raid Precautions Department of the Home Office and the Ministry of Health. To this end the Principal Medical Officer of the Emergency Medical Services was appointed Director-General of the Emergency Medical Services to both Departments.[6] It was agreed that administrative responsibility of each Department was not affected and that the Director-General would be responsible for medical advice on all matters regarding first-aid parties and the recruitment and individual training of personnel for the first-aid posts which had hitherto been the responsibility of the Air Raid Precautions Department.

REGIONAL HEADQUARTERS STAFF

In the Regions during July additional Hospital Officers were recruited by the selection board for the three most important Regions outside London, Lt. Col. C. L. Dunn, C.I.E., I.M.S. (ret.) for the North-Western Region, Dr. R. Tudor Hart for the Midland Region and Col. H. T. Bates for the Northern Region. Wing Commander A. J. Brown, Medical Branch, R.A.F. (ret.) was appointed in addition to Dr. Dobbie for the London Region. On September 1, 1939, several medical officers were seconded from the National Health Insurance Branch of the Ministry to the staffs of the Regional Hospital Officers as Assistant Hospital Officers, the numbers varying in accordance with the size of the Regions. Regional Nursing Officers were also appointed to the staffs of each Hospital Officer.

At the same time lay administrative, executive and clerical staffs were appointed to each of the Regions from the Ministry of Health under a Senior Regional Officer to whom many of the powers of the Minister were delegated and who was to act with all the powers of the Minister under the Regional Commissioner in the event of communications being cut off from Whitehall by enemy action.

MEDICAL PERSONNEL OF THE EMERGENCY MEDICAL SERVICES

The Ministry also took up with the Central Emergency Committee of the British Medical Association the question of the appointment, status and remuneration of the medical personnel who would be required to staff the Emergency Medical Services. It was generally agreed that the grades and remuneration should approximate to those of the Royal Army Medical Corps, and there was naturally a considerable difference of opinion as to how the Service should be organised. At first it was suggested that the Service should form part of the military organisation. Such an arrangement would have made it very convenient for the switch-over of men from civilian to military duty, but there were obvious disadvantages in taking doctors wholesale out of civilian practice. Eventually it was agreed in July 1939, that the service would be a civilian one directly administered by the Ministry of Health and that it should be established at once but would function only in the event of an emergency. It was to be divided into two classes of officers under which there would be sub-divisions as follows:

Class I. Whole-time Officers of the Emergency Medical Service:
(a) Whole-time Consultant Advisers . £1,400 p.a., plus allowances
(b) Group Officers . . . . £1,300 p.a., plus allowances
(This was a standard rate subject to variations in individual cases)
(c) Medical Superintendents of Hospitals . £800—£1,000 p.a., plus allowances
(d) Medical and Surgical Specialists . £800 p.a., plus allowances
(e) Medical Officers . . . . £550 p.a., plus allowances
(f) Junior Medical Officers . . . £350 p.a., plus allowances

Class II. Part-time Medical Officers on Sessional Fees:
(a) Consultants . . . . . £2 12s. 6d. for work up to two hours
(b) Practitioners . . . . . £1 11s. 6d. for work up to two hours

House officers were at first included among junior medical officers, but on representations being made by the British Medical Association and the voluntary hospitals, it was decided shortly after the outbreak of hostilities that house officers would not be recruited by the Emergency Medical Services but would be engaged by the hospital authorities on rates of pay varying from £120 to £200 p.a. In the event of these house officers being specially recruited in excess of the normal establishment of a hospital for Emergency Medical Service purposes, their pay and emoluments would be reimbursed to the hospital authorities by the Ministry, officers paid on the lower rate being graded by the British Medical Association as A appointments and those on the higher rate as B2 appointments. The British Medical Association agreed to all appointments higher than B2 up to the status of medical registrar or its equivalent being graded as B1. These included medical officers on a rate of pay of £350 to £550 p.a. plus allowances, in the Ministry's grading. The enrolment of a considerable number of medical officers was proceeded with at once from lists which had been submitted to the Central Emergency Committee of the British Medical Association for their scrutiny and registration, and forms of contract were issued for signature by the medical officers concerned. The contracts were to take effect from the date of calling up.

From time to time as medical officers serving with the Emergency Medical Services were called up to the Services, vacancies were filled from the house officers who had completed their contracts with hospitals and from available practitioners.

Difficulties that arose from time to time and the methods of dealing with them will be found in the chapter contributed by the British Medical Association and by the Medical Personnel (Priority) Committee which was set up at a later date to adjudicate between the demands of the civil and combatant services. (Chapter 14).

THE WHITE PAPER, 1939

In July 1939, a White Paper[7] was issued on the Emergency Medical Hospital Organisation, first-aid posts and ambulances. It set out for the information of Parliament the steps which had been taken up to date to bring the Emergency Medical Services into being, the stage which had been reached and the decisions which had been sanctioned for the provision of additional hospital accommodation in the way of hutted annexes, etc.

It also included a summary of the financial arrangements agreed between the Government and the local authorities. These provided that local authorities should bear three-tenths of the cost of making any premises under their control suitable for a hospital for the treatment of casualties (i.e. 'upgrading' and executing works for the purpose of protecting persons in hospital) subject to the proviso that no local authority's share of the cost should exceed one-tenth of a penny rate in any one year. If the cost exceeded that rate the Government would bear the whole of the excess. As to the voluntary hospitals, the Government agreed with the British Hospitals Association that the cost of approved protective work should be borne in the proportion of three-tenths by the hospitals and seven-tenths by the Government, subject to the proviso that no individual hospital's share should exceed £1 per bed. If it exceeded this amount the Government would bear the whole of the excess. Any 'upgrading' done at voluntary hospitals would be borne wholly by the Government.

After the outbreak of hostilities it was laid down that the Government would be responsible for the cost of the treatment of casualties by hospitals and that arrangements to this end were being negotiated with local authorities and the British Hospitals Association.

OPERATIONAL ORDERS FOR THE OUTBREAK OF WAR

As the international situation gave rise to increased anxiety it was considered desirable to draw up instructions as to the steps to be taken should a definite state of tension or one of emergency arise. Hospital Officers of Regions were supplied with instructions[8] which they were to issue to the medical officers of health of counties and county boroughs and Group Officers in their Regions as follows:

When a state of tension arose a telegram would be sent with the warning 'stand by'. On receiving this the officers concerned were:

(i) To ask all hospitals other than mental or infectious diseases hospitals—

(*a*) to restrict admissions to acute cases;

(*b*) to render daily a statement of the number of vacant beds;

(*c*) to maintain a daily record of patients who could be sent home within twenty-four hours and, in evacuation areas, to maintain a daily record of children in hospital who were unfit to be sent home but fit to be transferred to hospitals in the outer areas;

(*d*) to earmark daily, patients fit to be transferred within the next twenty-four hours at those hospitals from which it had already been agreed that a specific number of patients should be transferred;

(*e*) to accelerate protective work at hospitals;

(*f*) to set up the extra beds already received;

(*g*) to prepare for use any additional accommodation for which arrangements had been made;

(*h*) to review the adequacy of the staffing, medical equipment, stores and other arrangements required in the event of an emergency arising, including transport for sending patients home.

(ii) To distribute stretchers to those hospitals from which transfers were to be made and supplies of the official forms such as E.M.S. 105 for recording casualties, the Ministry of Pensions' forms and others which would be required during the treatment of casualties in hospital.

(iii) To supply the Hospital Officers with a summary of the vacant beds in hospitals and the number of children to be transferred.

(iv) To review the ambulance transport arrangements.

(v) To convey a preliminary warning to medical and other staff whose transfer to other hospitals had been arranged.

When a state of emergency had been declared Hospital Officers would issue a telegram to the officers concerned to 'clear hospitals'; on receipt of this these officers would put into active operation all those steps for which they had already prepared during the state of tension.

The orders issued to London and the Home Counties varied somewhat from those issued to the provinces and took account of the special circumstances of the Sector arrangements in the former.

In the last week of August it was obvious that war could not be postponed for many days and on August 25 instructions were received from the responsible Ministers to issue the code telegram 'stand by' to Hospital Officers. On August 27 it was agreed that the initial steps should be taken to clear those institutions which were to be completely evacuated and the Board of Control, the L.C.C. and Hospital Officers were given instructions to proceed with the transfer of the mental cases. At the same time warnings were issued to carry out the plan for decanting a fixed number of stretcher cases from certain designated hospitals to institutions in outer areas.

On August 31, it was decided that though a state of emergency must now be regarded as existing the clearance of hospitals should only partly be carried out; therefore, the code telegram having been sent to the provincial Hospital Officers, instructions were given to them to transfer on the following day those sick patients in respect of whom warning had already been given, including children. No general clearance of hospitals, apart from these two specified categories was in the meantime to take place. In London the Ministry took the following action to put into effect the evacuation of the London patients:

> (i) Warning was sent to the medical officers of health of the eight towns which were to receive patients from the initial evacuation of London on September 1.
> (ii) The London Passenger Transport Board were warned to bring into use as ambulances 180 coaches and report to the specified hospitals at 9 a.m.
> (iii) The 34 hospitals to be evacuated were warned that evacuation would commence at 9 a.m.
> (iv) The railway companies were instructed to have 21 evacuation trains ready at the stations at 9 a.m.
> (v) The L.C.C., who were to provide the medical officers for the evacuation, were warned of the time of leaving; the St. John Ambulance stretcher parties and the local authority and voluntary special children's hospitals were also warned.

All these moves were carried out on September 1 smoothly and efficiently in London and in the provincial Regions where evacuation from the large towns had been arranged.

THE EMERGENCY MEDICAL SERVICES AT OUTBREAK OF HOSTILITIES

(i) In the Emergency Hospital Service there were in England and Wales 2,370 hospitals Classes IA, IB and II containing 108,143 beds in the London Region and 384,427 in the provincial Regions, a total of 492,570 beds. Of these 309,554 were estimated to be available for casualties: 54,772 in the London Region, 254,782 in the provinces. It was estimated that by 'crowding' 146,953 additional beds could be provided—32,111 in the London Region and 114,842 in other Regions.

(ii) On September 3, 163,500 beds suitable for the reception of casualties in Class IA and IB Hospitals had been made available. These figures rose to 187,000 by September 7 and dropped to 181,000 on September 30.

(iii) A considerable amount of extra equipment had been distributed to the hospitals and more had been ordered for the purpose of 'crowding' and 'upgrading' of hospitals selected for expansion.

(iv) Considerable numbers of nurses and trained nursing auxiliaries had been enrolled by the medical officers of health of the scheme-making authorities, and others were under training and either had been appointed to the hospitals at which they were required to work, or were standing by for instructions.

(v) Extra medical personnel had been allotted to the hospitals in accordance with the pre-arranged scale.

(vi) Centres for special treatment had been established at certain hospitals possessing the equipment and the specialist staff.

(vii) Adequate administrative staffs had been appointed to headquarters of the Ministry and to the Regions.

(viii) The London Sector Scheme had been drawn up and was fully functioning.

(ix) In the provinces Group Officers had taken up their duties and had put into force their pre-arranged Group Schemes.

(x) Thirty-four ambulance trains were ready and partly equipped, but not fully staffed by September 5.

(xi) 2,180 first-aid posts had been approved, a few of which were still under construction because suitable buildings were not available, but most of them were functioning in suitable buildings adapted for the purpose; 783 mobile units had been approved and were mostly ready. The staffs of approximately 150,000 for these fixed and mobile posts had been enrolled. Of these about 10,000 men and 35,000 women were whole-time and the rest part-time. A large number of first-aid points had been chosen and supplied with the standard equipment.

(xii) In London 220 bus-ambulances, which were converted Green Line coaches containing ten stretchers each, were ready, and in the provinces 870 containing from eight to ten stretchers each had also come to hand. As regards local authority ambulances, in London 1,600 whole-time and about 150 part-time vehicles were ready, and in the provinces 5,300 whole-time and 5,200 part-time.

(xiii) Structural precautions at many hospitals and first-aid posts had been completed or were far advanced.

(xiv) The hutted annexes to hospitals which had been ordered were under construction and many of them were expected to be completed during the autumn.

REFERENCES

[1] *Emergency Medical Services Memorandum No. 1. Structural and other Precautions against Air Raids in Hospitals.* Issued by the Ministry of Health and the Department of Health for Scotland. H.M.S.O., 1939.

[2] *Emergency Medical Services Memorandum No. 2 (England and Wales). Emergency Hospital Organisation.* Issued by the Ministry of Health. H.M.S.O., 1939.

[3] *Emergency Medical Services Memorandum No. 3 (England and Wales). Procedure on the Admission, Transfer, Discharge or Death of Casualties, and for the Provision of Out-patient Treatment.* Issued by the Ministry of Health. H.M.S.O., 1939, and (2nd Edn.) 1940.

[4] *Parliamentary Debates, Official Report, House of Commons, Fifth Series*, Vol. 342, Cols. 349–50 (342 H.C. Deb., 349–50).
[5] *Emergency Medical Services Memorandum No. 4 (England and Wales). Memorandum for the Guidance of Medical Officers and other Personnel at First-aid Posts.* Issued by the Ministry of Health. H.M.S.O., 1939.
[6] Home Office (A.R.P.) Notice 4, December 8, 1939.
[7] *Statement Relating to the Emergency Hospital Organisation, First-aid Posts and Ambulances* [Cmd. 6061]. H.M.S.O., 1939.
[8] Emergency Medical Services Instructions 27 and 27(a), June 9, 1939. Instructions on action to be taken on declaration of (a) State of tension, (b) State of emergency.

CHAPTER 3
FURTHER EXPANSION AND ORGANISATION
September 1939 to April 1940

WAR on Germany was declared by the British Government at 11 a.m. on Sunday, September 3, 1939, and the Emergency Medical Organisation was at once mobilised for action.

MOBILISATION

POWER TO GIVE DIRECTION TO HOSPITALS

Under Section 32 of the Defence Regulations[1] made under the Emergency Powers (Defence) Act, 1939, powers were conferred on the Minister of Health to issue formal direction to hospitals in connexion with the treatment of casualties and other classes of patients. These powers were delegated by the Minister, within the limits set out, in an Instrument issued on September 2 to the Hospital Officers. They were only intended to be exercised if any hospital authority refused to obey the Hospital Officer's instructions.

HOSPITAL CLEARANCE

On September 2 all Hospital Officers were instructed to complete the clearance of hospitals, which had been partly carried out on September 1, and fully to put into force the instructions contained in the operational orders. The Group Officers in the London Region and in the provinces took over their duties.

By the evening of Sunday, September 3, the pre-arranged movement of civilian sick from the danger areas and the initial clearance of hospitals to provide casualty beds was completed. From the 34 London hospitals some 3,000 cases had been transferred to their destinations in 18 of the 21 improvised ambulance trains and between 1,800 and 1,900 children were evacuated from the children's hospitals in the inner zone to four L.C.C. hospitals in the outer areas in Green Line ten-stretcher bus-ambulances. In the provinces, some 18,000 cases were evacuated from hospitals in the large towns, nearly all in bus-ambulances. One improvised ambulance train was used to transfer cases from Birmingham to Cheltenham and Gloucester and two to evacuate the children's hospitals in Manchester and Salford to the Calderstones Emergency Hospital near Blackburn. The result of these moves and clearance of hospitals on September 3 had made 163,500 beds available for casualties, of which about 51,000 were in the area of the London Sectors. By September 7 the number had increased to 187,000 of which 56,000 were in the London area; of the latter 15,000 were in the London County Council area. The increase in available beds was due to further discharges from hospitals and restriction of admissions. These figures did not include the beds in the hospitals in the inner zone, in which it had been arranged that a proportion of the beds should be 'frozen' owing to their vulnerability and to the withdrawal of many of the staff to the hospitals in the outer zone.

Regional Hospital Officers and Sector Group Officers all reported that they were satisfied that the machine was coming satisfactorily into operation. By September 5 the 34 civilian evacuation trains were all ready and berthed at their appointed stations.

MEDICAL PERSONNEL

By Sunday, September 3, 1939, some 2,500 doctors in all categories mentioned in Chapter 2 had been enrolled in the E.M.S. Each doctor to be employed whole-time had received an intimation as to what he was to do, if a state of emergency was declared, but in order that there should be as little misunderstanding as possible the following broadcast was read in the six o'clock news on Sunday night:

> Those doctors who have been enrolled in the Ministry of Health Emergency Medical Services for hospital duty for the treatment of casualties, and who have been asked in their formal letters of enrolment to report automatically for whole-time duty at a specified hospital at the outset of an emergency, should now report accordingly. Doctors who have been enrolled for part-time hospital service, or who have been enrolled for whole-time hospital service, but have *not* been asked to report at the outset of an emergency, must await further instructions.

In spite of this many doctors, perhaps because they had not heard the broadcast, misinterpreted this instruction, and many more reported for duty than had been warned to do so. Many also, who had not been allotted duties, assuming that the war was going to follow the course predicted, namely, immediate and intensive air attack on London, shut up their houses and evacuated themselves and their families, thus bringing their practices and incomes to a sudden end and causing great loss and inconvenience to themselves and to their patients. They then appeared to think it was the duty of the Government to provide them with work and an income, apparently unable to appreciate that it was their own action which had largely contributed to their loss of income, and that their profession was by no means the only one which would suffer loss from the war.

After a time, enrolled practitioners, mostly specialists, were complaining either of having no work to do and having to watch their private patients going to other doctors, or of having to attend them and hand the fees received over to the Government. After some discussion, it was agreed to offer to release a large number of these doctors where the circumstances permitted and to require of them part-time duties only, the terms being that they would receive a salary of one-third of what they had been receiving for whole-time duty and would agree to work the equivalent of four days a week for the State, if and when required. This met with very little response, but after the matter had been discussed by a committee set up by the Central Medical War Committee and with the Royal Colleges, it was agreed to offer to specialists a part-time salary of £500 a year in place of a whole-time salary of £800 to £950, their services to be available to the Government to the extent required from time to time, without further remuneration. This offer proved to be more acceptable, and of the 758 specialists and consultants to whom the offer was made over 60 per cent. accepted, these being designated as Class II Officers and practitioners on sessional fees only were designated as Class III Officers. The numbers accepting the new terms increased as time went on, until only those not permitted to transfer to part-time work by the Ministry remained on full-time duty.

POOL HOSPITALS

Another change was made at this time in the method of payment of the honorary staffs of some of the voluntary hospitals. At the suggestion of the Central Medical War Committee it was agreed that, instead of paying sessional fees to the members of the honorary staff in hospitals where no whole-time staff was employed except house officers, the Ministry would pay hospitals at the rate of 1s. 6d. per patient per day for in-patients and 6d. per patient per day for out-patients treated. Voluntary hospitals into which this system was introduced were called 'pool' hospitals, as the money was pooled and handed over to the medical board to divide among the honorary staff in any manner they considered suitable. A large number of the voluntary hospitals in the country were paid on this 'pool' system; other hospitals with whole-time officers remained on the sessional fee system. These differences in the method of paying the medical staffs of hospitals meant that in certain hospitals there were many inequalities of payment for work done, as obviously some of the honorary staff did little or no work for E.M.S. patients, while others did a great deal. No change, however, in this dual system of payment was made.

MOBILE SURGICAL TEAMS

As it was impossible to predict with any accuracy the places where enemy attacks would be most severe, and because of the greater demands likely to be made on surgeons during the war, it became necessary to provide for the mobility of medical personnel in the Emergency Hospital Scheme. Instructions were therefore issued to all Regions to form as many mobile surgical teams as possible, each consisting of a surgeon, a sister trained in theatre duties, an anaesthetist, and a male assistant or orderly, based on the large hospitals. These surgical teams were to be instructed to be available for duty at their hospital when required. A rota of these teams was kept so that the teams next for duty on any particular day would always be available. It was also arranged that hospital authorities requiring the services of one or more mobile surgical teams should communicate with the Hospital Officers in Regions or the Group Officers in the London Sectors, who would be responsible for despatching a team from one of the hospitals on which they were based. These teams were not to be considered to be in watertight compartments as, although normally they would be available within a Region or Sector, if necessary they could be called upon for duty outside their Region or Sector. Transport, if not available from ordinary sources, was obtained from the nearest A.R.P. ambulance depot.

MEDICAL ESTABLISHMENT OF HOSPITALS

Owing to the great diversity in the types of hospitals included in the E.M.S. it was not considered practicable to lay down any fixed medical establishment for hospitals, but because a strong desire was expressed by the London Group Officers, a scale for the various sized advance base and base hospitals was suggested.:

No. of beds	200	400	600	800	1,000
Surgeons	2	4	6	7	8
Physicians	1	2	4	4	5
Anaesthetists	1	2	4	4	4
Radiologist	*1	1	1	1	1
Aural Surgeon	*1	*1	1	1	1
Ophthalmic Surgeon	*1	*1	1	1	1
Dental Surgeon	—	1	1	1	2
Medical Superintendent	—	1	1	1	1
Housemen	3	6	8	10	12
	10(3*)	19(2*)	27	30	35

* Part-time.

Pathologists were omitted from these scales as the pathological arrangements were being dealt with separately.

It was recognised that these establishments were purely hypothetical, and that it would be more or less impracticable in advance to picture fully the staff that would be required in any individual institution, and that therefore, quite apart from the numbers of staff who would ultimately be available, its exact composition could not be gauged. In the provinces, in most expanded and *ad hoc* hospitals, the necessary staff was appointed from time to time as the beds came into use. Even during the period dealt with in this chapter there were certain difficulties in

FURTHER EXPANSION AND ORGANISATION

obtaining suitable staff owing to the demands of the Services. These difficulties became acute later on in the war from the further expansion in the Services and the wastage of personnel.

ALIEN DOCTORS

The question of employing alien doctors was discussed by a conference at which the Royal College of Physicians, the General Medical Council, the British Medical Association, and the Government departments concerned were represented. There were about 1,100 alien doctors residing for the time being in this country who were precluded from practising, and in addition there were 50 Austrian and 50 Czech doctors who had been given permission to qualify and subsequently practise in the United Kingdom. There were also alien doctors who had been given permission to obtain a British qualification on the understanding that they would leave the United Kingdom when they had qualified. The view was expressed that as yet there had been no true indication of an acute shortage of doctors and that no further alien doctors should be permitted to practise until there appeared to be a real demand for their services, when the matter could be reconsidered. Eventually, the shortage became very acute, and alien doctors were not only allowed to practise in E.M.S. hospitals, but were also allowed to enter general practices as assistants. Full details of the conditions governing the employment of alien practitioners are given in Chapter 14.

MEDICAL ESTABLISHMENT OF FIRST-AID POSTS

Mobilisation of the Civil Defence Services was completed during the winter of 1939–40, and suitable medical men were chosen by the local authorities to be in medical charge of first-aid posts and mobile units. In non-vulnerable areas these medical officers in charge were paid 20 guineas per annum, plus sessional fees when called upon for duty. They were only required to hold courses of training at intervals at first-aid posts and to attend when casualties were being admitted as a result of enemy action. In vulnerable areas the medical officers were paid £75 per annum, and were required to attend first-aid posts regularly for the purpose of carrying out exercises and collective training of the personnel, and to undertake responsibility for the stores and the general maintenance and administration of the post. They would still be eligible for the usual sessional fees when required to attend the post owing to an actual air raid.

CIVILIAN EVACUATION TRAINS

The medical officers in charge of the 34 civilian evacuation trains were paid on the scale for medical officers mentioned in Chapter 2, i.e. £550 per annum plus £100 a year in lieu of board and lodging. These medical officers were required to do whole-time duty at their trains, and to drill the staff in first aid, stretcher bearing, collective exercises, etc.

NURSING PERSONNEL

As mentioned in Chapter 1, steps had been taken to form a Central Emergency Nursing Committee on the same lines as the Central Medical Emergency Committee. This was set up in 1938, and during the spring of 1939, this committee, in conjunction with the local authorities, had organised local nursing committees to register and enrol trained nurses, assistant nurses and auxiliaries, and to organise training classes for these auxiliaries. This work devolved largely on the medical officers of health of the local authorities, aided by the British Red Cross Society and the Order of St. John of Jerusalem. By June 1939, 7,500 trained nurses and 2,900 assistant nurses had been enrolled, and 45,000 auxiliaries were under training. Also arrangements had been made with the War Office to release for duty in the emergency hospitals about 24,000 immobile trained auxiliaries who were on their registers. From these was formed a Civil Nursing Reserve, and during the whole period of hostilities the enrolment and training of all categories of nurses continued. The demand of the hospitals for trained nurses and auxiliaries on mobilisation for war was met by the allotment thereto of these various categories of nurses by the Local Emergency Nursing Committees. These nurses were, however, not called up for duty at hospitals until the Regional Hospital Officer concerned had accorded sanction.

In pursuance of this policy certain numbers of nurses were called up at the outbreak of war, but large numbers were not called up until later when many were found to have taken employment elsewhere, often outside the nursing profession altogether. This caused some difficulty during the spring of 1940 in obtaining suitable staffs for hospitals then being opened up for the purpose of receiving convoys of Service sick and casualties from base hospitals in France. Although hospitals in many parts of the country suffered from shortage of nursing staff, there was at the same time considerable unemployment among State registered nurses—largely due to movements of population at the outbreak of war and to the voluntary closing of many private nursing homes. A deputation from representative nursing bodies, received at the Ministry of Health in December 1939, suggested that one of the main causes of this unemployment was the substitution of nursing auxiliaries for qualified nurses in E.M.S. hospitals. To show that such was not the case, the deputation was informed that of a total nursing staff of 12,000 in London County Council hospitals, only 32 were auxiliaries. It was pointed out that there was an actual shortage of nursing staff in many parts of the country and that employment was available for qualified nurses although it might not be available in the hospitals near their residences where they wished to be employed.

It was, however, thought desirable to appoint a Regional Nursing Officer to the staff of each Region in order that the use of the Civil Nursing Reserve and its organisations should be under closer control. Also in January 1940, it was considered that the Central Emergency Committee for the nursing profession had so far completed the initial organisation of the Civil Nursing Reserve that its executive functions could be transferred to the Ministry, and the committee itself could be replaced by an advisory council of nurses and employing organisations, with the Parliamentary Secretary of the Ministry of Health, Miss Florence Horsbrugh, M.P., as chairman. Local Emergency Committees were to carry on as before, assisted now by the Regional Nursing Officers and their staffs.

Recruitment of Nurses. Progress in recruitment of nurses was slow; but by the beginning of January 22,000 trained and assistant nurses and 26,000 trained nursing auxiliaries had been registered with the Civil Nursing Reserve, while a further 14,000 nursing auxiliaries were in the final stage of their training. But the need for nurses in the hospitals at this stage was small, the number from the Reserve actually full-time in the E.M.S. hospitals being approximately 5,000. This state of affairs continued until the summer of 1940, after which the demand of the Services and hospitals increased to such an extent that there was throughout the remainder of the period of hostilities a considerable shortage of trained nurses and auxiliaries, although the proportion of trained nurses and auxiliaries was fixed at one to five, a standard much below that obtaining in the civil hospitals in peace-time.

In many hospitals the proportion of trained nurses was very large, and some hospitals were obstructing the transfer of their surplus nurses to other institutions; in others the nurses themselves would not go to the hospitals in which they were required. In the absence of enemy action the distribution of nurses resulted in there being actually more nurses than patients in some hospitals although in others it was becoming impossible to open wards for lack of nursing staff. These difficulties, however, were gradually overcome in the London Sectors by the Sector Matrons fully exercising the authority which had been given them over nursing personnel, and in the Regions by the Regional Nursing Officers and their staffs.

Full details with regard to the nursing service will be found in Chapter 15.

TREATMENT OF CIVILIAN SICK

RESTRICTION OF ADMISSIONS

The setting up of machinery which, in the absence of heavy casualties, was for some time not required to function as intended, had its repercussions in complaints from civilian sick as well as from the consultants and specialists of whose services they were to some extent deprived. Restrictions on admissions to hospitals, which would have been recognised as necessary had the war followed its expected course, were resented when many beds were known to be unoccupied.

Another cause of complaint was that many of the voluntary hospitals had closed their out-patient departments, although no instructions to this effect had been issued by the Ministry.

THE REFLUX OF CIVILIAN SICK

It had always been part of the scheme that the established hospitals would continue to admit urgent and acute cases. A reflux of patients into the evacuated beds had also been foreseen and had been taken into account in estimating the number of beds required. There was no reason, therefore, to expect that the shortage of beds for civilian sick would last very long. Even in Central London, where about two-fifths of the beds normally available in the large voluntary hospitals had been 'frozen', the rapid turnover of cases which had been arranged by the Group Officers by transferring blocks of cases to the outer zone hospitals, was designed to meet the requirements of those hospitals for fresh admissions.

As a result of public clamour and of misinformed statements in the lay and medical press, the Prime Minister in the House of Commons made it clear that hospitals should continue to admit acute cases.[2] Inquiries made at certain hospitals to ascertain the position revealed that there was no shortage of beds, but that some voluntary hospitals were keeping too many beds vacant and that this was causing extra pressure on the beds in the London County Council hospitals; but no evidence was found that any case recommended by a doctor had been refused admission. Voluntary hospitals were, however, instructed not to refuse any acute cases even if this entailed encroachment on the casualty quota of beds, and on September 16, 1939, the following statement was broadcast:

> Although the hospitals of the country have now been placed on an emergency footing and are ready to deal at a moment's notice with air raid casualties, they have not been closed against the ordinary needs of the population.
>
> Hospital accommodation for in-patients and out-patients is still available, both for the ordinary needs of the population and for all urgent cases though admissions should, of course, be regulated with discretion.

Complaints however continued and on September 23, 1939, the Minister again published a statement:

> As there still appeared to be some misapprehension on the part of certain hospitals about the admission of ordinary sick to beds which have been made available for casualties, the Minister of Health has taken

FURTHER EXPANSION AND ORGANISATION

further steps to make it generally known amongst the hospitals that patients whose medical condition necessitates in-patient treatment should be immediately admitted. This 'reflux' into the normal hospital accommodation was always provided for in the Ministry's scheme. To meet it, beds are continually being opened up in hospitals in various parts of the country, so that on balance the number of beds necessary to be held in reserve for casualties should not be seriously diminished. Figures of the beds in reserve for casualties received in the Ministry each day from the Regional Hospital Officers show that this is in fact taking place. The number of beds in reserve for casualties remains practically stationary. In other words beds equivalent to the new beds provided are being re-absorbed by ordinary civilian cases. Thus, more and more beds are now being used for the treatment of the ordinary sick.

Outpatients departments are continuing to function and are being re-opened at a number of hospitals where they have been temporarily closed.

RELAXATION OF RESTRICTIONS

The reflux of civilian sick continued and although 7,500 new beds and beds obtained by 'crowding', at the rate of about 1,000 a week, had come into use, the total available for casualties gradually decreased after September 7, 1939, to 181,000 at the end of the month, by which time the London voluntary hospitals had cleared off most of their normal waiting lists of patients.

It was decided that some relaxation of the restrictions imposed on hospitals was justifiable. Regional Hospital Officers were therefore instructed to inform all hospitals in their Regions that they could admit ordinary civilian sick up to 75 per cent. of their normal capacity. Subsequently, as hospitals received the beds and full equipment to bring them up to their agreed 'crowded' capacity, admissions up to the full extent of their normal capacity were authorised, provided that at least one bed per thousand of the population remained available for casualties in each of the areas concerned. As the 'up-graded' hospitals and the large base hospitals in mental and other institutions were rapidly coming into use during the autumn, and any excess of patients in central hospitals could be transferred to them, all causes of complaint on the score of lack of accommodation were removed. It was, of course, laid down that should the necessity arise a general clearance of the hospitals would again be required.

Some indication of the results of this relaxation is provided by the following figures of unoccupied beds in voluntary hospitals:

> During the first fortnight of the war the Ministry paid for 48,723 unoccupied beds in 778 voluntary hospitals. During the second fortnight there was little change, but during the third, fourth and fifth fortnights the numbers progressively dropped to 32,574, 10,837 and 5,833, so that at the end of ten weeks the position had nearly returned to normal.

The only remaining complaint from the public was that in the case of patients admitted to central hospitals being 'decanted' to outer zone hospitals, inconvenience was caused to relatives and friends in having to make considerable journeys to visit them.

In October 1939, the British Hospitals Association and other bodies suggested to the Ministry that the large London hospitals should be re-opened owing to the hardships alleged to exist among the poorer classes on account of the restrictions. It was considered that the risks to be run from air attacks would be the lesser of the two evils. In the discussions which followed, however, it became fairly obvious that this recommendation regarding the teaching hospitals was largely influenced by anxiety as to the efficiency of medical education. Had this proposal been acted upon it would have entirely upset the Emergency Scheme for London, for it would have meant bringing back to the central hospitals all the staff which had been transferred to the outer zones.

The representatives of the large hospitals thought that the allegations of hardship could not be substantiated. It was stated that there was no pressure on the voluntary hospitals' beds, and that in many places waiting lists had entirely disappeared. This was partly accounted for by the fact that in peace-time from a quarter to a third of all patients admitted to these hospitals came from outside London and that now they were avoiding London and were being treated elsewhere. The considered view of the London Group Officers was that not only were patients being adequately treated, but through the use of peripheral hospitals their number was greater than could have been accommodated before the war.

It was also considered that all teaching hospitals, some by using the peripheral hospitals and others by transferring all their students to provincial centres, had made adequate provision for maintaining the standard of teaching. As time went on examination results fully confirmed this view.

Eventually, the Ministry agreed that hospitals in the inner zone also should increase their accommodation for civilian sick, which could be done by utilising up to one-fifth of the number of beds set aside for casualties. In addition, hospitals could open as many closed beds as would bring the total of casualty and sick beds up to approximately two-thirds of their normal capacity. This step was facilitated by the reversion of some 400 specialists in the London area from whole-time to part-time service in the E.M.S. By December civilian sick were being admitted to hospital almost as freely as in peace-time.

TRANSFERRED SICK

In this month also the Ministry issued circulars 1938 and 1938A laying down the responsibilities which the Minister had undertaken for the treatment of 'transferred civilian sick'. These included any civilian

FURTHER EXPANSION AND ORGANISATION

sick transferred from one hospital to another in order to free beds for casualties or to receive treatment at a special centre. These patients became the sole responsibility of the Ministry for treatment, professionally and financially, subject only to the Ministry's being reimbursed to the extent, if any, that the patient was already entitled to hospital treatment under any contributory scheme and/or as a charge on the rates of local authorities. Under the terms of the above mentioned circulars a nominal roll of patients thus transferred was made on Form E.M.S. 116, one copy of which was retained by the receiving hospital on which it could base its claims to the Ministry for treating these patients.

The numbers of civilian sick transferred under the provisions of circulars 1938 and 1938A during the six years of war averaged over 86,000 per annum and are given in Appendix III. It will be realised that the transfer of civilian patients, both adults and children, on such a scale over a prolonged period was a measure of considerable sociological magnitude and one for which there was no precedent. These routine transfers were carried out without detriment to the patients—indeed often to their advantage. It was no small achievement. The advantages of fully equipped and staffed hospitals and special centres in rural surroundings, removed from the dangers of aerial attacks, were substantial and outweighed any dissatisfaction felt by patients in being a greater distance from their homes than in normal times.

TREATMENT OF OTHER CIVILIAN CATEGORIES

The E.M.S. hospitals were primarily provided for the treatment of civilian and Service casualties due to enemy action. As detailed above, they now also accepted responsibility for other patients transferred to freed casualty beds. In addition to these categories they accepted responsibility for the treatment of police sick, police casualties and casualties among all classes of civil defence workers occurring while on duty, and for the treatment of 'unaccompanied evacuated children'. Additions to the list of categories entitled to treatment in E.M.S. hospitals were made from time to time, until by the end of hostilities the list included many classes of civilian war workers and others for whom the best treatment available was considered essential to enable them to return to their duties as soon as possible. (The complete list of these categories will be found in Appendix IV.)

TREATMENT OF CIVILIAN CASUALTIES

TREATMENT OF WAR INJURIES

When the Ministry of Health took over responsibility for the initial treatment required by civilian air raid casualties, it had been assumed that cases for which the Ministry of Pensions had accepted liability would receive subsequent treatment under that organisation. On

September 5, however, it was stated at a conference that the Ministry of Pensions had insufficient provision for undertaking such treatment; and it was agreed that for the duration of the war the Ministry of Health should undertake responsibility for this as well as for the treatment of war service injuries. There were, however, two major questions on which no decision had been reached:

(1) what prostheses and appliances, if any, were to be authorised after treatment in hospital?

(2) what limit was to be placed upon the responsibility of the Ministry of Health for the treatment of civilians?

At a conference at which the Treasury was represented, their view was that it would be wrong for the Government to undertake the responsibility for treating civilian casualties—in some cases for the rest of their lives—and that logically there ought to be some limit to the period for which the Government should accept the responsibility for hospital and domiciliary treatment.

It was recognised, however, that the Ministry of Pensions would arrange after the war for the treatment of persons receiving pensions under the Personal Injuries (Civilian) Scheme, with a view to reducing their disability. After some discussion, it was proposed that the Government should accept responsibility for the treatment of civilian casualties as well as recipients of injury allowances during hostilities, and should provide and maintain any necessary appliances, including artificial limbs. Eventually, it was decided that, during the war, full responsibility would be taken and that the post-war policy should be left open until some clearer idea could be formed of what was likely to be involved. The limb-fitting facilities of the Ministry of Pensions would be used, the Ministry acting as agents of the E.M.S. for that purpose. (See Civilian Health and Medical Services, Volume I, Part II, Chapter 5.)

DOMICILIARY MEDICAL ATTENDANCE

Initial treatment of minor injuries due to an air raid was provided for as far as possible at first-aid posts, but further treatment was expected to be given at out-patient departments of hospitals. It was recognised, however, that in certain circumstances, where a casualty had been primarily treated at a first-aid post or at a hospital as an in-or out-patient, it might be impracticable to provide the necessary further treatment at a hospital for reasons such as remoteness of the patient's home, etc. Arrangements were therefore made to give domiciliary treatment in such cases at Government expense, the practitioner concerned receiving a capitation fee of 16s. per annum for each patient so treated, unless the patient was already entitled to medical benefit under the National Health Insurance Acts. The order for domiciliary treatment was issued at the hospitals on E.M.S. Form 114. The scheme did not work well. In some cases the hospital discharged the patient, considering that no further treatment of any kind was necessary; but subsequently the patient would go to a practitioner, complaining of ill-effects, and would receive treatment for which the practitioner would demand fees from the Ministry. In these cases it was necessary to get the hospital to look up its records and issue E.M.S. Form 114 to regularise the situation. In others the patient could present Form 114 to a practitioner and receive treatment, but would subsequently change his residence and call in another practitioner who also required reimbursement for the treatment given; this led to complications, as the Ministry would pay only one capitation fee in each year. Eventually, it was agreed that such cases should be dealt with in the same way as patients changing their doctor under the panel system. The provisions made above for domiciliary treatment did not cover cases in which a patient who, receiving an initial injury owing to enemy action, went direct to a private practitioner, and much heart-burning was caused when the Ministry would not accept responsibility for payment to the practitioner on the grounds that the patient should have gone to a first-aid post or a hospital. The Ministry only agreed to pay practitioners for the initial treatment of air raid casualties if the casualty occurred in an area situated a long way from a first-aid post, and in cases in which it would appear detrimental to the patient's health to delay treatment. In these cases the practitioner was paid sessional fees on the scale applied to Class III practitioners for attendance on air raid casualties in hospitals.

TREATMENT OF SHIPWRECKED SAILORS

From the outbreak of war, merchant seamen were being landed from mined and torpedoed vessels at ports all round the coast of Britain, and in most cases the arrangements made for their admission to E.M.S. hospitals, in which they were entitled to free treatment, worked smoothly and efficiently. In some instances, however, where large numbers were involved, misunderstanding and confusion arose through the failure of the local authorities to realise that the E.M.S. organisation was meant to deal with all classes of civilian war casualties, irrespective of the kind of enemy action that had caused them. (See Civilian Health and Medical Services, Volume I, Part II, Chapter 4.)

TREATMENT OF THE BLIND

In October the Ministry of Pensions informed the Ministry of Health that St. Dunstan's had undertaken to provide after-care and training for blinded serving officers and men on the lines they had followed in the last war. For this purpose they had offered the services of their new home at Ovingdean as a hospital for cases requiring medical or surgical treatment in the first stages before training could be commenced. There was no proposal or indeed intention, that these facilities should be extended to similar civilian or war service injuries. Eventually, however, an agreement was come to with St. Dunstan's whereby so long as accommodation was available civilian casualties, (including members of Civil Defence organisations injured in the course of their duties, who had become blinded, or were thought likely to become blind as a result of their war injuries) should also be eligible for admission to Ovingdean if they were over 16 years of age. Those under 16, it was considered, would be more appropriately and conveniently cared for by the special organisations who dealt with blind children. These arrangements not only enabled the civilian casualty to share the facilities available to the Services, but brought the procedure for transfer into line with that under the general scheme. At the same time arrangements were concluded for the Ministry to be responsible for the construction of a hutted annexe to Ovingdean for civil cases.

PHYSIOTHERAPY

How far it would be necessary for the Ministry to provide facilities for physiotherapy at the new and upgraded hospitals was becoming a matter for closer consideration. It was obviously necessary to avoid providing such facilities irrespective of the ultimate use to which an institution was to be put, but it was agreed that all first-class hospitals and certain convalescent hospitals should be provided with a standard equipment, in accordance with the number of beds, as advised by Sir Robert Stanton Woods, Consultant Adviser in Physiotherapy to the Ministry, and this policy was carried out. Later, in the light of experience, when the enormous importance of rehabilitation was realised, certain hospitals were earmarked for the issue of complete equipment for adequate rehabilitation to all cases so that the patients might be able to resume work of national importance at the earliest possible moment. This subject is dealt with fully in Chapter 13.

DENTAL TREATMENT

In peace-time dentistry was not included in the work of most civilian hospitals, such treatment being confined to hospitals with dental schools. It was decided that responsibility for dental treatment could not be accepted by the Ministry in the E.M.S. hospitals except in so far as it might be necessary as a result of direct injury to the face or jaws or as part of the actual medical and surgical treatment. Hospitals were therefore instructed that, apart from the treatment of maxillo-facial wounds, fractures, etc., dental treatment could only be provided under the E.M.S. for:

(a) the relief of pain;
(b) the elimination of oral sepsis;
(c) the eradication of dental foci of infection;
(d) the restoration of efficient mastication in cases in which it was so impaired that substantial improvement in the patient's condition, with a view to hastening discharge from hospital, could not otherwise be expected.

Only in this last case could artificial dentures be supplied—and then only on the authority of the Regional Dental Officer—and patients were not to be detained in hospital for the provision or completion of dental treatment. Dental cases in hospitals lacking the necessary facilities for dental treatment were, if not fit for discharge, to be transferred to the nearest E.M.S. hospital with these facilities.

SPECIAL CENTRES

In addition to provision for the above categories, special centres had already been provided for in all Regions, and are fully dealt with in Chapter 2.

TREATMENT OF GAS CASUALTIES

From the time the Ministry of Health took over the administration of hospitals and first-aid posts, the policy laid down by the Home Office in the years 1935–8 for dealing with gas casualties had been carried out as far as possible. By the outbreak of the war the provision of facilities for the cleansing and treatment of gas casualties at first-aid posts was well in hand, though a great deal of work still remained to be done; but in hospitals the work of providing adequate arrangements for the reception of gas casualties had tended to lag behind. One reason for this was the difficulty of providing suitable accommodation for the reception, undressing, cleansing and anti-gas treatment of casualties, most of whom might be expected to be more or less seriously wounded and on stretchers, therefore requiring not only anti-gas treatment but probably resuscitation and often early operation. The ideal aimed at was that there should be a separate reception unit for gas casualties, with its own resuscitation wards, but if this was not practicable, the suite for anti-gas treatment had to be so placed that the flow of casualties through it would have ready access to the general casualty receiving rooms in the hospital. This was found extremely difficult to provide for in many hospitals.

Accommodation for the interchange and disposal of contaminated stretchers and blankets had also to be provided at entrances for gas casualties.

Another cause of delay was the difference of opinion among the medical staffs of hospitals as to the degree of cleansing and anti-gas treatment, which could safely be applied to casualties whose condition demanded immediate medical attention. The prevailing feeling was that the rapid removal of contaminated clothing, by cutting if necessary, and of obvious liquid contamination of the skin by means of swabs, was all that should be attempted in serious cases, and that after such action the danger of the introduction of gas into the hospitals was negligible. The Ministry of Health, however, took the view that adequate provision for cleansing and anti-gas treatment must be made at all Class I hospitals unless it had been found that such facilities could not be made available, or that there was another hospital with adequate facilities close by or, in exceptional cases, a first-aid post which was able to deal with contaminated stretcher cases as well as walking cases and to which patients could be sent. The Ministry considered that the medical staffs of hospitals should use their own discretion as to the degree of cleansing and anti-gas treatment, if any, which should be applied, according to the urgency of the case, before proceeding to medical or surgical treatment. In view of all these considerations it is not surprising that satisfactory arrangements were not completed in all hospitals until late in 1941.

Mobile Cleansing Units. In areas where hospitals were few, and as a reserve for fixed cleansing units which might be put out of action, the Ministry in the autumn of 1941 provided a considerable number of self-contained mobile cleansing units. These were distributed to all local authorities desiring them. In combined training exercises these units were found to function exceedingly well and, although never used as gas cleansing units, they were found extremely useful by local authorities in providing hot water rapidly when the usual sources of supply were out of action.

RADIUM: PROTECTION AND TREATMENT

Among the precautionary measures to be considered under the threat of war, those concerned with radium were not least in importance.

When, in December 1938, the Ministry of Health was approached by the Royal Cancer Hospital on the subject, it was recognised that the omission of practical steps to conserve stocks of radium and to regulate its use under war conditions might have serious and far-reaching consequences in material loss and human suffering.

Measures to safeguard a substance of unique value and potency must be such as to command the confidence and assent of those chiefly concerned with its use. The question was therefore referred to the National Radium Commission, who arranged a representative conference, held on March 24, 1939, at which proposals submitted in a paper by Professor S. Russ, representing the King Edward VII Hospital Fund for London, were discussed and generally endorsed.

Though the preservation of existing stocks and the welfare of patients undergoing treatment were obviously of great importance, the conference also emphasised the necessity for taking steps to protect the public from the effects of radium should any considerable quantities be violently dispersed. It was held that in the event of dispersal of radium in a building by high explosive action, not only the building concerned but also its immediate surroundings would be rendered uninhabitable for many years to come. The inhalation of even as small a quantity as a hundredth part of a milligram might have fatal consequences.

FURTHER EXPANSION AND ORGANISATION

The conclusion was reached that the only way to store radium in safety from bombing was to deposit it in boreholes of 8 in. diameter and not less than 50 ft. deep.

Of the estimated total of 60 g. of radium in London, 15 g. were held at the Radium Institute and amounts up to 7 g. at the Middlesex Hospital, the Royal Cancer Hospital and St. Bartholomew's Hospital, and it was proposed that safe borehole deposits should be provided at each of these four centres. Considerable amounts were also held in provincial centres, such as Manchester, Sheffield, etc., for which similar provision was recommended.

The expenditure on sinking these boreholes was sanctioned as part of the structural measures required to safeguard E.M.S. hospitals from the results of enemy action, but the Minister of Health, though anxious to co-operate in impressing upon all concerned the need for taking adequate precautions, rejected as unnecessary and unlikely to prove effective, the recommendation that all owners and holders of radium should be compulsorily registered.

Meanwhile the National Radium Commission had begun to compile a register on a voluntary basis, appeals to register being made through the medium of medical, scientific and trade journals. The response, however, was disappointing, and the commission decided to concentrate its efforts on securing safe deposits at the large hospitals, to which holders were advised to send their stocks for storage.

Thus in London and in certain provincial centres insurance against loss of radium was provided. The preservation of radium for future application, however, involved withholding it from immediate use. At the outbreak of war radium treatment in vulnerable storage areas may be said to have come to a sudden stop, and thus for a time a premium was paid in suffering which radiotherapy might have avoided or alleviated.

In certain regions treatment centres were established in comparatively safe rural areas, to which cancer cases were transferred; but as weeks went by without bombing attacks it was felt that even in vulnerable areas persons suffering from cancer should no longer be deprived of treatment, the general resumption of which was approved as recommended by a further representative conference, convened by the Ministry of Health and held on October 18, 1939, subject to the following safeguards:

(1) The provision of a deep borehole deposit or, for quantities not exceeding 350 mg., the alternative of an approved bomb-proof steel container (designed by Mr. Greatbatch of the Research Department, Woolwich Arsenal).

(2) Substitution of radon for interstitial radium.

(3) Withdrawal of surface radium or intracavitary containers in the case of imminent danger and their return to borehole or bomb-proof container.

Centres for the manufacture of radon had already been established in safe areas.

The county centres organised by Sheffield and Manchester enabled these clinics to continue to treat an increasing number of patients throughout the war. By the end of 1943, two somewhat similar organisations were in working order at Mount Vernon, Northwood, and Warren Road Hospital, Guildford, where most of the radiotherapy normally carried out at London hospitals was concentrated.

In the light of later information regarding the distribution of radium among doctors and certain trade interests, a pamphlet was prepared by the Ministries of Health and Home Security and circulated to local authorities by the Ministry of Health with instructions to bring it to the notice of all known holders of radium.[3] It contained details of approved types of boreholes and steel containers and laid down that:

(a) all radium exceeding 1 mg., if not actually in use, should be kept in a borehole or steel container of the approved type;

(b) not more than 350 mg. of radium should be kept in one steel container;

(c) in a hospital situated in a vulnerable area not more than 350 mg. should be in use at any one time;

(d) radon should be used instead of radium where this was possible without loss of therapeutic efficiency;

(e) patients should not remain under treatment by radium during an air raid unless accommodated in a basement or ground floor room strengthened up to the approved A.R.P. standard for a shelter;

(f) radium should not be transported through the medium of the post office, but should be conveyed either by special messenger or sent by passenger train under the care of the guard. Radium so conveyed should be specially protected as laid down in the circular.

In the event of actual or suspected dispersal of radium during an air raid incident, holders or users were instructed immediately to inform the medical officer of health, who would have the danger area cordoned off pending examination of the site by experts from the National Physical Laboratory, Teddington. If the presence of radium was detected they would locate and recover it if intact in its container, or if dissipated, indicate the extent of the contaminated area and advise on the action to be taken.

These measures for safeguarding the public from the effects of radium were first put to the test on May 4, 1942, as a result of the last of the 'Baedeker' raids on Exeter. In this incident the circumstances were peculiar; 85·58 mg. of radium in a nest of drawers protected by lead were stored in a steel safe in the basement of a house which was completely burnt down. The safe was exposed to a very high temperature, and after the fire was removed to a store room in a hospital in Exeter and opened by a doctor. It was found that the lead protecting the radium had melted and the radium had been dissipated; the safe was then closed up. The prescribed procedure for notifying the Ministry of Health and the

National Physical Laboratory was not carried out, and it was only in the middle of July, nearly two months later, that the Medical Officer of Health heard anything about the radium. He took immediate action and representatives of the National Physical Laboratory examined the safe and found that its contents had become highly radioactive. They arranged for these to be removed so that the radium might be recovered by experts, as their tests showed that 61 of the 85·58 mg. of radium could be accounted for in the safe. It was stated that these values might be expected to increase until radioactive equilibrium was reached. The safe itself was dumped into the sea. Examination of the store room in which the safe had been for several weeks showed no signs of contamination. The missing lead was located among the debris at the site of the fire and found not to be radioactive, nor was any sign of radioactivity found on the site. This incident seemed to indicate that, in the circumstances detailed above, this quantity of radium had not become a public danger.

Another incident, which occurred on February 18, 1944, is also of interest. A 500-kg. bomb exploded in the operating theatre of the Marie Curie Hospital at Hampstead. This operating theatre was in a semi-basement, and in an adjoining room were two steel containers of the approved standard pattern, one containing 365 mg. and the other 100 mg. of radium. On this occasion the procedure laid down was strictly followed, and representatives from the National Physical Laboratory began a search for these containers within thirty-six hours. As the radium was in containers 3 in. thick, buried in debris, it was estimated that the gamma rays would not indicate the presence of radium unless the testing instruments could be brought within 5 ft. of the containers. After excavating until February 24, the instruments indicated radioactivity and the container in which there were 365 mg. of radium was found on the 28th, 14 ft. from its original situation. On opening the container, although the radium had not been securely packed in the cavity, no evidence of dispersal was found. The search was then continued for the second container, excavation going on daily, but it was not until March 23 that gamma rays were again detected, and the second container was located 50 ft. from its original place on March 30. Again the radium was found intact and there were no signs of dispersal. This incident confirmed the efficacy of the steel container designed to protect the radium (see Plates II, III and IV).

On the advice of Sir Edward Appleton, Director of its Scientific and Industrial Research Department, the National Physical Laboratory and also the Cavendish Laboratory at Cambridge were exempted from the conditions laid down for hospitals and other users of radium. Both held and used large quantities, for which the 350-mg. container would be useless, and their existing protective arrangements were thought to be more suitable to their special circumstances.

TREATMENT OF SERVICE SICK AND CASUALTIES

DISPOSAL OF SERVICE SICK AND CASUALTIES IN ENGLAND AND WALES

On the outbreak of war the E.M.S. became responsible for the treatment of all Service sick and casualties where admission to Service hospitals was not possible or practicable, with the exception of cases of infectious diseases (including tuberculosis and venereal diseases) and mental diseases. (See Army Medical Services, Volume I, Chapter 2.) Cases in these categories were admitted to special hospitals under the peace-time procedure, by direct communication between the military authorities and the hospitals concerned, or to Service hospitals. Patients suffering from minor complaints requiring admission to hospital for only a few days were treated in the established Service hospitals, in a small number of extra military hospitals mobilised in this country and in camp reception stations. By 1942 about 70 of these hospitals (mostly small, including a few hospitals for special diseases), containing about 17,000 beds, and about 300 camp reception stations containing about 8,000 beds were administered by the War Office. The Navy had about 30 hospitals of various sizes to take about 6,500 patients, and the Royal Air Force 26 hospitals with about 8,000 beds, excluding small detention hospitals at aerodromes, etc. Details will be found in the Service volumes of the Medical History. These provisions, of course, were not meant to supply the needs of the greatly expanded establishments of the Services. From the outbreak of war, owing to the rapid expansion of the Services, involving the setting up of training centres all over the country, the majority of Service sick and casualties of all kinds were treated in E.M.S. hospitals, which also dealt with all cases of sickness and injury among families of Service personnel entitled, under Service rules, to treatment in families' hospitals in peace-time. At the end of November 1939, 4,100 Service sick and casualties were occupying beds in the E.M.S. hospitals and over 16,500 by the end of January 1940.

At first the Services were prone to send cases requiring more than a few days treatment rather long distances to their own hospitals; there were even instances of military hospitals having long lists of men awaiting operation although large numbers of beds in surgical wards of E.M.S. hospitals, with highly competent surgeons on the staff, were empty. But with the improvement in liaison between the Hospital Officers of the Regions and the Service Commands this uneconomic procedure became rare, and the facilities provided by adjacent E.M.S. hospitals of all grades came regularly into use for Service cases in accordance with the intentions of the Government.

The improved liaison was largely due to the early appointment by the Service Commands of military medical officers to the offices of the

Regional Hospital Officers to act as liaison officers. These officers were whole-time in the case of the Army and part-time in the case of the Navy and R.A.F. and they fulfilled many useful functions.

DISPOSAL OF SERVICE SICK AND WOUNDED FROM OVERSEAS

On September 15, 1939, the War Office drew the attention of the Minister of Health to the undertaking given by him in 1938 that, the Army Council having agreed to forego the mobilisation of all but four of the Territorial Army General Hospitals, he would place hospital bed accommodation at the disposal of the Army at forty-eight hours' notice when required in time of war. (See Chapter 1.) Circumstances had now arisen which made it necessary for the Army Council to give such notice; convoys of sick and wounded might be expected at any time and, in view of the great expansion of the Army, the existing military hospitals in this country would be unable to accommodate them. Ships carrying about 280 patients each were expected. The Army Council, therefore, requested that six blocks of 300 beds should be placed at their disposal in such civil hospitals as the Minister of Health might decide. (See Army Medical Services, Volume I, Chapter 2.)

The original undertaking was given at a time when the Minister had been advised that accommodation for civilian casualties would be required chiefly during the first six weeks of enemy attack, after which the number of casualties would steadily decline, and that during this period there would be hardly any military casualties.

But the war had taken a different course; air attacks on this country were still awaited and might occur at any moment. To implement the original agreement would be to incur the risk of depriving civilian casualties of accommodation. The Minister therefore informed the Army Council that he was quite prepared to receive and treat in E.M.S. hospitals the numbers of military sick up to the total suggested, and even in excess of that number; but that there would be serious difficulties if the request of the Army Council implied that a number of separate blocks of beds were to be handed over exclusively for the Army. He hoped that this matter would not be pressed while we were still unaware of the effects of air attacks which might be delivered. Meanwhile, Regional Hospital Officers were instructed to submit a daily return of hospitals in their Region, containing 200 and upward vacant beds suitable for the reception of convoys of male military patients, so that the military liaison officer might keep a priority list of such hospitals for the information of the War Office. The first of the military convoys of sick from overseas arrived on October 25, 1939, and was dealt with without any difficulty under these arrangements. The patients unfit for further travel were admitted to the nearest military or E.M.S. hospital. Special cases were sent direct to hospitals with special centres, and the rest to a large base hospital, Park Prewett Emergency Hospital,

Basingstoke. Further convoys as they arrived were similarly dealt with.

But this arrangement, while unassailable as regards treatment, was criticised by the Army Council from the point of view of administration and discipline. It was argued that to preserve Army discipline and a soldierly spirit, even in hospital, for the distribution of soldiers' pay and to maintain fighting strength by the strict avoidance of unduly prolonged detention in hospital, definite blocks of beds for Service patients were essential. Early in November 1939, the Minister agreed in principle to this proposal and blocks of 300 beds were allotted in six large base hospitals.

The preliminary allocation of blocks of beds was regarded as temporary, because with the progress of the hutting scheme, more appropriate accommodation might become available in a few months. These blocks of beds were termed 'military wings' of the E.M.S. hospitals and R.A.M.C. medical registrars, a clerical staff, and a staff of military police were appointed to each. (See Army Medical Services, Volume I, Chapter 2.) The registrars were to advise medical superintendents of hospitals and civil staffs on all matters pertaining to Army procedure, but would in no way relieve the medical superintendents of any of their existing responsibilities. It was specifically laid down that registrars would have nothing to do with the medical care of patients and later on, owing to the increasing shortage of medical personnel, the medical registrars were replaced by combatant officers. Offices, and in most cases board and lodging, were provided for the registrar and his staff, and in hospitals likely to become permanent convoy hospitals the provision of pack stores and clothing stores for the Army patients was undertaken. At first, there was some misunderstanding and friction between the hospital authorities and the registrars, most of whom were temporary R.A.M.C. officers, but, when the spheres of each were thoroughly understood, little or no trouble was experienced in the large number of convoy hospitals which were eventually brought into being all over the country. By the end of February 1940, thirteen of them were in full use. At first, each convoy hospital had its own military registrar and staff, but later on, to effect economy in personnel, registrars were allotted to groups of hospitals including convalescent hospitals for Service cases, and had their headquarters in one of the large hospitals in the group. This system was found to work satisfactorily, from the point of view of both the War Office and the Ministry of Health. These hospitals were afterwards called Registrar Hospitals and arrangements were made to concentrate as far as possible all Service cases in them. If Service cases likely to be in hospital for more than a few days were in the first instance admitted to other hospitals, as frequently happened in the case of Service sick from home stations, they were transferred to Registrar Hospitals as soon as possible.

EXPANSION OF THE CONVOY HOSPITALS

The immediate needs of the War Office for bed accommodation having been met, it was thought necessary to take up the question of their probable requirements in the future. The 250,000 beds which it was expected could at any time now be made available would probably suffice to meet the estimated civilian casualties alone, but already by the end of January 1940, 16,000 of these beds were occupied by Service patients. The actual civil requirements were still a matter of conjecture and might have been overestimated, as proved to be the case. A conference was held with the War Office, Department of Health for Scotland and H.M. Office of Works on February 1, 1940, at which the War Office representatives stated that in the not too distant future they might be called upon to handle a peak figure of 16,000 casualties a week, but that this would not be expected to be maintained for more than a few weeks. For the current year they estimated their requirements at 70,000 beds altogether, and relied on the original assurance that the civil and Service hospitals were to be pooled and hospitals handed over to the War Office, if and when necessary, to provide more beds. The War Office had in hand no provisions for new hospitals, and their present hospitals had been expanded to their maximum capacity by crowding, and by building huts. Their peace-time provision of just over 3,000 beds had been expanded to 10,500 and was expected to reach 15,000, apart from 3,500 beds in camp hospitals and reception stations. These figures included, in addition to their peace-time hospitals, four Territorial Hospitals for Home Service, eleven General Hospitals and four Casualty Clearing Hospitals of 150 to 300 beds each, which were for overseas but would be replaced by fresh units. The Army had also made special provision for cases of psychosis in certain military hospitals and in portions of civil mental hospitals taken over from the Board of Control, and for venereal diseases.

The conclusion was reached that the military needs could only be met by fresh building of *ad hoc* hospitals, and it was agreed that the Ministry of Health and the Department of Health for Scotland should construct additional accommodation required and be responsible for the administration of the new hospitals; but if the War Office needed a whole new hospital, instead of an allocation of beds in military wings which had already been agreed on, it should be handed over and administered by them. As a result, authority was asked for and received by the end of February to construct hutted hospitals with 40,000 beds in England and Wales and 5,000 in Scotland (Block C) to be provided gradually as material and labour became available. This programme was subject to review in the light of experience as accurate estimates of requirements were not possible at that time. The Ministry of Pensions also received authority to extend their hospitals by 2,500 beds in accordance with a programme prepared in 1938 which had been held up in view of the E.M.S. hutting schemes. A review of the position in March revealed that out of the beds which were immediately available by evacuation, by crowding of hospitals with the 100,000 new beds which had been issued, and by new accommodation, 100,000 beds would be available forArmy sick and wounded, and in April the War Office were supplied with a list of 75,000 beds suitable and available for military patients in 112 hospitals. (See Army Medical Services, Volume I, Chapter 2.)

SEGREGATION OF SERVICE CASES IN E.M.S. HOSPITALS

Inspection of E.M.S. hospitals had brought to light the fact that the medical superintendents of various hospitals had different views as to the way Service cases should be accommodated in their hospitals. Where more than a small number of Service patients were in hospital, it was the general intention that the men should be segregated as far as possible in a definite portion of the hospital. This was both for the patients' comfort and to enable the military authorities more easily to carry out their responsibilities in connexion with discipline, pay, clothing, etc. In some hospitals this intention was being carried out, but in others Service and civilian cases were mixed up and in some of them officers were found in the general wards. In most cases this mixing was intentional, the medical superintendents being of the opinion that it was desirable for medical purposes. It was therefore emphasised that this matter was not one for the exercise of discretion, but that wherever the number of Service cases warranted it they should be given separate accommodation, and, except in emergency, civilians should not be admitted to Service beds.

HOSPITALS WITH WARDS FOR OFFICERS

Since officers had been found in some hospitals in general wards, hospitals were asked to inform Regional Hospital Officers of the hospitals in their Region which had separate accommodation suitable for officers, and it was found that a considerable number of hospitals had, or could provide, suitable separate accommodation. Lists of such hospitals with the number of beds available in each were sent to the appropriate military authorities in each Region.

CONVALESCENT DEPOTS

Large convalescent depots were established by the War Office in each Command to which military patients who were ambulatory and on full diet were sent from the convalescent hospitals, either for boarding or for graduated physical exercises before being returned to duty. Only patients who had been in hospital for more than twenty-one days—known as 'Y' cases—were disposed of in this manner. Patients who had been in hospital for less than twenty-one days could be sent back to their units direct if considered fit for full duty.

MEDICAL BOARDS

Part of the duties of the military registrars at hospitals, or groups of hospitals, was to arrange medical boards for all Service patients reported by the medical superintendents as likely to be unfit for further service for a considerable time. The names of such patients were furnished weekly. Arrangements were also made for reports to be sent to the various Services on all patients who had been under treatment in hospital for more than one month. Each Service had its own regulations for holding these boards, which are dealt with in the Service portions of the Medical History. (See Army Medical Services, Volume I, Chapter 11.)

TRANSPORTATION OF MILITARY CASES

Another question that arose was the method by which military sick or casualties should be brought to hospitals or first-aid posts. The military authorities were informed that it was the responsibility of the E.M.S. to provide whatever transport was necessary for all casualties due to enemy action whether they were civilian or Service casualties, but that where the Service authorities had their own transport available, instead of communicating with the nearest control centre for transport, they should in the obvious interests of the patients use their own transport to the extent available. As regards ordinary Service sick, the Services concerned were supposed to provide their own transport, but if none of their transport was available, civilian transport would be supplied on application to the appropriate authority in each area.

Military Stretcher Bearers. On the arrival of ambulance trains with military sick and casualties, certain difficulties were experienced in some Regions in providing an adequate number of stretcher bearers to unload cot cases from trains and to load them into ambulances for transport to hospital. In many places also a sufficient number of stretcher bearers was not available at hospitals to unload these cases. After discussion, the War Office accepted responsibility for supplying military stretcher bearers at detraining stations and at hospitals from the nearest military depots, the civil authorities supplying the necessary transport. The numbers to be supplied at detraining stations and at hospitals were one N.C.O. and twenty-four men, but, if the convoy was a large one, considerably larger numbers were always supplied by the local military authorities.

SPECIAL CENTRES

In addition to the above general provisions for the treatment of Service casualties and sick, the special centres for specialised treatment referred to in Chapter 2 and detailed in the booklet 'E.M.S. Instructions Part I' were fully available for the Services. Blinded Service patients had priority for admission to St. Dunstan's, and special centres for Service cases of effort syndrome at Mill Hill Hospital and of non-articular rheumatism at the Royal Devonshire Hospital, Buxton, were constituted on the recommendation of Professor F. R. Fraser (afterwards Sir Francis Fraser), Consultant Adviser to the Ministry on General Medicine. In December 1941, a further centre for the treatment of other rank Service patients was opened at Bath, viz. the Royal National Hospital for Rheumatic Diseases.

INVESTIGATION OF GASTRIC CASES

One of the most notable features of the military sick had been the high proportion of gastric cases. This high incidence in the Armed Forces of a disabling disease was a matter of such importance that Colonel Tidy (afterwards Major General Sir Henry Tidy), Consulting Physician to the Home Forces, persuaded the Royal College of Physicians to organise an investigation into its nature and cause. For this purpose Dr. Charles Newman and Mr. Reginald Payne were seconded by the Ministry and by the British Postgraduate Medical School for three months in order to devote their full time to the work. They investigated Service cases in both E.M.S. and military hospitals and found that this dyspepsia in the Forces was not any new disease brought about by military service, but was in fact only a reflection of the breakdown under Service conditions of peptic ulcers from which the patients had suffered, in many cases for many years in civil life. Eventually a special unit for the treatment of gastric cases was formed in White Lodge Emergency Hospital, Newmarket, under the charge of Dr. A. Morton Gill, and large numbers of patients were dealt with in this unit. (See Medicine and Pathology, Chapter 2.)

RECORDING CASUALTIES

CIVILIAN CASUALTIES

The Ministry's scheme for recording casualties treated at first-aid posts or as in- or out-patients at E.M.S. hospitals is given in detail in E.M.S. Memorandum No. 3[4] already referred to in connexion with the setting up of casualty bureaux in Chapter 2. The forms required are given in the appendices to that memorandum. A civilian casualty for the purposes of their records was defined as:

(1) a case of injury (physical or otherwise) caused by enemy attack, or by repelling enemy attack;
(2) a case of physical injury to a member of the Civil Defence organisation in the course of performing his duty.

Members of the Mercantile Marine, as well as passengers in ships, suffering from injury as the result of enemy action were recorded as civilian casualties, as were foreign seamen unless they were prisoners-of-war. The admission of a casualty to hospital was notified on E.M.S. Form 105 in duplicate, one copy being sent to the appropriate casualty bureau, and one copy sent to the nearest relative direct. On transfer to another hospital, E.M.S. Forms 105 were again submitted to the casualty bureau, and to the relative by the admitting hospital but not by the discharging hospital. On final discharge from hospital, these forms were also submitted by the discharging hospital. On the death of a casualty, only the form to the casualty bureau was sent, the medical superintendent of the hospital sending to the relative an appropriately worded intimation of the death, with an expression of the sympathy of the Minister of Health on behalf of the Government. E.M.S. Form 105 contained full information as to the cause and nature of the injury. Any patient placed on the seriously or dangerously ill list was included in daily lists of such patients submitted to the casualty bureau by the hospitals, which also notified the nearest relative by telegram, at the same time intimating that if any relative wished to visit the patient and could not afford the expense, a return railway warrant for two persons would be issued at the nearest police station on production of the telegram.

Casualties reached hospital in one of the following ways:

(*a*) on the recommendation of a medical practitioner;
(*b*) from first-aid posts;
(*c*) direct from incidents;
(*d*) normal sick from the Defence Forces;
(*e*) transfers from other hospitals.

For the purpose of medical statistics and for use in clinical treatment on transfer, the Ministry of Pensions supplied all hospitals and first-aid posts with Ministry of Pensions casualty forms as follows:

M.P.C. 42 Classification of injury schedule
M.P.C. 43 Discharge certificate to any injured person
M.P.C. 43/1 Receipt from the casualty for the discharge certificate
M.P.C. 43/2 Duplicate of the above returned to the hospital
M.P.C. 44 Record of first-aid treatment at a first-aid post to be made out in triplicate, one to be retained by the first-aid post, and two to be sent to the medical officer of health, who forwarded one to the Ministry of Pensions Casualty Record Office.
M.P.C. 45 Record of out-patient treatment only at a hospital, made out in triplicate, one to be retained by the hospital, and two to be sent to the medical officer of health, who forwarded one to the Ministry of Pensions Casualty Record Office.
M.P.C. 46 Casualty card. Prepared at the first-aid post or dressing station in respect of any casualty transferred to a hospital and sent with the patient.
M.P.C. 47 A cover envelope for medical history documents and for M.P.C. Forms.

Form M.P.C. 47 and its contents were forwarded on the patient's final discharge from hospital or death to the Casualty Recording Offices of the Ministry of Pensions by the hospital authority concerned, a complete record of the case of each casualty thus being available for statistical and other purposes. The envelope M.P.C. 47 was endorsed in the top left hand corner 'civilian casualty'. (See Civilian Health and Medical Services, Volume II, Part II, Chapter 2.)

In addition to the recording of casualties on E.M.S. Forms 105 and M.P.C. Forms, each hospital in the E.M.S. was advised to keep a separate admission and discharge book of all civilian casualties.

SERVICE CASUALTIES AND SERVICE SICK

The procedure for recording Service casualties and sick was precisely similar to the above except that the Forms E.M.S. 105 were made out in triplicate and two copies were sent by the casualty bureaux to the appropriate Service Record Office. These record offices notified the next-of-kin of Service casualties and the hospitals notified the next-of-kin of patients seriously or dangerously ill. The M.P.C. Forms for Service casualties were endorsed on the top left hand corner with the name of the Service, i.e. Navy, Army, R.A.F., and those for Dominions or Allied troops with the name of the country, such as New Zealand, Poland, etc.

The notification of death of casualties or sick to the next-of-kin was made by the Service Records Office concerned and not by the hospital.

Full details of the procedure on the admission, transfer, discharge or death of casualties, and for the provision of out-patient treatment are to be found in E.M.S. Memorandum 3 above referred to.

RECORDING AND NOTIFICATION OF AIR RAID CASUALTIES IN LONDON

For some months before the outbreak of war, consideration had been given to the question of what arrangements should be made for the recording and notification of casualties in London. It was the original intention that when air raid casualties were taken to hospital, or their bodies removed to mortuaries, notification should be posted to the home address of the casualty, and if these notices were not delivered they should be forwarded to the Town Hall or Council Office of the district. The latter would act as a 'dead letter' office and as an inquiry bureau for relatives and friends of those believed to be injured or killed by enemy action.

The Commissioner of the Metropolitan Police was not satisfied with the proposed scheme, chiefly because of the time that would elapse before information about casualties would reach the persons concerned. He took the view that after a raid many people would naturally be anxious as to the safety of their relatives or friends. This feeling of anxiety would inevitably be widespread because a fairly large number of people in the Metropolis, particularly in the central area, are there for business or pleasure, but reside in some other part of London or outside London altogether. A further material factor was the possibility of delays in transport or in communications. In these circumstances, it was felt that immediately after a raid many persons would not be content to wait, but would make inquiries by telephone or by personal call at the local police station or possibly at the scene of the incident.

To meet these conditions the Commissioner was of the opinion that arrangements should be made which would ensure that after a raid the information about all casualties treated at hospitals or taken to mortuaries would be at once collected; that in identified cases the friends or relatives would be informed; and that particulars of all casualties would be available at certain centres easily accessible to any part of the London area. For fairly obvious reasons, the Police were in the best position to undertake this vital work, and, after consultation with the Ministry of Health, the following plan was adopted:

(a) As soon as practicable after an air raid, police would call at hospitals and mortuaries and collect returns giving in the case of identified casualties, their names and addresses and those of the persons to be informed, and, for unidentified casualties, the descriptions of the bodies. These particulars would be circulated by teleprinter to all police stations in London and the local police would thereupon inform the relatives and friends. Notification to relatives and friends resident outside London would be effected by arrangement with the provincial police force concerned.

(b) Ten casualty bureaux would be established in the London Region by the Ministry of Health; hospitals would be required to notify casualties to these bureaux and, inform the next-of-kin of civilian casualties by post. Superintendents of mortuaries would notify deaths to the local authorities who would inform the next-of-kin by post.

With regard to (a) it was realised that the early information collected by police from the hospitals and mortuaries might at times be incomplete or faulty, but the prime consideration was speed rather than accuracy. The compilation of more reliable information was undertaken at a later stage and took the form of a printed list prepared in two parts, viz. Part I, Identified casualties in alphabetical order by name, and Part II, Unidentified casualties, with descriptions of the bodies (and photographs where these were likely to be helpful).

This printed list was compiled by a central casualty bureau established at New Scotland Yard, from information supplied by (a) the Town Clerks of the local authorities as regards dead bodies, and (b) the Ministry of Health casualty bureaux for the cases dealt with at hospitals.

The central casualty bureau referred to was set up as a result of a meeting held on April 25, 1940, at the Ministry of Health, to decide which authority should be responsible for the preparation of complete casualty lists. The Commissioner of Police agreed to do this, and also to supply statistics of air raid casualties to the Ministry of Home Security, and to London Region Headquarters and local authorities for public information.

As the institutions supplying the information fell within the jurisdiction of the Ministry of Health, a Ministry official was designated to work in liaison with Scotland Yard. The Commissioner of the City Police also agreed to work in conjunction with Scotland Yard in this matter. These arrangements were found to work very well during the heavy raids on London; fuller details of the organisation are given in the chapter on these raids. (See Volume II, Part III, Chapter 1.)

CASUALTY BEDS

HOSPITAL RETURNS

In accordance with the provisions laid down in E.M.S. Memorandum 3,[8] each hospital in the Emergency Medical Scheme was required, from the outbreak of hostilities, to prepare a return at least twice daily, stating the number of:

(a) Casualties in hospital:
   (i) Service Cases ;
   (ii) Others ;
(b) Service cases other than casualties ;
(c) Vacant beds and the number of additional beds in reserve which could be set up when required.

This return was amended from time to time as it was found that additional information was necessary. Hospitals were asked to give occupied beds, and for a time the 'discharge' beds, i.e. the beds which could be made available within twenty-four hours by accelerating the discharge of patients to their homes. Reserve beds were subsequently divided into Reserve A and Reserve B beds. Reserve A beds were those already set up, or which could be set up immediately, and for the attendance on which sufficient medical and nursing staff was available. It was considered that every hospital should be able to provide medical and nursing attendance on patients up to 20 per cent. in excess of the normal capacity for which staff was provided.

Reserve B beds were those not necessarily set up in the hospital, but available in store with full equipment, in which no patients could be treated until additional medical or nursing staff were provided.

These returns were submitted to the casualty bureaux when necessary. In practice the returns were made by telephone to the casualty bureaux as a rule once daily, but during lulls a statement of the returns was sent by post. Returns of vacant and occupied beds were not required from hospitals temporarily released from the E.M.S. Scheme. The only returns required from such hospitals were Forms 105 for casualties or

FURTHER EXPANSION AND ORGANISATION

Service sick admitted owing to urgency, and the necessary Ministry of Pensions M.P.C. Forms. The casualty bureaux in each Region informed the Hospital Officer by telephone daily of the number of occupied and vacant beds, etc., in each hospital, giving the hospital code number before the figures, and each Region informed the Ministry of Health in Whitehall by telephone, telegram or letter in accordance with the instructions in force at the time, giving the Regional totals. A complete picture of the hospital bedstates was therefore always available in the Regions and at Headquarters.

VARIATIONS IN THE NUMBERS OF CASUALTY BEDS AVAILABLE

The number of beds available at any time after the outbreak of hostilities varied according to the normal factors of the admission and discharge of civilian sick and civilian and Service casualties and Service sick, but also in the first few months of the war to the following factors:

(1) the reflux of the civilian sick dispersed in the initial clearance of hospitals;

(2) the extent to which beds became available by 'crowding' in existing hospitals;

(3) the progress made in 'upgrading' Class II hospitals to Class I;

(4) the rate of delivery of the equipment necessary for beds and for the treatment of the patients;

(5) the provision of the necessary medical and nursing staff;

(6) the rate of construction of hutted annexes to hospitals and *ad hoc* hutted hospitals;

(7) the suspension of large numbers of small Class I and Class II hospitals;

(8) the withdrawal of certain hospitals at first included in the E.M.S. Hospital Scheme, but afterwards found to be unsuitable for casualties, or for other reasons;

(9) transfer to the Services of whole hospitals from time to time.

CROWDING AND UPGRADING

The additional beds to be made available by crowding were ready in the autumn of 1939, and by upgrading in the spring of 1940; these were fully equipped, and in most cases adequately staffed, though in some of the larger base hospitals the staff was augmented from time to time as required.

HUTTED ANNEXES AND HUTTED HOSPITALS

Beds in hutted annexes of Blocks A and B became available as shown below:

```
Up to January 1, 1940      2,240 beds in  6 hospitals
 ,,  ,,  May 1, 1940      10,240  ,,    ,, 30    ,,
 ,,  ,,   ,,  1, 1942     30,080  ,,    ,, 92    ,,
```

In Block C, beds gradually became available, as follows:

By January 1, 1941	120 beds in 1 hospital
,, ,, 1, 1942	3,880 ,, ,, 12 hospitals
,, ,, 1, 1943	*7,600 ,, ,,*26 ,,

* Including 1,200 beds in 2 *ad hoc* hospitals.

CHILDREN'S HOSPITALS

The extensive evacuation of children from vulnerable areas necessitated hospital provision for them in reception areas. In hospitals in the outer zones of each of the London Sectors, special children's units, varying from 15 to 70 beds, were set up. In provincial hospitals also, extra accommodation and treatment were arranged to meet the needs expected to arise from the evacuation of all children from certain specified areas. As equipment was transferred from the evacuating central hospitals, the total number of beds available was not affected.

An example of a children's unit in the London Sectors was the one provided at Cuckfield in Sector 9, in order to serve the part of London south of the Thames. The East Sussex County Council's Public Assistance Institution at Cuckfield had been handed over to the Emergency Medical Services as a general hospital at the outbreak of the war and huts were built to contain about 400 beds. The main building was selected to house a children's unit of 100 beds. Full-time medical and surgical services were available and a pathological laboratory was also housed in the unit. The nursing staff was provided from the training school of the Hospital for Sick Children, Great Ormond Street. The patients came partly from the London area and partly from other E.M.S. hospitals in the southern area and from hospitals and clinics in the East Sussex Coastal area. An out-patients clinic was also provided. The unit functioned at Cuckfield until the whole hospital was handed over to the Canadian Army in August 1942, when it was transferred to Elfinsward Auxiliary Hospital at Haywards Heath. There it continued to function until August 1945.

HOSPITALS SUSPENDED OR WITHDRAWN

In the autumn of 1939, a large number of the smaller hospitals and some of the larger hospitals which were considered unsuitable, except in an emergency, were suspended or withdrawn from the Emergency Hospital Scheme. These were chiefly Class 1B hospitals containing less than 70–80 beds and Class II hospitals. The latter were chiefly maternity homes; homes for convalescent children; and for special categories, such as seamen, miners and police. Sanatoria required for tuberculosis cases were withdrawn from the Scheme. These were the chief factors affecting the numbers of beds available during the period dealt with in this chapter. In later periods, of course, the beds available were affected by the numbers rendered temporarily or permanently unusable by enemy action. The following table gives the number of vacant beds in hospitals in the E.M.S. from time to time during the period ending April 30, 1940, together with the numbers of casualties, civilian or Service, in hospitals:

SUMMARY OF BEDSTATE RETURNS

September 3, 1939 to April 30, 1940

Date	Vacant beds	Civilian casualties	Service casualties	Service sick
1939 September 3	163,500 London 51,000			
,, 7	187,600 London 56,000			
,, 30	181,000			
October 31	170,000	100	461	2,513
November 30	151,000	234	500	3,600
December 31	152,450	124	476	4,000
1940 January 31	123,250 including Res. 13,000	120	520	16,000
February 28	125,100 including Res. 30,000	120	470	13,200
March 31	131,000 including Res. 37,000	100	550	10,400
April 30	136,900 including Res. 38,000	100	1,280	11,500

It will be noted that there was a gradual reduction in the numbers of beds available up to the end of January. This was chiefly due to the suspension and withdrawal of hospitals from the Scheme, and to reduction of the actual number of beds in some hospitals as accommodation at first allotted for beds had been found unsuitable or required for the expanded ancillary services of the hospital. The increase from February was chiefly due to beds becoming available in hospitals that were being upgraded and to the completion of numbers of hutted annexes.

Between October 25, 1939 and April 30, 1940, military patients from overseas were admitted to E.M.S. hospitals from the base hospitals in France, chiefly owing to the periodical clearing from those hospitals of patients likely to require prolonged hospital treatment or invaliding from the Services.

THE EMERGENCY MEDICAL SERVICES ON MAY 1, 1940

1. The period of eight months of inaction on the Western Front had given the Ministry of Health much valuable time during which to consolidate the emergency services in accordance with the 'long-term' policy in the following respects:

(*a*) To complete the organisation at Headquarters to enable it to deal with all probable calls on the Emergency Medical Services following attacks by air raids on the civilian population, or from the fighting Services.

(*b*) Similarly to complete the Regional organisation.

(*c*) To complete the equipping and staffing of between 30,000 and 40,000 beds in the parts of mental hospitals which had been taken over, chiefly to act as base hospitals.

(*d*) To equip and staff the hutted hospitals or hutted annexes, as they were taken over from the Office of Works on completion.

(*e*) To complete the 'upgrading' of the selected hospitals.

(*f*) To reduce bed accommodation in the larger hospitals in unsuitable portions of the buildings which had been equipped as wards as a 'short-term' emergency measure.

(*g*) To expand the provisions for the ancillary hospital services, and provide day rooms, pack stores, etc. in the military wings of convoy hospitals.

(*h*) To equip and staff the special centres already selected and add further to their numbers.

(*i*) To suspend or withdraw from the Emergency Medical Services large numbers of the smaller hospitals which would be of little value except as a reserve in very grave emergencies.

By the end of April, 930 hospitals with a bed accommodation of 71,247 had been suspended, and 125 hospitals with a bed accommodation of 14,711 had been withdrawn. The suspended hospitals were mostly those in rural areas with no resident medical staff, or small private hospitals in urban areas; the hospitals withdrawn were mostly maternity hospitals, homes for incurables, etc. which were never likely to be available for casualties.

2. As a result of these measures the numbers of hospitals remaining in the Emergency Medical Services on May 1, 1940, were:

	Hospitals	*Total beds*	*Casualty beds*
Class 1A	667	281,985	189,184
” 1B	104	6,814	4,746
” II	436	117,813	68,929
Total:	1,207	406,612	262,859

FURTHER EXPANSION AND ORGANISATION

This represents a diminution of 1,163 hospitals and 85,958 beds since September 1, 1939.

3. The numbers of ambulances and first-aid posts were:

	In London (Standing by)	In the Provinces (Standing by)	(On call)
Inter-hospital ambulances with eight or ten stretchers each as at 1.1.40	219	838	136
Fixed first-aid posts (31.3.40)	408	1,498	
Mobile Units: (31.3.40)	171	682	
Local Authority Ambulances (1.1.40): whole-time	1,902	5,181	
part-time	215	5,945	
Sitting-case cars: (1.1.40) whole-time	1,310	1,022	
part-time	1,122	11,402	

4. Structural precautions to nearly all the hospitals had been completed and were well advanced as regards the first-aid posts.

5. In hutted hospitals and in the hutted annexes 12,480 beds were in use and about another 10,000 were nearing completion.

REFERENCES

[1] *Defence Regulations (being Regulations made under the Emergency Powers (Defence) Act, 1939), printed as amended up to and including March 19, 1940.* H.M.S.O., 1940.

[2] *Parliamentary Debates*, Fifth Series, Vol. 351, *House of Commons Official Report*, September 13, 1939, Col. 661 (351 H.C. Deb., Col. 661).

[3] Air Raid Precautions to be taken by holders and users of Radium. Issued by Ministry of Home Security, October 1941 (Min. of Health Circular 2489, October 22, 1941).

[4] *Emergency Medical Services Memorandum No. 3 (England and Wales). Procedure on the Admission, Transfer, Discharge or Death of Casualties, and for the Provision of Out-patient Treatment.* Issued by the Ministry of Health. H.M.S.O., 1939 and) 2nd Edn.) 1940.

CHAPTER 4
THE PERIOD OF ACTIVE OPERATIONS IN BRITAIN
May 1940 to July 1941

THE HOSPITAL SERVICES

HOSPITAL ACCOMMODATION

THE invasion of Holland and Belgium on May 10, 1940, naturally led to some speculation as to its effect on the medical arrangements in this country. The estimated requirements of the War Office for casualty beds in this country during active operations on the Continent had been agreed upon at the conference held on February 1, 1940, referred to in Chapter 3, viz. 70,000 beds in E.M.S. hospitals. These requirements had been met by the provision by April 1940, of 75,000 beds in 112 hospitals. Since about 20,000 new beds in huts were now either in use or ready for occupation and another 15,000 would be ready in the near future, little further action was thought necessary. The military wings in E.M.S. hospitals were, however, increased to 32, and others had been selected to meet future requirements. This increase was made because a further 21 convoys had been received from overseas (bringing the total number of convoys admitted to E.M.S. hospitals to 57) and in anticipation of an early campaign on the Western Front. Some 173,000 beds were thus immediately available, a figure which could have been largely increased at any time by clearing hospitals.

There was also the following accommodation available in Service and Ministry of Pensions hospitals:

	Hospitals	Total Beds	Occupied Beds	Vacant Beds
Royal Navy	7	4,485	2,225	2,260
Royal Air Force	13*	2,674	1,604	1,070
Army	66	8,991	6,389	2,602
Ministry of Pensions	8	2,244	995	1,249

* Includes R.A.F. hospitals in Scotland and Northern Ireland.

The situation at this time naturally gave rise to various suggestions for action, not all of which were considered to be either practicable or necessary. One such, as the then Director-General, Sir John Hebb, records in his notes on the early history of the E.M.S., was to the effect that all hospitals east of London Bridge should be closed. It was said to have emanated from the Civil Defence Committee. 'The suggestion', wrote Sir John, 'in itself was disturbing since if taken at its face value it would have affected some 46,000 beds, but really still more disturbing was the inference that a situation had arisen which was sufficiently critical to make necessary such drastic recommendations to the Ministry from a body on which the Ministry had no representative and from which it had received no previous warning'. The suggestion was dropped, probably as a result of representations made informally, of which there appears to be no further record.

Action was taken, however, on another suggestion, which reduced the number of available beds. The Air Ministry advised closing any hospital within 1,000 yards of an aerodrome, which distance was regarded as likely to be within the margin of error in bomb aiming. Only four hospitals of any size were affected at this time. These were closed, entailing a loss of 1,631 total beds and 603 casualty beds in three Class I hospitals and 60 total beds and 25 casualty beds in one Class II hospital.

With aerodromes springing up rapidly all over the country, the potential danger to existing hospitals was somewhat disquieting. By close liaison and discussion with the R.A.F., however, further loss of beds in essential hospitals was avoided.

Service Tuberculosis Cases. Having regard to the rapid expansion of the Fighting Services after the outbreak of war, it was inevitable that—despite the most careful examination of recruits by medical boards—a small percentage of tuberculous cases, with no authenticated history or physical signs of the disease, were passed fit for service. When, under the rigours of training and weather, unsuspected quiescent foci of the disease became active and their tuberculous condition came to light, such cases were dealt with for the most part in Service hospitals. Some, however, were sent to E.M.S. hospitals, usually by the military medical authorities, undiagnosed or suffering from other complaints. As the policy laid down for E.M.S. hospitals excluded provision for tuberculous cases, they were transferred to military hospitals as soon as a positive diagnosis was made, but, occasionally, patients had to be retained in E.M.S. hospitals, sometimes for prolonged periods, because of lack of accommodation in the Service hospitals. These patients were examined by Service medical boards in the E.M.S. hospitals; but when invalided, difficulty was often found in obtaining their admission to sanatoria, these being mostly full because of the general increase of tuberculosis among the civil population and because, although 6,000 of the beds which had been earmarked for casualties in sanatoria had been released, a considerable number had been retained. It was therefore found necessary early in May 1940, to allot beds for military cases in ten sanatoria, in different parts of the country.

When cases were diagnosed in E.M.S. hospitals, applications were made for their admission to one of these sanatoria. This was found to involve considerable delay while a vacancy was being sought. In March 1941, therefore, the procedure was amended and thereafter applications for accommodation were made to a central clearing office at the Ministry of Health, Whitehall, under Dr. Norman Smith, who was responsible for allotting beds in sanatoria to cases awaiting transfer. These regulations applied only to tuberculous cases in the Army and the R.A.F., the naval cases being treated by the naval authorities in their own hospitals.

The following provisional figures of Army personnel invalided on account of pulmonary tuberculosis since the outbreak of hostilities were supplied by the War Office:

	Males	Females	Total
September 1939—December 1940			2,827
1941			3,689
1942	2,606	173	2,779
1943	2,613	365	2,978
1944	3,436	377	3,813
1945 (Jan.–August)	1,955	182	2,137
1945 (Sept.–Dec.)	1,251	123	1,374

a total of 19,597 males and females.

These figures represent a very small percentage of the very large numbers recruited.

Later on in 1941, finding that the numbers of casualties as the result of air warfare and from overseas had not thrown any pressure on E.M.S. beds, the Ministry released a certain number of wards in selected hutted hospitals for civilian tuberculous cases. This relieved the pressure on sanatoria, especially as the general incidence of tuberculosis began to take a downward course in the year 1942; but difficulties were still experienced in dealing with tuberculous cases owing to shortage of nurses and domestic staff in the sanatoria.

Service Mental Cases. There was also during this period an increasing demand for accommodation for psychosis patients. A number of cases admitted to E.M.S. hospitals for neurosis were found to be psychotic and, as there was insufficient accommodation for them in existing military hospitals and they could not be admitted to mental hospitals without certification, such cases had to be sent to the observation wards of public assistance institutions. Eventually, in December 1940, 1,277 additional beds in six military mental hospitals were made available, to which such cases could, under Army regulations, be transferred without certification.

Resuscitation Wards. All Class 1A hospitals had already been provided with resuscitation wards, fully equipped for resuscitation and blood transfusion, and arrangements had been made for mobile resuscitation teams, based on the larger hospitals, to be available on call. It was intended that these teams should carry the necessary equipment, but as an additional precaution it was now decided similarly to equip all Class 1B hospitals, since it was expected that these small hospitals would also be brought into use.

Special Centres. Special centres for the various types of injury having been established all over the country, it was found necessary to appoint Regional Consultants to inspect and report on their equipment and staffing, and to direct the special treatment required. Orthopaedic centres in one or more hospitals had been set up in all the Regions and London Sectors, because a large number of orthopaedic cases, probably amounting to 60 per cent. of all casualties, would have to be dealt with. Special centres were set up for neurosis, chest injuries and for head injuries in ten hospitals, and in certain of these, provision had been made for dealing with peripheral nerve injuries. There were also twelve centres for plastic surgery and jaw injuries. The treatment of burns had also become of great importance and for this purpose three special centres had been established. In addition all Regions were provided with centres for the treatment of skin diseases.

Instructions were again issued to the medical superintendents of all hospitals emphasising that the earliest possible transfer of cases to special centres was essential, it having been found by experience that hospitals, especially some of the larger ones, were very reluctant to part with these special cases.

Lists of special centres and of Regional consultants on special disabilities, and the arrangements for use of these special centres were issued in June 1941, in a booklet *Emergency Medical Service Instructions, Part I: Medical Treatment and Special Centres.* (See Chapter 2 and Appendix II.)

Ministry of Pensions Hospitals. As a temporary measure, arrangements were made in June by which the Ministry of Pensions was prepared to take into seven of their hospitals, Service surgical cases of a severe type likely to be boarded out as invalids requiring prolonged hospital treatment. Such admissions were restricted to (*a*) patients with disabilities already attributed to war service and (*b*) gunshot wound and burn cases, these being *prima facie* attributable and therefore likely to become the responsibility of the Ministry of Pensions.

REGIONAL ADVISERS

In addition to Regional Consultant Advisers for the special centres, Regional Advisers in general medicine and surgery were appointed, to report to Regional Hospital Officers on the clinical provisions and efficiency of E.M.S. hospitals and make recommendations to ensure as high a standard as possible. In some of the smaller Regions these appointments were held by consultant physicians or surgeons to the Army Command covering the area concerned.

GROUP ADVISERS

In December 1940, it was found that the areas allotted to Regional Advisers were too large for them to have an intimate knowledge of the working and personnel of each hospital. It was therefore decided that in addition to the groups of hospitals based on large cities in the provincial regions to which Group Officers had been appointed, the remaining E.M.S. hospitals, including the auxiliary hospitals, should be formed into suitable groups. To each of these groups, medical officers of consultant rank, resident in the group, were appointed as Class II officers (i.e. on a part-time basis). Their main function was to ensure that all the facilities provided by the Emergency Medical Service for the efficient treatment of patients should be known to hospitals and their medical officers. Group Advisers were asked to pay particular attention to the following points:

(*a*) The arrangements for the reception of casualties and for resuscitation;

(*b*) the immediate transfer, where necessary, of patients to hospitals with special treatment facilities;

(*c*) the use, whenever possible, of convalescent homes and depots;

(*d*) the calling in of specialists for consultative advice;

(*e*) the employment of Class III (sessional) surgeons and physicians for the care and treatment of the patients.

EVACUATION OF THE BRITISH EXPEDITIONARY FORCE FROM FRANCE

CASUALTIES ADMITTED TO E.M.S. HOSPITALS

The general evacuation of the British Expeditionary Force from Dunkirk and other ports in France which began at the end of May 1940 resulted in a sudden flow of casualties into Service and E.M.S. hospitals. Most of these casualties were landed at South Coast towns, though some of the later ones were landed as far north as Liverpool. They came in hospital ships and other vessels of various kinds and all sizes. Most of them were distributed from the ports in ambulance trains to hospitals in various parts of the country, the more serious cases being sent in ambulances to the nearest hospital equipped for dealing with them. Others went by ordinary trains with batches of men not requiring hospital treatment and were then sent to hospital after examination at their destinations. There were also small numbers of French, Belgian and Polish casualties. (See Plates V and VI.)

The total number of Army casualties admitted to E.M.S. hospitals during this period from 47 ambulance trains was 28,354. In addition 3,487 naval ratings were admitted.

The London Sector hospitals received a large proportion of the serious cases, but considerable numbers, of which about half were stretcher cases, went to the large base hospitals in the north-west and north of England. A small proportion of these cases became serious because gas gangrene supervened. The flow of casualties from France had practically ended by June 10, but a few more arrived in small parties later in the month.

Of the London Sector hospitals, Sector 10 received many serious cases either directly or through local hospitals on the coast, to which they had been taken from small craft which had landed them at ports, piers and beaches round the coasts of Kent and Sussex.

The military authorities had posted a number of R.A.M.C. officers, stretcher bearers and ambulances at all the small ports in Kent and Sussex at which casualties were likely to be landed and the R.A.M.C. had undertaken to transport these casualties to the E.M.S. hospitals. Some serious cases requiring immediate attention had to be admitted to the nearest local hospitals, where they were retained only until they were fit to be transferred in ambulances to the larger Sector hospitals.

But in some places, the flow of casualties was greater than these small detachments were equipped to deal with. In Ramsgate and Margate there was a shortage of stretcher bearers and in Ramsgate some of the cases had to be temporarily provided for in private houses. To relieve the congestion the Group Officer of Sector 10, Professor T. B. Johnston, arranged for an ambulance train which cleared 112 cases from Margate and over 100 from Ramsgate to Guildford. A number of ten-stretcher inter-hospital ambulances were also sent to collect the casualties from the train and to take some direct to Sector hospitals.

In Dover, on May 29, the flow of casualties was so great and the proportion of serious cases so high that the staff of the Dover Emergency Hospital were unable to cope with them and at the request of Dr. R. O. C. Thomson, Hospital Officer, Region 12, Professor Johnston sent to their assistance a mobile surgical team under Mr. Hedley Atkins, Assistant Surgeon, Guy's Hospital. On May 30, at the request of Mr. Atkins, two house surgeons, a senior student and five trained nurses, together with a certain number of essential instruments and equipment were sent to Dover. Mr. Atkins handled a difficult task with great efficiency and the situation was well in hand by June 1. In all 190 operations had to be carried out. The Dover Hospital was never intended to deal with large numbers of seriously injured casualties, being only meant to deal with local air raid casualties. There was therefore a shortage of trained nurses accustomed to serious cases. Mr. Atkins commended the work of the local surgical teams and stated that the need for outside help was wholly due to the large number of patients and the severity of their wounds which threw too great a strain on the organisation of the hospital.

Apart from this and a few other minor setbacks, the collection of casualties from the ports and their transport to hospitals was carried out smoothly, rapidly and efficiently. Perfection could not be expected, as it was impossible to forecast with any accuracy the number of casualties which would arrive at any port or pierhead, or the time at which they would arrive. In these difficult circumstances, the way in which cases were dealt with was highly creditable.

Major Gen. J. F. Martin, late R.A.M.C., who was attached to the headquarters of Region 12 on special duty, inspected the Dover Hospital on June 1, and found that everything was working in an orderly manner. On subsequent days he inspected a number of the other hospitals in the area and reported that all patients were well looked after and comfortable. In his opinion the temporary breakdown at Dover was due to the Regional Hospital Officer's not having received early ifnormation of the state of affairs at the hospital, which was too small and poorly equipped to receive all the seriously wounded disembarked at that port. He did not consider that the case mortality was affected by the breakdown. In all 354 patients were admitted to the one hospital at Dover, of whom 51 died, while at Brighton three hospitals admitted 211 cases with 53 deaths—a greater case mortality than at Dover. This is only a rough comparison and does not in any way reflect adversely on the treatment given at Brighton.

Professor Johnston had foreseen the probability that the outer zone hospitals of his sector would be required and had ensured that some 2,000 empty beds were available in the southern portion of Kent and Sussex and about 5,000 in south-east London and northern Kent.

Many of the cases received in the Sector were those wounded on the beaches at Dunkirk and on the way over; many had burns from incendiary bombs. One group had been sunk twice and had been immersed in the sea for two and a half hours before they were finally rescued. As the flow of casualties continued, hospitals in Tunbridge Wells and Maidstone were working day and night though they still had many vacant beds. Other hospitals were therefore used to ensure the rapid surgical treatment of all cases.

As there was no exact means of estimating when the flow of casualties would stop, cases were evacuated from the sector hospitals by civil evacuation trains to other parts of the country to provide for the accommodation of further cases. Four such evacuations by train were carried out, and ensured that ample accommodation was constantly available.

The flow of casualties came to an end after twelve days, and during this period 1,873 cases were dealt with in the Sector hospitals. Although nearly half of these patients had received no treatment other than first aid and had travelled in ambulance coaches for distances between thirty and sixty miles only 33, 1·7 per cent. of the total number, died.

The ambulance service worked with the greatest smoothness and efficiency; the W.V.S. worked day and night providing refreshments, cigarettes and other comforts at railway stations; and the railway authorities went out of their way to make the journeys as comfortable and expeditious as possible.

The advantages of transporting serious cases in bus ambulances direct to large hospitals efficiently equipped to deal with them, and the distribution of the cases among a number of hospitals to ensure early active treatment, were two of the valuable lessons learned.

This, its first experience of the war, proved that the Sector scheme could work just as efficiently in reverse, i.e. from without inwards as from within outwards as had been planned and that 'base' and casualty clearing hospitals in the E.M.S. system could function equally well for either purpose.

Notwithstanding the flow of casualties from overseas during the Dunkirk period, the number of recorded military admissions to E.M.S. hospitals for the second quarter of 1940 showed no spectacular rise when compared with those of the preceding and succeeding quarters. The explanation lies in the fact that admissions during the first quarter were greatly swollen by influenza and rubella epidemics, and in the greatly increased size of the Army by the third quarter.

The total number of military personnel admitted during the quarter ended March 31, 1940, was approximately 41,000, the larger proportion of which consisted of local sick, but there were also many admissions of sick from the base hospitals in France. Admissions of Army personnel to E.M.S. hospitals in April, 1940, amounted to some 7,000 rising to some 20,000 in May and falling to 13,000 in June, the total for the second quarter thus being approximately 40,000. No reliable returns of admissions were made for the next two quarters, during which improved methods of recording were adopted. From the second quarter of 1941 until the end of 1942 the average number of Army cases admitted remained at about 40,000 per quarter.

EMERGENCY HOSPITALS COMMISSION

CONSTITUTION OF THE COMMISSION

After the collapse of France and the memorable evacuation of the British Expeditionary Force from the Channel ports, enemy preparations for an attack on this country by air and by sea were becoming increasingly evident, and it seemed more than probable that further accommodation for casualties would be required in the immediate future. In these circumstances it was essential that the Emergency Hospital Service should be enabled to meet its obligations as rapidly and efficiently as was humanly possible, and that all causes of delays in administration, building, adaptations and the supply of equipment and personnel which reduced efficiency, should be eliminated.

To advise him in the attainment of these objects, the Minister of Health early in June 1940, appointed a commission, afterwards referred to as the Emergency Hospitals Commission or the Colville-Chatfield Commission. At first it consisted of the Rt. Hon. (afterwards Sir) John Colville, M.P., formerly Secretary of State for Scotland, Mr. E. G. Bearn, Principal Supply Officer of the Ministry of Health, and Mr. (afterwards Sir) Ernest Rock Carling, F.R.C.S., but on July 12, Mr. Colville was succeeded by Admiral of the Fleet Lord Chatfield, P.C., G.C.B., as head of the commission. The terms of reference were stated in the House of Commons by the Minister of Health, to be entirely unlimited.[1] They were concerned with the administration of the Emergency Hospital Scheme itself, the relation of that administration to the regional administration, the supply of beds, equipment, nurses, doctors—every relevant question was within their terms of reference.

The commission visited various Regions, inquiring into the working of the Emergency Hospital Scheme, its regional administration and the possibilities of its expansion, and made a number of recommendations to the Minister, of which the following were the most important:

INCREASE OF HOSPITAL ACCOMMODATION

In order to provide extra bed accommodation in the Emergency Hospital Scheme for the large number of casualties which might have to be dealt with during an invasion, Regional Officers should be urgently instructed:

(*a*) To make an immediate survey of buildings likely to prove suitable as annexes to existing large hospitals wherever they could be found;

(*b*) To extend the survey to all buildings in the Regions which might be suitable for conversion into *ad hoc* hospitals which could be adapted and equipped without undue delay and earmark them as 'shadow' or 'reserve' hospitals, and

(*c*) In addition to consider the provision of a number of auxiliary hospitals for convalescent patients.

Hospital Annexes. The Ministry accordingly instructed the Regional Authorities urgently to inspect all buildings which might be suitable for rapid adaptation as hospitals in close proximity to large base hospitals, which could supply the necessary staff to administer them as part of the parent hospitals. These annexes were to be used for the accommodation of suitable patients who could be transferred to them and so free beds in the parent hospital for more acute cases. As the result of this survey roughly some 10,000 extra beds were provided, most of them in large country houses and some in schools. The largest of the latter was The Leys School, Cambridge, capable of accommodating 350 patients, which was taken over by Addenbrookes Hospital, Cambridge, and administered as part of that hospital. This annexe afterwards functioned as a Class 1A hospital, the greater portion of it accommodating a fully-equipped Fracture 'A' department.

'Shadow' or *'Reserve' Hospitals.* In addition, an urgent inspection of many other buildings in the Regions, not necessarily in close proximity to hospitals, was put in hand. This inspection was carried out primarily by the lay staff of the Regions; the buildings recommended were then inspected by the Regional Hospital Officers or their medical staff and lists of those considered suitable for conversion into hospitals were submitted to the Ministry of Health, who earmarked a selected number in each Region. A few of these were designated 'key' hospitals and at once adapted and equipped. The total number of reserve hospitals eventually selected was 407, estimated to provide accommodation for 69,301 beds, and of these 68 were 'key' hospitals, accommodating 9,778 beds. (See Army Medical Services, Volume I, Chapter 2.)

Auxiliary Hospitals. The need for the provision of convalescent hospitals and homes for Service personnel as an intermediary stage between their discharge from first-class hospitals and their return to duty, or their admission to convalescent depots for graduated physical exercises before returning to duty, had not been adequately met in the E.M.S. organisation or by the War Office. Class II E.M.S. hospitals were unsuitable for Service cases requiring separate accommodation and military supervision, and arrangements were made to provide, as an integral part of the E.M.S. hospital scheme, 10,000 beds in suitably placed country houses to be adapted and equipped for the purpose by the Joint War Organisation of the British Red Cross Society and the Order of St. John, who also agreed to provide for each such auxiliary hospital a part-time medical officer and Red Cross and St. John personnel. In return the Ministry of Health would pay the Joint War Organisation a capitation grant of £10 per bed to cover the cost of adaptation, plus 6s. per day for each occupied and 4s. per day for each unoccupied bed for running expenses. These auxiliary hospitals, to each of which the War Office would attach a R.A.M.C. corporal or sergeant for discipline, etc. were to be included in groups under the group system for military registrars. No military patient was to be sent to them for any period likely to exceed twenty-one days without permission of the Regional Hospital Officer. These hospitals, some of which were later provided with physical training instructors and special rehabilitation equipment, fulfilled their functions in a most satisfactory manner and in most Regions were fully used.

DECENTRALISATION

The commission were of the opinion that much of the work which had previously been thrown on the Hospital Officers and their staffs could have been done by the lay staffs of the Regions and they recommended that Regional administration should be reorganised to permit this. They also recommended very considerable decentralisation of the Ministry's powers to Senior Regional Officers especially for financial sanction and the acquisition and adaptation of buildings for use as hospitals. The adoption of these recommendations was amply justified by the resultant progress. But the commission continued to view with concern the shortage of bed accommodation, notably in Regions 1, 3 and 7, and urged rapid construction of hutted hospitals by the Office of Works. Meanwhile, difficulties were being met with in staffing the hospital annexes already provided.

MEDICAL ARRANGEMENTS IN THE COASTAL BELT CONSIDERED LIABLE TO INVASION

EVACUATION OF THE POPULATION

The areas in which an attempt at invasion seemed probable extended from Great Yarmouth down the coast of East Anglia to Southend-on-Sea, and from Margate round the coast of Kent to Hythe; it was considered by the Government that as complete an evacuation as possible of certain towns in these areas should be arranged. The object was to evacuate the whole of the civil population except the estimated 10 per cent. engaged in essential services, such as the police, fire services, the maintenance of water supplies, drains, lighting, food supplies, etc. Plans were made accordingly, but, as a preliminary measure, a voluntary evacuation of about 60 per cent. of the population was aimed at, and full arrangements for this evacuation were made.

EVACUATION OF HOSPITALS

In pursuance of this policy, the Ministry of Health issued instructions[2] to the Regional authorities to arrange for the evacuation of the sick from all E.M.S. hospitals in these areas and advised local authorities similarly to arrange for the evacuation of the chronic sick from institutions housing this class of patient, and also domiciliary chronic sick, who desired to take advantage of the Ministry's scheme. It was also necessary to ensure that sufficient medical practitioners would remain in these areas to deal with casualties and sick among the remaining civil population. Similarly, arrangements had to be made for sufficient dentists, nurses, pharmacists, and other technical staff to remain, the rest, not required in these areas, would be permitted or directed to leave.[3]

ALLOCATION OF MEDICAL PERSONNEL

It was estimated that for a town with say a hundred hospital beds, from six to eight practitioners would be required for each 2,000 of the population remaining, and Regional authorities were directed to consult the Civil Defence Services, local medical officers of health and local medical war committees as to which practitioners should be retained for duty in each town. Those chosen to remain were to be enrolled in the

E.M.S. and, since it was expected that they would lose all but a small proportion of their practices, it was agreed with the Central Medical War Committee that they would be paid on a whole-time basis—those of consultant rank £800 per annum, general practitioners £550 per annum, plus board and lodging or £100 in lieu thereof in each case. It was to have been a condition of the contract that all other fees received, whether from private and panel practice or from other appointments held, were to be paid over to the Ministry of Health; but the Ministry agreed to modify this condition on the lines of the protection of practices arrangements which had already been made for practitioners called up to the Fighting Services, whereby practitioners who attended the patients of those called up retained for themselves 50 per cent. of the total fees received, and the whole of the allowances for drugs and travelling permitted under the National Health Insurance Act, and paid the balance to the absentee practitioner. A scheme was put into operation accordingly, but further representations were discussed with the Central Medical War Committee, as a result of which the following conditions were finally agreed and embodied in the contracts issued by the Ministry to the 'designated' practitioners:

1. That the enrolled practitioner should aggregate all fees received from his own private and panel patients, together with the sums payable under the National Health Insurance Act for the supply of drugs and travelling, retain half of the total, and pay the other half, less 25 per cent. for expenses, to the Ministry of Health.

2. He should retain 25 per cent. of all sums received as 'acting' practitioner for absent practitioners and hand the balance to the Ministry.

As regards the practitioners not required to be enrolled in the E.M.S., the local medical war committees were to submit their names to the Central Medical War Committee, who would endeavour to place them in private practice or in hospitals in other areas or, if of military age, in the Fighting Services.

Accordingly, the Regional authorities, medical officers of health, and local medical war committees reviewed the whole situation and made their representations to the Ministry, who thereupon 'designated' the medical practitioners required to remain and issued to them forms of contract.

THE WORKING OF THE SCHEME

In the meantime the scheme for the voluntary evacuation of the population had been put in force and from 19 towns with a pre-war total population of 493,935, 304,375 persons were evacuated. Of the 189,560 persons remaining 50,665 were considered to be essential workers. Seventy-three doctors were designated to remain in these towns and a sufficiency of dentists, nurses and technicians.

Voluntary evacuation of these towns began in June 1940, by persons who wished to leave and could make their own arrangements, the general evacuation of the sick was carried out in August and September, and was more or less complete by the end of the first week in September. 2,352 patients were transferred in 15 civil evacuation trains. The chronic sick from public assistance institutions in certain East Coast towns, such as Great Yarmouth, Lowestoft, etc., had already been evacuated early in July, on account of the vulnerability of these institutions.

As the threat of invasion became less acute during the autumn, it was never necessary to undertake the compulsory evacuation of these towns up to 90 per cent. of the population, and with the advent of winter small numbers began to return, although discouraged to do so by the authorities.

EXTENSION OF THE SCHEME

In September it was considered by the Government that similar arrangements for evacuation should be prepared for a further area[4] to include the towns of Colchester and Ipswich in East Anglia and Canterbury and Ashford in Kent, together with a further strip of the South Coast west of Hythe from New Romney to Newhaven, which included, of course, Hastings and Eastbourne. Arrangements were therefore prepared and the necessary medical personnel, etc., were 'designated', 'deferred' contracts being issued under which practitioners were required to report for duty when called upon. In these towns also, it was never found necessary to put into force the arrangements for evacuation.

During the winter there was some relaxation of restrictions on the return of the inhabitants to these coastal belt towns, but E.M.S. hospitals were still required to keep half their beds empty. This rule was extended to hospitals in areas as far north as the Wash in East Anglia and as far west as Weymouth, and subsequently in 1942, to Plymouth on the South Coast. To give effect to these restrictions and at the same time to permit of adequate hospital treatment being available for the civil population, especially in the towns where no large evacuation of the civil population had taken place, the authorities of these hospitals were required to notify the Regional Hospital Officers daily, when submitting their bed states, the number of admissions in excess of 50 per cent. of their accommodation and the number of civilian patients fit for transfer out of the area in order to bring the bed occupancy down to 50 per cent. again.

At first many objections were raised by the relatives of these civilian patients to their being moved, sometimes considerable distances, from the hospital to which they were originally admitted and most hospitals took the precaution of informing relatives that such moves were liable to take place and that under war conditions they must be prepared for such contingencies. Eventually, these inconveniences were accepted by the civil population without further difficulty. As time went on, during 1941 these restrictions were greatly relaxed and the hospitals in these towns were only required to keep 25 per cent. of their casualty beds vacant for emergencies.

THE 'GREEN BELT' SCHEME

In 1942 in an area termed the 'green belt' in the rear of the 'coastal belt', a number of hospitals were selected to function as advanced base and base hospitals in which arrangements were made for a partial evacuation of patients at the same time as the 'coastal belt' scheme was brought into force, in order that beds would be available for casualties evacuated from the coastal belt hospitals during hostilities. The partial evacuation aimed at 60 per cent. of the beds in these hospitals being available for casualties.

ADMINISTRATION AND PERSONNEL

CHANGES IN HEADQUARTERS STAFF

The inception and evolution of the Emergency Medical Services owed much to its first Director-General, the late Sir John H. Hebb, C.B., K.H.P., who after his distinguished service as an organiser and administrator in the capacity of Director-General of Medical Services of the Ministry of Pensions, was seconded to the Ministry of Health. To Hebb fell the arduous task of organising the Emergency Medical Services, and he carried it through its early stages until his health broke down and Professor (afterwards Sir) Francis R. Fraser, M.D., succeeded him in May 1940. On relinquishing his work, Hebb undertook to write the story of the evolution of the Emergency Medical Services for the Medical History, and much of the early part of this narrative has been prepared from the material collected by him. He died, while engaged on this work, on February 16, 1942.

Some further changes took place in the headquarters staff. Dr. Murchie, who had been acting as Director, Emergency Medical Services, London and Home Counties, was appointed Director of Medical Personnel in August 1940, *vice* Lt. Col. Potts, who took over the post of medical officer in supervisory charge of the first-aid services. Mr. (afterwards Sir) Claude H. S. Frankau, C.B.E., D.S.O., F.R.C.S., succeeded Dr. Murchie as Director, Emergency Medical Services, London and Home Counties. Dr. Lethem who had been Director, Emergency Medical Services for the Regions outside London and the Home Counties was succeeded by Colonel A. B. Ward on June 6, 1941. Colonel Ward was afterwards succeeded by Dr. W. J. Gill, F.R.C.S., on April 1, 1942, and Dr. Murchie was appointed Deputy Director-General on March 10, 1942.

LIAISON WITH THE FIGHTING SERVICES

(a) *At Headquarters*. To the office of the Director-General of the Emergency Medical Services, at the Ministry of Health, there was attached a special military liaison officer, whose sole function was to keep in close touch with the Fighting Services on all questions of mutual interest. Weekly meetings between representatives of the Services, the Ministry's liaison officer and other officers of the Ministry whose presence might be desirable, were held and at these meetings all current questions affecting civilian and Service medical interests were discussed and appropriate recommendations made when required.

(b) *In the Regions*. Military medical liaison officers had also been appointed to the staffs of the Regional Hospital Officers. The Army representatives were whole-time but for the Navy and Royal Air Force part-time officers were considered adequate. The chief functions of the military liaison officer were to keep in touch with the D.Ds.M.S. and A.Ds.M.S. of the local military commands, and where necessary, to advise and assist on all matters relating to military patients and military medical arrangements generally.

(c) *In Hospitals*. More detailed liaison between the military authorities and the E.M.S. was secured by the appointment of military registrars to certain E.M.S. hospitals and groups of hospitals. At first, at the end of 1939, R.A.M.C. officers were appointed to military wings of E.M.S. hospitals, as already mentioned in Chapter 3. Later on, these officers were made responsible for many of the non-clinical needs of military patients in groups of hospitals, and in 1941, owing to the shortage of medical personnel, they were replaced by non-medical military registrars. The duties of these officers were to advise the medical superintendents and staffs of hospitals in their groups on all matters relating to Army procedure, pay, leave, kit, service conditions, etc. and to deal with such statistical work as the Army might require in connexion with hospital cases. (See Army Medical Services, Volume I, Chapter 2.)

ORGANISATION CHANGES IN THE LONDON REGION

As the result of further recommendations of the Emergency Hospital Commission, certain changes in the London Region were introduced on September 1, 1940.[5]

It was decided that:

(1) In each Sector, the Sector Group Officers would perform duties corresponding to those of a Regional Hospital Officer as far as the hospital services were concerned. The Hospital Officer, London Region, would continue to supervise first aid, the ambulance services and the inter-hospital transport. His title would be unaltered.

(2) The Sector Group Officers would be responsible for planning among themselves the movement of casualties in various circumstances

between the Sectors and with the Hospital Officers of Regions 4, 6 and 12, into which the Sectors projected, between the Sectors and the Regions. The Group Officers would be responsible for the administration of the Sector Hospitals situated in these Regions, but would consult with the Hospital Officers concerned and agree on plans for their use by the Regions when necessary.

(3) The Sector Group Officers would work under the control of Mr. C. H. S. Frankau, Director, Medical Services, London and Home Counties Regions, instead of under the Hospital Officer of the London Region. Dr. Gill and Dr. Bonham Carter were appointed deputies to Mr. Frankau to deal with local authority hospitals in the London Region and with voluntary hospitals respectively.

(4) As the Hospital Officers of Regions 4, 6 and 12 would not be responsible for the Sector hospitals in their Regions, which became known as 'fringe' hospitals, county and county borough medical officers of health would not act as their agents for these hospitals or as agents to the Sector Group Officers.

(5) No changes were required in the functions of the various officers attached to Sector headquarters.

These new arrangements were made after full consultations with the local authorities concerned and represented the general agreement which was reached.

Certain matters such as bedstate returns, the work of the casualty bureaux, the control of inter-hospital transport and the provision of certain surgical appliances were still at this time controlled from the London Region, but eventually the Director, Emergency Medical Services, London and Home Counties Regions, took over the control of these matters.

The reasons given by the commission for the above recommendations were as follows:

(a) The commission found that, except for the supervisory control of the Civil Defence Services and relatively unimportant matters connected with the hospitals, the Sector Group Officers were functioning fully as Hospital Officers. They had direct access to the Director-General, Emergency Medical Services and even to the Secretary, Ministry of Health, and it was to Whitehall that they normally referred any matter of difficulty.

The Hospital Officer, London Region, had little knowledge either of the hospitals in the Sectors or of their personnel. He collected bedstates (copies of which were sent to Whitehall), generally supervised the inter-hospital transport, which in practice was controlled by the Regional Ambulance Officer, and dealt with questions of the supply of certain medical and surgical requisites. The commission therefore saw no reason for continuing this post in the London Regional Office as far as hospital organisation was concerned.

(b) They found that the medical staff available in the London Region as a whole was unevenly distributed, some of the Sectors based on larger hospitals at the apices being much better staffed than other Sectors with more beds in the periphery. They therefore advised that the whole personnel available should be treated as a single pool in order to obtain greater flexibility, and that the machinery at the headquarters of the Ministry should be strengthened so as to control the allocation of the staffs of the Sector hospitals and their distribution in the event of an emergency.

It was also considered of the greatest importance that the controlling authority should be one in which all hospital authorities should have absolute confidence and that its powers would be exercised with complete impartiality.

This re-organisation functioned well and met all requirements even under the greatest strain.

ALTERATION IN REGIONAL BOUNDARIES

In March 1941, the Emergency Medical Services in the County of Dorset were transferred from Region 7 to Region 6. This involved 26 hospitals containing 1,882 total beds and 808 casualty beds and the Civil Defence Services. At the same time the Civil Defence Services in the part of Surrey previously in Region 6 were transferred to Region 12. It did not involve a transfer of hospitals as all the hospitals in Surrey were already included in the London Sectors south of the Thames.

CONSCRIPTION OF PRACTITIONERS

In April 1940, the National Service (Armed Forces) Act, (1939) was applied with certain exceptions to practitioners up to the age of 41 and the Central Medical War Committee was entrusted with the responsibility of advising the Government on the call-up of doctors to the Forces in the light of the medical needs of the civil population. For this purpose the Central Medical War Committee made arrangements with the local medical war committees for the preparation of lists of eligible practitioners for submission to the medical authorities of the Forces.[6]

This Order resulted in many junior members of the medical staffs of E.M.S. hospitals being called up, their places as far as possible being filled by newly qualified medical men, but as medical men at that time could not be 'directed' for duty to E.M.S. hospitals, some difficulty was experienced in obtaining staff for the large base hospitals which had been established outside the large centres of population. This difficulty was accentuated after the fall of France, when the demand for medical men, to replace casualties and to provide medical personnel for the rapid expansion of all branches of the combatant Services, became much greater.

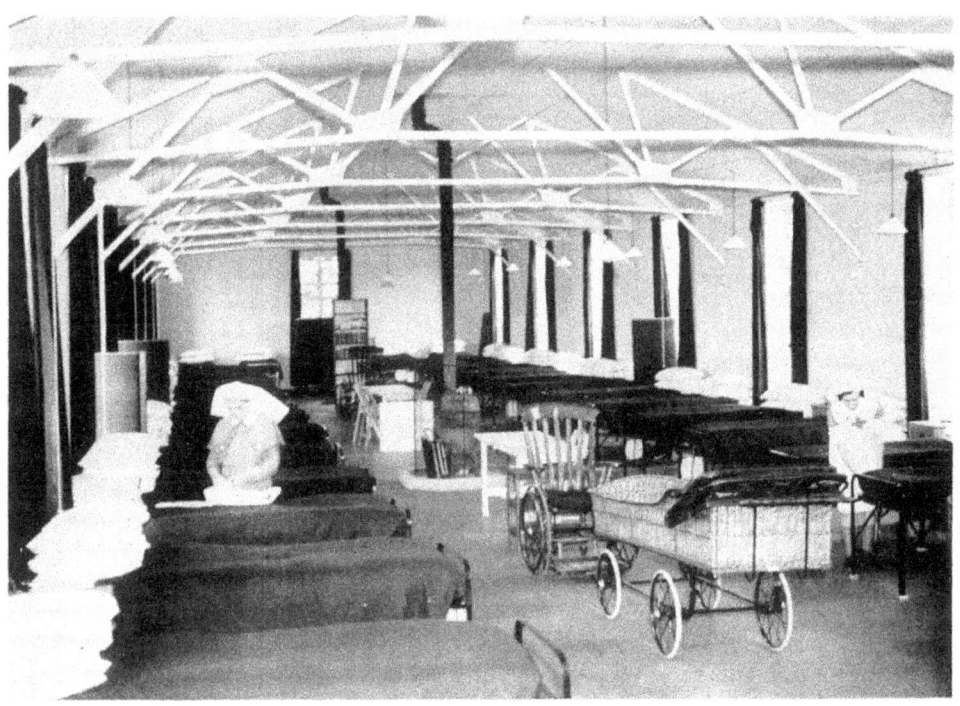

PLATE I. A ward in a hutted hospital

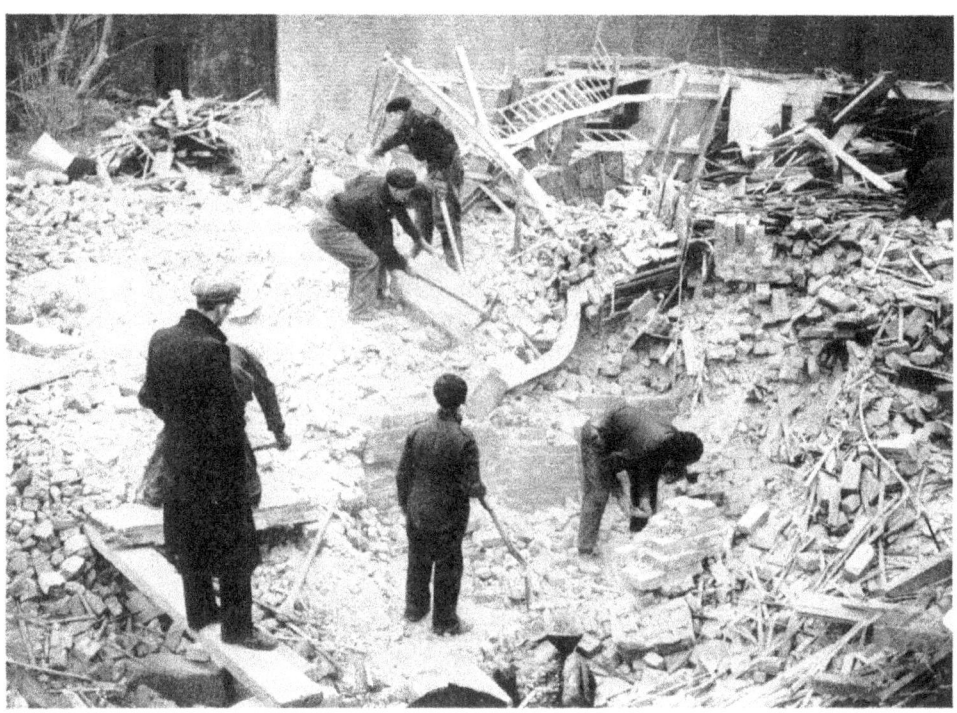

PLATE II. Searching for radium—Marie Curie Hospital, Hampstead

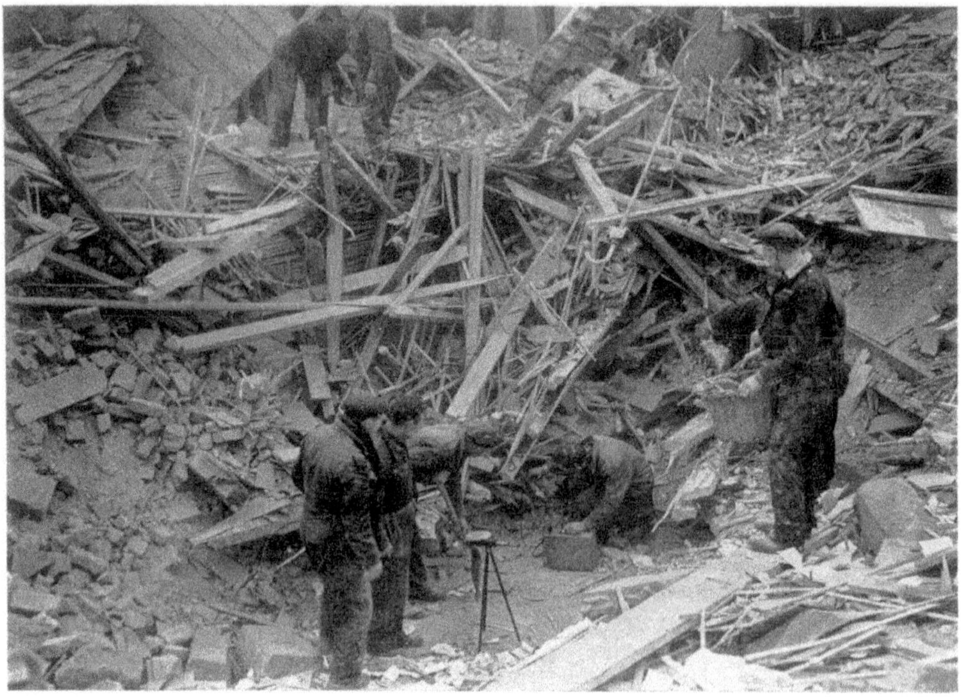

[Daily Mail

PLATE III. Marie Curie Hospital, Hampstead. Mr. H. E. Smith of the National Physical Laboratory searching for radium with a detector.

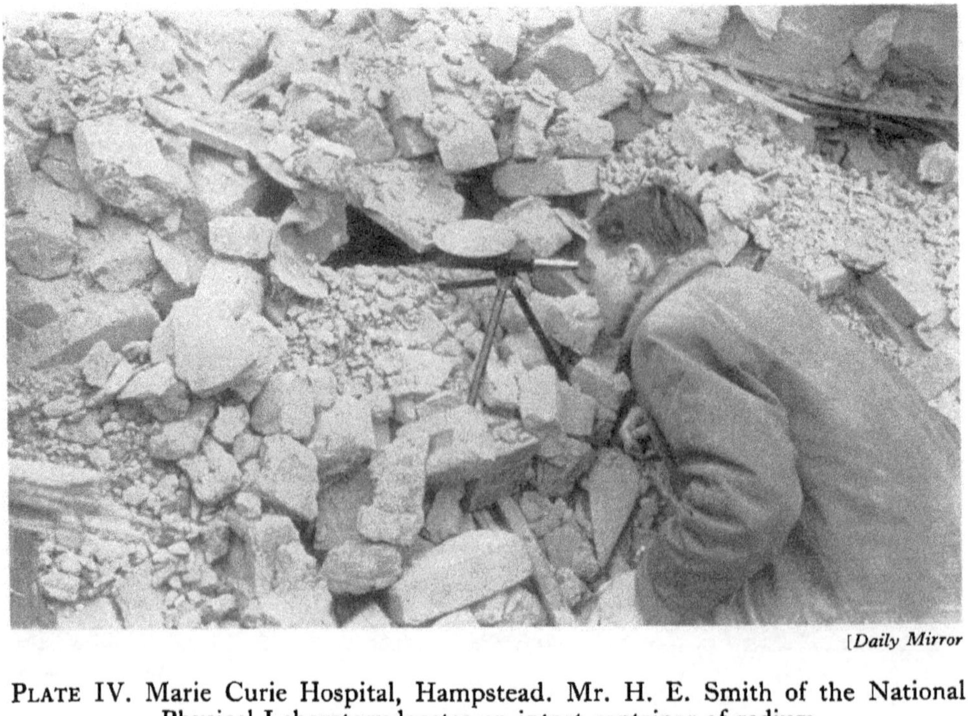

[Daily Mirror

PLATE IV. Marie Curie Hospital, Hampstead. Mr. H. E. Smith of the National Physical Laboratory locates an intact container of radium

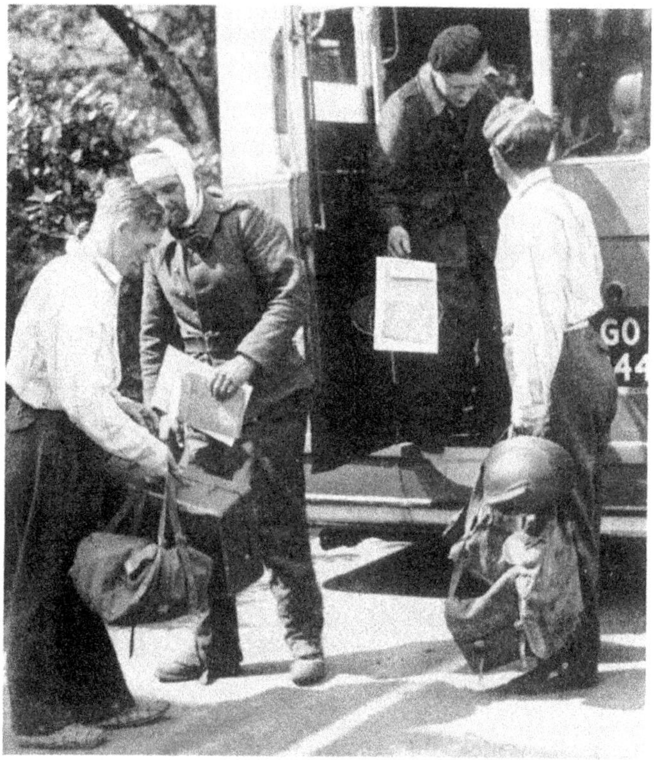

PLATE V. Casualties from Dunkirk

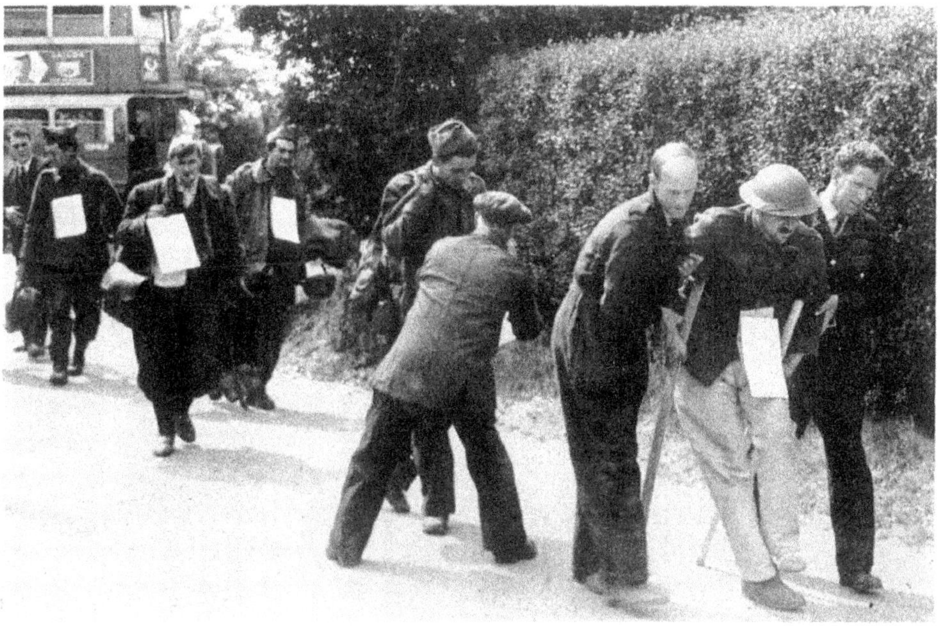

PLATE VI. Casualties from Dunkirk

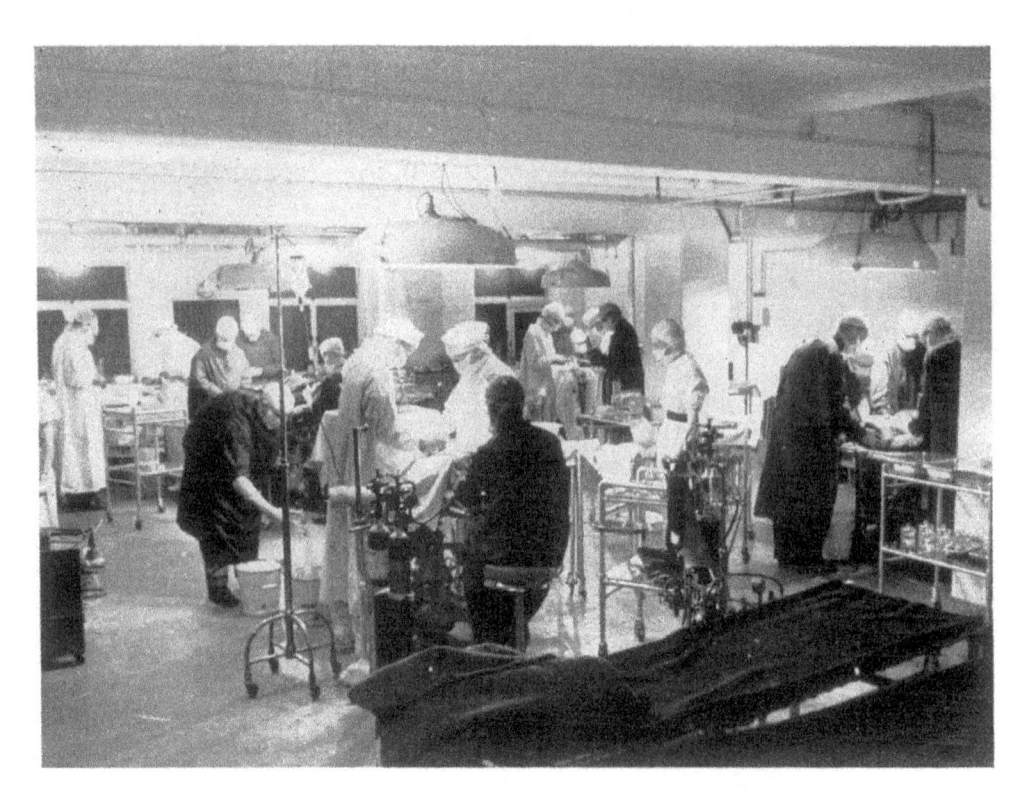

PLATE VII. Guy's Hospital underground operating theatre

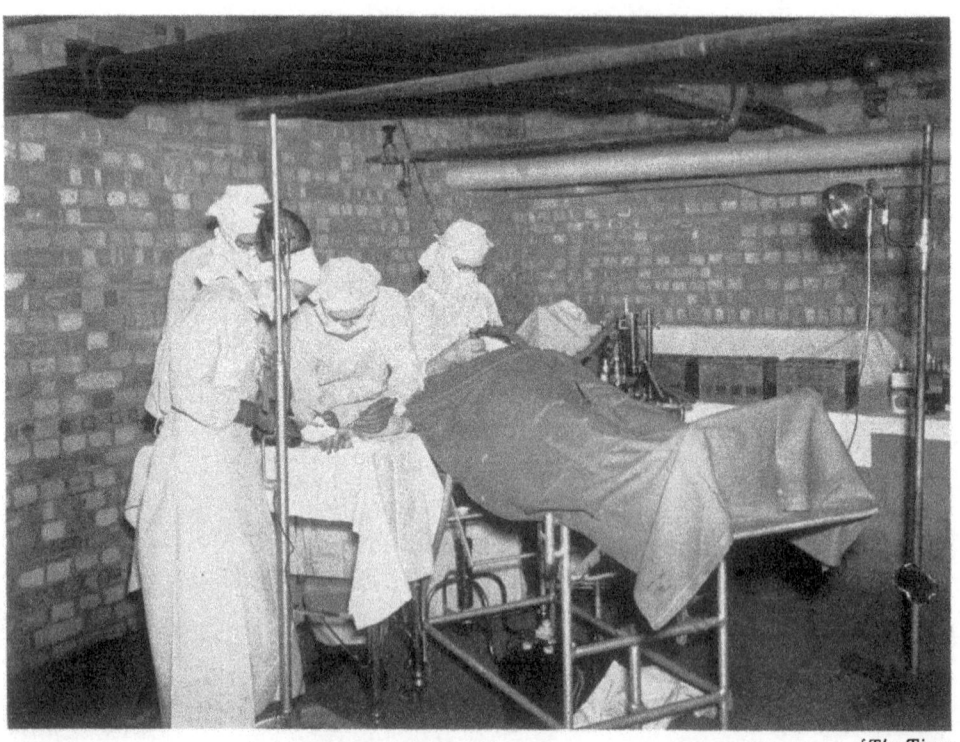

[The Times

PLATE VIII. Middlesex Hospital, underground operating theatre

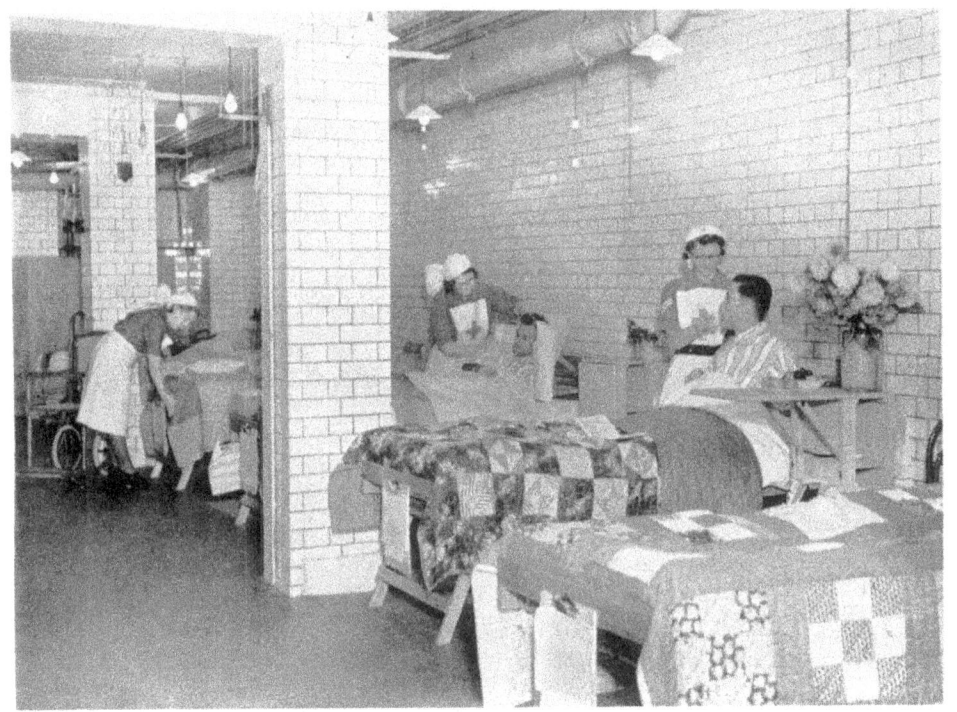

[*Pictorial Press*

PLATE IX. City Corporation Hospital, Cheapside. Underground male ward

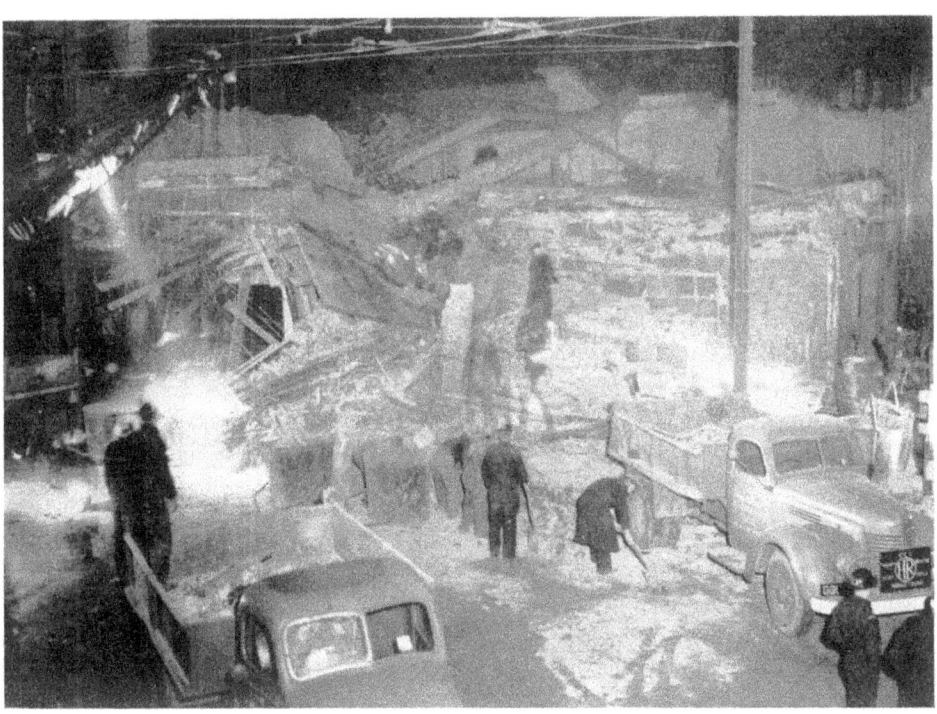

Associated Press

PLATE X. Rescue scene after a Putney dance hall had been struck, November 7, 1943. Many casualties were caused

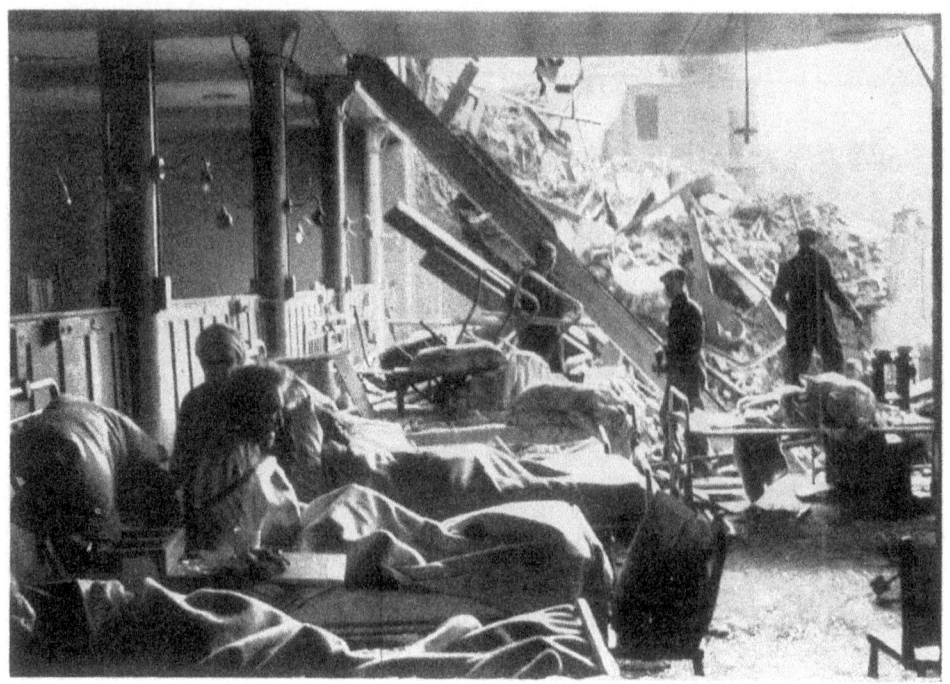

Imperial War Museum

PLATE XI. A pilotless plane crashes into a hospital. Rescuers at work with patients still in bed. June 17, 1944

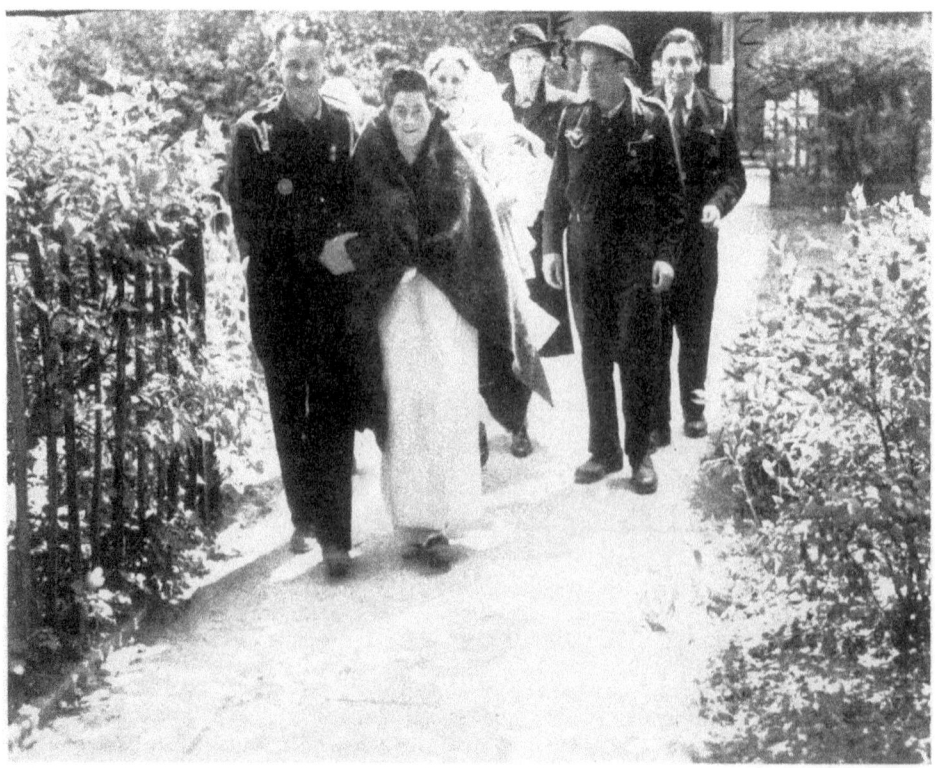

Imperial War Museum

PLATE XII. Walking patients being removed to ambulances. June 17, 1944

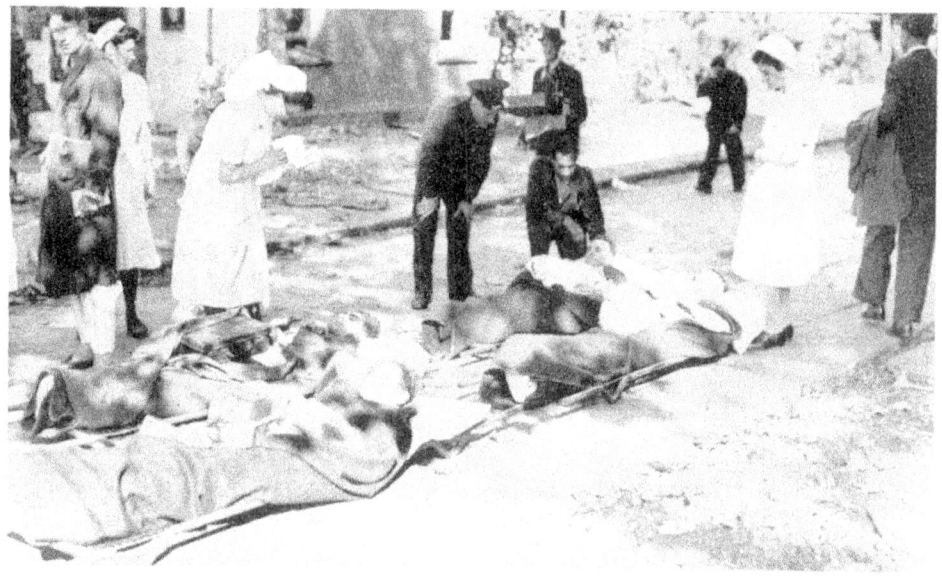

Imperial War Museum

PLATE XIII. Checking the bed patients after evacuation of a hospital hit on July 6, 1944

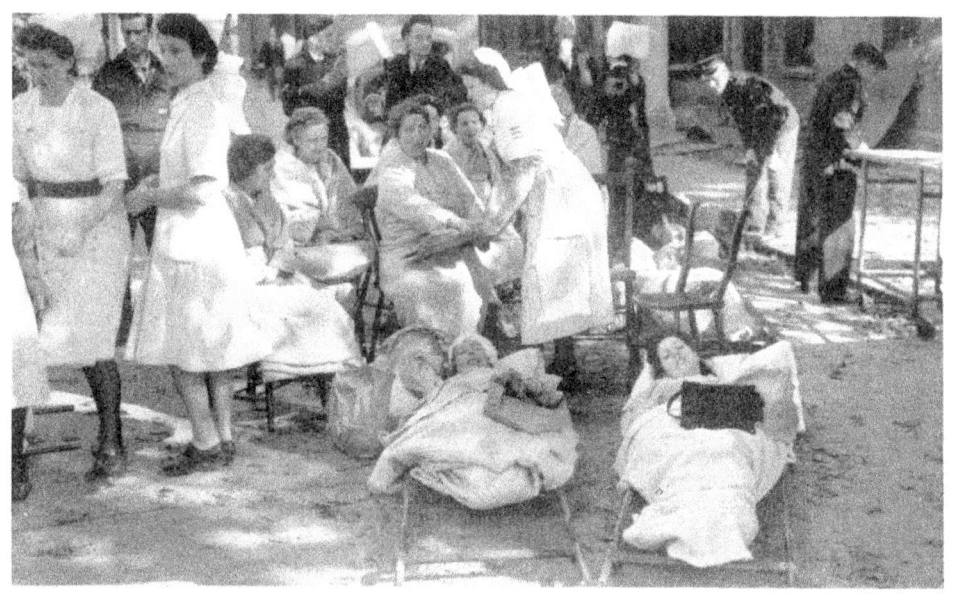

Imperial War Museum

PLATE XIV. Evacuation of patients from a damaged hospital. July 6, 1944

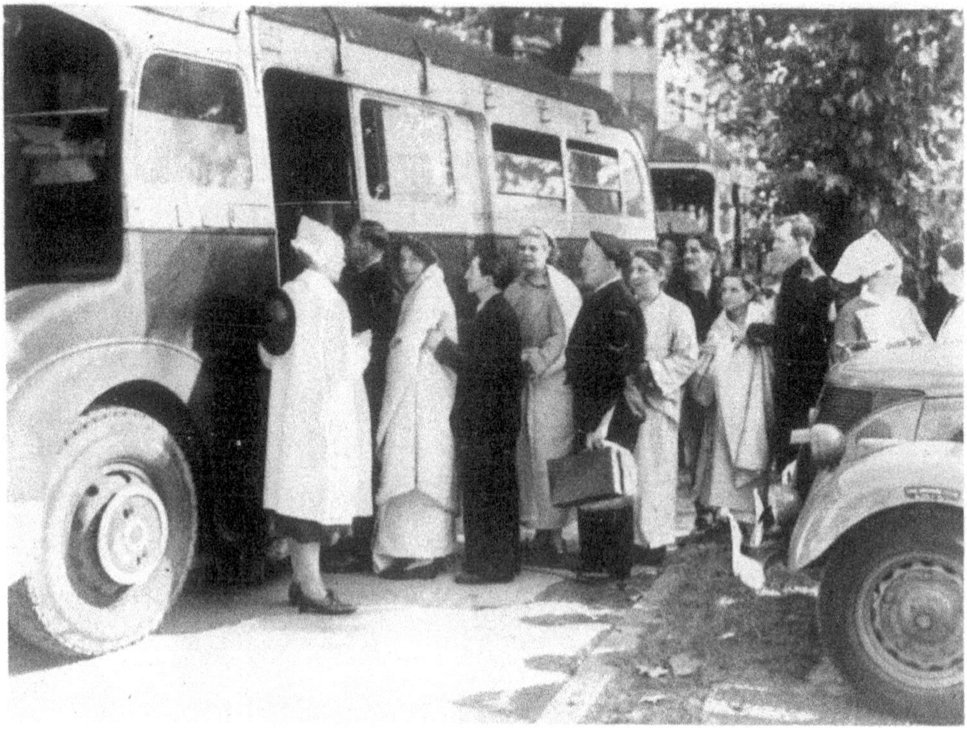

Imperial War Museum

PLATE XV. Patients entering a bus ambulance during the evacuation of a hospital, July 8, 1944

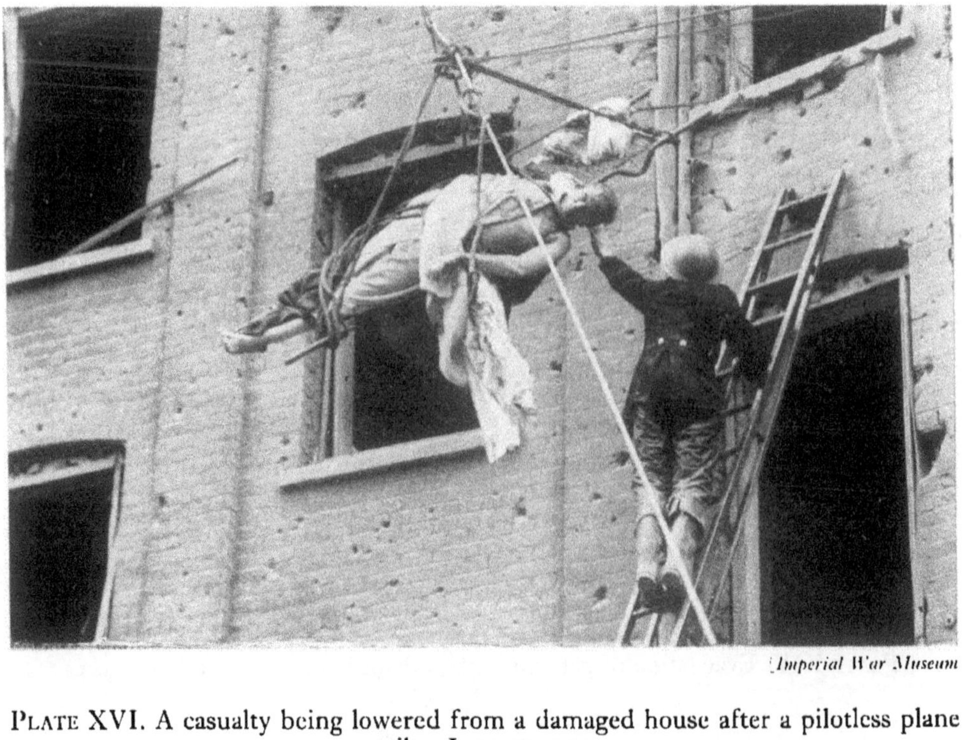

Imperial War Museum

PLATE XVI. A casualty being lowered from a damaged house after a pilotless plane strike. June 29, 1944

As time went on, the demands of the Services could only be met by depleting the personnel of the E.M.S. hospitals and general practitioners to such an extent as to cause anxiety for the efficiency of these services, especially should any serious epidemic arise.

Full details of the measures taken by the authorities to deal with this and other urgent matters regarding the supply of medical personnel will be found in the special chapter on the subject (Chapter 14).

REGIONAL BLOOD TRANSFUSION SERVICE

The need for an organised service capable of providing whole blood, blood plasma, serum and also dried plasma to every part of the country had been under consideration for some time. As stated in Chapter 2, a comprehensive blood transfusion service for London had already been set up under the auspices of the Medical Research Council and was working satisfactorily, but in the provinces the supply of blood and blood plasma had been left to local efforts, except that financial assistance had been sanctioned for certain populous areas in connexion with the grouping of donors. In July 1940, however, a Regional Blood Transfusion Service to cover the whole country was sanctioned and brought into being. This organisation and its working is fully described in the special chapter on the Blood Transfusion Services (Chapter 11).

BEDSTATE RETURNS

In October 1940, instructions were issued to all hospitals in the Emergency Hospital Scheme amending the bedstate returns.[7] Hospitals were now required to divide their reserve beds into Reserves A and B. The Reserve A beds were those fully equipped and available for patients during a short emergency of a few days' duration without any additions to the medical or nursing staffs. Reserve B beds were those fully equipped but not available for patients without an increase of the medical and nursing staffs.

THE BATTLE OF BRITAIN

THE DAYLIGHT RAIDS ON PORTS AND AERODROMES

The Battle of Britain may be said to have begun in May 1940, when it is estimated that about 100 bombs were dropped, all on England, but only three seriously injured casualties due to enemy action were reported. Before this there had been sporadic bombing in Scotland and on the north-east coast of England. Concerted attacks were, however, not experienced until June, after the evacuation of the British Expeditionary Force, during which month it was estimated that 880 metric tons of bombs fell. These attacks were at first mostly on convoys and on naval ports. Mass attacks were made on Chatham, Portsmouth, Plymouth and other South Coast towns, and at the same time a planned series of attacks of increasing severity on aerodromes went on. These attacks, the object of which was to put the R.A.F. out of action in order to pave the way for an invasion of this country, were mostly by daylight and they reached their peak early in September.

Weight of the Attacks and Casualties. The following table gives the approximate weight of bombs recorded in the United Kingdom and numbers of civilian casualties in England and Wales caused by these attacks up to the end of August:

| | U.K. | England and Wales | |
Months	Weight of bombs recorded (tons)	Killed	Seriously injured
1940			
June	880	40	49
July	2,170	230	285
August	6,770	1,140	1,524
Total:	9,820	1,410	1,858

Note.—Casualties in Scotland during the above period were: killed 81, and seriously injured 76. (See E.M.S. Volume II, Part I.)

The greatest number of civilian casualties in one day occurred at Portsmouth on August 24, 1940, when 117 people were killed and 99 seriously injured as the result of the dropping of 64 H.E. and 3 oil bombs. This was the only day on which more than 100 fatal casualties were caused. These figures were supplied by the Research and Experiments Department of the Ministry of Home Security.

THE NIGHT RAIDS ON INDUSTRIAL CENTRES

Weight of the Attacks and Casualties. In September the beginning of heavy night raiding on London and the larger provincial towns overlapped the end of the daylight raiding. In this month 9,980 metric tons of bombs were recorded in the United Kingdom causing 6,964 deaths and 9,472 seriously injured casualties in England and Wales. Thus less than a 50 per cent. increase in the weight of attack as compared with August caused more than a 500 per cent. increase in casualties, the increase being due to main attacks on thickly populated areas, whereas in the previous period the majority of the attacks were on ports and aerodromes. This month was the peak period in weight of attack and for casualties, both of which gradually decreased until February 1941; rose again up to May 1941, and then died away to negligible figures in June and July. The table below (also supplied by the Ministry of Home Security) gives the figures for each month:

| | U.K. | England and Wales | |
Months	Weight of bombs recorded (tons)	Killed	Seriously injured
1940			
September	9,980	6,964	9,472
October	6,910	6,296	7,933
November	6,120	4,966	6,217
December	4,110	3,988	4,862

Months	U.K. Weight of bombs recorded (tons)	England and Wales Killed	Seriously injured
1941			
January	2,460	1,648	2,037
February	1,420	831	1,036
March	4,220	3,336	3,896
April	5,410	5,581	6,015
May	4,690	4,900	4,424
Total:	45,320	38,510	45,892

Note.—Casualties in Scotland and N. Ireland during the above period were: killed 2,964; seriously injured 2,578. (See E.M.S. Volume II, Parts I and II.)

The heaviest attack on London during this period was on the night of April 16–17, 1941, when 1,720 people were killed and 2,030 seriously injured. The estimated weight of bombs dropped that night was 450 tons and the number of bombs of various sizes, excluding incendiaries, was estimated to be 1,603. In the provinces the highest figures recorded for one night were on the night of November 14–15, 1940, when 554 people were killed and 865 seriously injured in Coventry. No exact figures were available regarding scale of attack, but it is estimated that between 1,200 and 1,600 bombs fell.

The full story of the night raids on London and the large provincial towns is given in the special chapters in Volume II, Part III.

Damage to Hospitals. With such heavy raiding it was only to be expected that there would be considerable damage to hospitals and first-aid posts by direct hits and near misses, or blast from large bombs. In London and large towns very few hospitals were put completely out of action, although some were untenable for varying periods: others carried on with a reduced number of beds, and some established operating theatres in convenient basements which enabled them to continue to carry out useful emergency operations. On no particular night of heavy attack were sufficient hospitals put wholly or partly out of action to reduce the number of available beds below those required. Some large hospitals in London and in large provincial cities were damaged several times. In London, St. Thomas's Hospital was particularly unfortunate, receiving no less than six direct hits during the period of the night raids. The only large voluntary hospital in London which was not damaged sufficiently to cause a reduction in the number of available beds was St. Mary's Hospital, Paddington.

Details of damage to large hospitals and the measures that were taken to deal with them will be found in Volume II, Part III.

Hospital Occupancy. It is obvious that no undue strain, except perhaps for a few hours in a small number of hospitals, was thrown on the E.M.S. hospitals throughout the country, in dealing with 45,892 seriously injured casualties over a period of nine months. The number of civilian air raid casualties in hospitals during the whole period of the Battle of Britain and the night raids rose gradually from under 100 in May to 7,181 on December 1, 1940. The figures fell to 6,369 on January 1, 1941, and then progressively fell to 3,516 on July 1, at the end of the period of heavy attacks, after which they further fell to an average of about 1,000 for the period ending January 1, 1943. The approximate number of occupied beds in E.M.S. hospitals—including all ordinary civilian cases, civilian casualties, Service sick and casualties—which was 160,000 in May, 1940, gradually rose to 176,000 on March 1, 1941, and then fell to 166,000 by July 1, 1941, afterwards falling and remaining below that figure to the end of 1942.

The numbers of beds available for casualties in E.M.S. hospitals never dropped below 120,000 during the whole period and it is to be particularly noted that no reduction whatever in admissions of ordinary civilian cases was necessary. The only difficulty that would have been experienced as the result of a much larger inflow of casualties was the shortage of medical and nursing personnel already referred to.

The number of patients in E.M.S. hospitals on February 1, 1941, was 31,770 excluding ordinary civilian sick and transferred civilian sick, evacuees, munition workers, etc., for whose treatment the Ministry had accepted responsibility. This was the peak figure for this period, as was also the total of Service sick (22,102) in E.M.S. hospitals on the same date. Service casualty patients were highest, at 5,640 on November 1, 1940. It should be noted that the returns of Service casualties at that time did not differentiate between war service injuries and injuries due to enemy action.

Types of Casualties. From analyses made by the Research and Experiments Department of the Ministry of Home Security, based on data collected for certain specific periods during the night raids, it appears that of total casualties in urban areas fatal cases were about 21 per cent. seriously injured and slightly injured each about 30 per cent. and cases of shock only, about 20 per cent.

The following table giving the anatomical distribution of injuries was compiled from the results of inquiries made in sample areas:

	First-aid post Cases per cent.	Hospital Cases per cent.
Arms or Hands	31	27
Legs or Feet	22	22
Head or Face	35	32
Eyes	6	5
Spinal column and Pelvis	2	4
Chest	3	8
Abdomen	1	2

It will be noted that there was no marked difference in distribution as between the mainly lightly injured treated at first-aid posts and the seriously injured treated in hospitals, except in cases of spinal, pelvic, thoracic and abdominal injuries—the hospital ratios of which were double those of the first-aid posts, because casualties with these more serious injuries were taken direct to hospital.

Casualty Rates in Relation to Weight of Attack. The numbers of killed and injured per bomb or metric ton weight of bombs dropped, naturally varied according to the density of the population. Analyses made in the London area showed much higher casualty rates in the thickly populated metropolitan boroughs, the rates gradually diminishing from the centre of the area to the perimeter, as did the rate per thousand of the population. Another interesting conclusion indicated by these researches was that the casualty-causing capacity per ton weight of bombs of various sizes was practically the same, i.e., the casualty-inflicting capacity of ten 50-k.g. bombs was about equal to one 500-k.g. bomb. Later surveys however showed that the 50-kg. bomb was the most efficient size for causing casualties.[14] In urban areas the rate approximated to one person killed and one seriously injured per bomb, and 3·8 killed and seriously injured respectively per metric ton.

As regards the numbers of males, females and children who became casualties, it was noticeable that during day raids more males were killed than females, whereas during night raids the numbers were about equal. The children formed about 10 per cent. of the casualties in both day and night raids.

EXPERIENCES AND LESSONS OF THE RAIDS

HOSPITALS

On the whole, the hospitals, improved in accommodation and equipment as experience of their working dictated, adequately fulfilled the purposes for which they were established.

Reception arrangements worked smoothly and well in large hospitals with fully equipped out-patient departments accustomed to receiving streams of casualties, but at others—e.g. some of the large advance base, and base hospitals in upgraded and mental institutions—difficulties were experienced which necessitated structural changes and additional equipment to regulate the flow of patients. In some of these, separate reception rooms were prepared for stretcher and walking cases and resuscitation facilities were provided in special resuscitation wards through which patients requiring such treatment on arrival were passed on their way to the casualty beds or operating theatres. In most hospitals adequate apparatus for the transfusion of blood or plasma was available, but in others additional equipment was necessary to bring them up to the required standard of efficiency. It was found also that the routine procedure for the rapid transfer of cases requiring treatment at special centres had to be tightened up, as in some hospitals these cases were not transferred after the necessary initial treatment so promptly as they should have been. Again, in some hospitals it was essential to provide large fixed X-ray plants, in place of the plants originally supplied, for the examination of serious abdominal, chest and head injuries.

The arrangements under which casualty receiving hospitals during and after air attacks were to notify the control centres when their bed accommodation was nearly exhausted, did not always function well. It was found that casualties requiring immediate operation were often in excess of the number with which the surgeons could adequately deal without unreasonable delay. Thus some of the seriously injured had either to wait for periods which might endanger their lives, or be transferred to another hospital, which might involve the same risk. In June 1941, instructions were issued that casualty receiving hospitals should regulate the admissions of casualties, not by the number of empty beds available, but by the number of operating tables and operating teams which the hospital could call upon.

From experience it was known that about 50 per cent. of all casualties sent to hospital required operative treatment. It was therefore laid down that if the receiving hospital had four operating tables and four teams, the limit of casualties that could be admitted would be 75, if they had three tables, 50 and if they had two tables, 35. These figures were arrived at on the basis that one operating team could adequately deal with not more than 15 to 20 cases, allowing about half an hour for each case, with the necessary interval between the removal of one case and the commencement of operation on another. After operating from six to eight hours it would not be justifiable, in the interests of either patients or surgeons for that team to continue.

Underground Operating Theatres. Emphasis was laid upon the advantages of having, especially in London, operating theatres and a small number of beds in suitable rooms in the basements of hospitals, adequately strengthened to support the weight of the building above should it be demolished by blast, etc., in order that operations could be conducted on urgent cases, whose lives might otherwise be endangered by transfer to other hospitals.

Emergency theatres were set up during the raids at St. Thomas's Hospital, Great Ormond Street Children's Hospital, Guy's Hospital, St. Bartholomew's Hospital, The Middlesex Hospital, etc. (see Plates VII, VIII and IX), and many serious cases requiring immediate operation were successfully dealt with in these theatres. By providing comparative quiet and a feeling of some remoteness from the distractions of the battle raging outside, they enabled the surgeons and staff to concentrate on their important duties without the conscious effort which would otherwise have been necessary. Attached to these theatres from 20 to 100 emergency underground beds were provided so that the patients could remain in the hospital until sufficiently recovered to be safely transferred from the areas under attack. In some of the larger provincial towns similar arrangements, either under hospitals or other suitable buildings in thickly populated areas, were made. In Birmingham one was opened in Lewis's departmental store, with four operating tables and over 100 beds, and later another was opened at Aston. Others were opened in other large towns and in some of the 'coastal belt' towns, notably in Yarmouth, Southend, Lowestoft and Ipswich. The emergency theatres and wards in Birmingham dealt with over 100 cases during the heavy raids in April 1941, and in Norwich four tables provided under the Norfolk and Norwich Hospital were fully used when other operating theatres were put out of action in April 1942.

Dispersal System. The provision of basement hospitals did not, however, commend itself to certain local authorities. They preferred what was called the 'dispersal system' which was adopted by the Coventry authorities after the heavy raids. This consisted in upgrading certain first-aid posts on the periphery of the city by adding operating theatres and a number of beds to these posts instead of to the highly vulnerable hospitals in the centre of the city, from which cases had to be removed as soon after operation as possible to base hospitals in the rural areas. In Coventry, which is not a large straggling city like Birmingham, the adoption of this policy had undoubtedly much to recommend it, especially in view of their experiences during heavy raids directed almost entirely on or near the centre of the city.

CIVIL DEFENCE SERVICES

First-aid Posts. In the central areas the distribution of patients was found to be reasonably good, very few serious cases being sent from 'incidents' to first-aid posts, instead of direct to hospital, but it occasionally happened that walking or sitting cases were found to be serious on examination at the first-aid posts; cases of this kind were passed on to hospital on stretchers. As the access to some of the first-aid posts was narrow and tortuous some difficulties were experienced, and structural alterations were required.

Organisation at Incidents.* At incidents it was found in most towns that the first-aid party leaders fulfilled their functions of directing first aid and the distribution of casualties to hospitals and first-aid posts in a most efficient manner. As the distances which casualties had to travel were short, little attempt was made at elaborate splinting, which would have had to be done in the dark. Immobilisation of the injured parts by sandbags or by bandaging limbs was found sufficient,

---

* Sites where enemy missiles fell causing casualties or damage.

the chief object being speed in obtaining expert treatment by doctors. Similarly tourniquets and digital pressure to stop haemorrhage were seldom used, the application of pressure by dressings and bandages being usually sufficient. In some cities and boroughs it was considered an improvement to use a rota of practitioners residing in the area, who had volunteered to attend incidents on being called by wardens or summoned by telephone from the central controls, to supervise the preliminary treatment of casualties, thus ensuring that the more seriously injured would be dealt with first, and that all cases requiring hospital treatment would be sent direct to hospital. Further, the presence of a doctor at an incident ensured the administration of morphia, when necessary, at the earliest possible moment.

Mobile First-aid Units. Heavy mobile units provided in towns were seldom used for the purpose for which they were originally intended, as they found it difficult to open out in a building in a blitzed area in the dark, and unnecessary delay was thereby caused. In towns, these heavy mobile units were later gradually reduced in number and light mobile units consisting of a doctor, trained nurse and an attendant, with a supply of necessary instruments, were substituted. These teams could be readily sent to an incident in an ordinary sitting-case car. In some cases, where first-aid posts had received direct hits and their equipment had been destroyed, mobile units functioned as first-aid posts in the neighbourhood, but as a rule such arrangements could not be brought into being until after the raid was over.

As a result of all these experiences it was decided at a later period to reorganise the Civil Defence Services in the country as a whole and to institute simpler forms of training for all civil defence personnel. A full description of the changes in the Casualty Organisation will be found in the special chapter on the Civil Defence Casualty Services. (Chapter 7.)

It was also found that the large staffs which had been laid down for first-aid posts were not required and a reduction in the establishment of these posts was afterwards effected.

Ambulance Services. Nearly all the local ambulance services were found to function adequately, even in the heaviest raids and, even when telephones were broken down and messenger services had to be substituted, very few delays were caused. One defect emphasised by control centres was that it was difficult to estimate, from the reports received from wardens, the numbers of civil defence personnel and ambulances which would be required at an incident, as it was sometimes impossible to estimate the numbers of casualties which would be found. This usually meant that more personnel than necessary was sent to incidents, with the result that ambulances which might be more urgently required elsewhere were for varying periods not available. But these cases were few and far between, and in most of the London boroughs and provincial towns the mutual aid organisation from neighbouring areas had very seldom to be used.

Another criticism was that there might be casualties suitable for transportation in sitting-case cars but that only stretcher ambulances were available. This defect was subsequently removed by conversion of stretcher ambulances in accordance with specifications laid down, so that the upper stretchers could be slung up and the lower ones used for sitting cases.

The defects noted and criticisms made by the local authorities will be found fully described in the special chapters contributed by the medical officers of health of towns subjected to heavy enemy attacks from the air. (See Emergency Medical Services, Volume II, Part III.)

EVACUATION OF CHRONIC SICK

It had not been the policy of the Ministry of Health to evacuate special institutions for the chronic sick in the same way as maternity hospitals and children's hospitals had been evacuated, but on consideration of representations made by local authorities and by the general public the evacuation of large numbers of chronic sick and shelter derelicts from the London area was decided upon and between October 10 and November 14, 1940, 7,612 chronic sick and infirm persons were evacuated by 34 Civil Evacuation Trains primarily to large E.M.S. base hospitals outside the large towns. Evacuation of the chronic sick was also carried out in Southampton, Plymouth, Cardiff and elsewhere. This measure, although it was in their own interests, was much resented by many of the aged, infirm and shelter derelicts, many of whom would rather risk being bombed in the big towns than be removed far from their friends and relations, and some complained bitterly of the accommodation and medical attention provided for them in their new surroundings. Many complaints were addressed to the mayors of the towns from which these patients had been evacuated, to Members of Parliament and to the Minister of Health. All these complaints were most carefully investigated by the Regional Hospital Officers concerned and only in a very few cases was there found any justification for them, the sole object of the complainants being to influence the Ministry to return the evacuees to their homes. The Regional Hospital Officers were instructed not to help these persons to return, but a few actually did return at their own expense although they were strongly advised not to.

The evacuation of the chronic sick was not only in the interests of the patients but was also of considerable help to the civil defence organisation in towns subjected to heavy attacks because when the institutions in which these patients, and aged and infirm persons were housed had to be evacuated, greatly difficulty was experienced in removing them on stretchers from chronic wards in upper floors down winding and narrow staircases, such as are to be found in many of the older types of public assistance institutions, which were by no means constructed for such a purpose.

THE EMERGENCY MEDICAL SERVICES IN JULY 1941

ACCOMMODATION FOR CASUALTIES

Summarised below are the numbers of beds available for casualties of all kinds not only in the E.M.S. hospitals but also in the British and Canadian Service Hospitals, and in the Ministry of Pensions Hospitals. These are included on account of the arrangements which had been agreed upon to pool all hospital resources in the United Kingdom. Casualties occurring in any part of the country could thus be primarily accommodated in the nearest suitable hospital as a matter of expediency or in grave emergencies. Similar reciprocal arrangements were subsequently made between E.M.S. hospitals and United States military hospitals (see Chapter 6).

Owing to the considerable numbers of Allied military personnel who were evacuated from the Continent after invasion of their countries by enemy forces, arrangements, had to be made for the treatment of their sick and wounded, mainly in E.M.S. hospitals. An account of these arrangements has been compiled from the limited sources of information available and will be found in Chapter 6.

1. *Hospitals*

    (a) *Bed Accommodation in Emergency Medical Services Hospitals.* A number of hospitals had been added to the 'suspended' list and others had been withdrawn from the scheme altogether. Accommodation had been further reduced by increasing the minimum space between bed centres from 5 ft. to 6 ft. in estimating 'crowded' capacity. The number of E.M.S. hospitals remaining was 1,008, containing 310,150 beds including 195,985 casualty beds, in the following categories (see Army Medical Services, Volume I, Chapter 2):

	E.M.S. Hospitals	Total Beds	Casualty Beds
Class IA	669	240,581	164,969
,, IB	81	3,139	2,187
,, II	258	66,430	28,829
	1,008	310,150	195,985

In addition to civilian sick and other categories for the treatment of which the Ministry had accepted responsibility, such as transferred sick, evacuees, munition workers, etc., the occupied beds included:

Service sick . . 17,187
Service casualties . . 4,243
Civilian casualties . . 3,516

(b) *Auxiliary Hospitals:* Under the arrangements made between the War Office, the Ministry of Health and the Joint War Organisation of the British Red Cross Society and the Order of St. John of Jerusalem, 185 auxiliary hospitals containing about 8,000 beds had been opened. About 50 per cent. of these beds were normally occupied by convalescent Service cases.

During the year ending September 1, 1941, 38,462 British and 1,163 Allied 'other ranks', and 3,516 civilian patients were admitted to the auxiliary hospitals, while 1,110 British and 69 Allied officers and 573 British and 9 Allied 'other ranks' were treated at the six convalescent homes for officers.

(c) *Service Hospitals:* The bed accommodation in Service hospitals on May 1, 1941, was as follows:

	Hospitals	Total beds	Occupied beds	Vacant beds
Royal Navy	8	4,104	1,946	2,158
Royal Air Force	20*	5,920	3,907	2,013
Army	79	17,662	10,244	7,418
Canadian Army	4	1,773	1,356	417

* Includes R.A.F. Hospitals in Scotland and Northern Ireland.

(d) *Ministry of Pensions Hospitals:* The Ministry of Pensions hospital accommodation on May 2, 1941, was as follows:

Hospitals	Total beds	Occupied beds	Vacant beds
12	4,293	1,864	2,429

Returns at July 1, 1941, showed that there were 97,554 vacant and Reserve A beds and 32,645 Reserve B beds in E.M.S. hospitals. In addition to these there were also as shown above 12,006 vacant beds in Service hospitals and 2,429 in Ministry of Pensions hospitals, a total of 144,634 beds in England and Wales immediately available for casualties without a clearance of civil hospitals, such as was carried out in September 1939.

2. *Personnel.* Conscription of medical personnel had been introduced and the Medical Personnel (Priority) Committee was carrying out very useful work in advising the Ministry on the distribution of available medical man-power between the Civilian and Service hospitals.

3. Complete plans had been prepared in an area known as the 'Coastal Belt' for the mobilisation of the civil medical practitioners and plans for co-ordinating the work of the Emergency Medical Services with the Military Authorities had been approved.

4. A complete Blood Transfusion Service for the whole of the country had been established and was functioning satisfactorily.

5. The Emergency Medical Services organisation in the hospitals and the Civil Defence Services had been fully tested during the heavy enemy raids and had not been found wanting. The hospital services had had no difficulty in dealing with the comparatively small number of air raid casualties, and the civil defence organisation, although occasionally put to considerable strain, had adequately fulfilled its functions.

6. As was only to be expected, certain minor defects became evident during this period of heavy enemy attacks, and by the re-organisation of the Civil Defence Services, steps were taken to eliminate such defects as were found.

REFERENCES

[1] Parliamentary Debates, 5th Series, Vol. 361, House of Commons Official Report, June 13, 1940, Cols. 1426–7 (361 H.C. Deb., 1426–7).
[2] Circulars 2060 and 2061, June 21, 1940.
[3] Circular 2076, June 29, 1940.
[4] Min. of Health Circular 2141, September 9, 1940.
[5] Emergency Medical Services Instruction 222, August 30, 1940.
[6] Min. of Health Circulars 2014 and 2015, May 11, 1940, and Emergency Medical Services Instruction 148, May 14, 1940.
[7] Emergency Medical Services Instructions 228, 228A and 228B, October 15, 1940.

CHAPTER 5
PERIOD OF CONSOLIDATION AND IMPROVEMENT
July 1941 to December 1943

ADMINISTRATIVE CHANGES

WITH the cessation of mass attacks the Ministry of Health was able to devote more attention to improvements in the organisation of the Emergency Medical Services in view of the increasing scope of their work for the civilian population and for the Armed Forces. In the light of experience, certain administrative changes were made.

London Region. From July 1, 1941, Sector I was abolished and all the hospitals in the County of Essex outside the Metropolitan Police District, with the exception of four hospitals in what was called the 'Brentwood Island', affiliated to the London Hospital, were transferred to Region 4. These comprised 15 Class IA hospitals containing 5,694 total beds and 3,417 casualty beds, 5 Class IB hospitals containing 156 total beds and 85 casualty beds and 5 Class II hospitals containing 947 total beds and 364 casualty beds. As Region 4 had previously a comparatively small number of hospitals, no increase in the Regional establishment was entailed by this re-arrangement except the attachment of another medical officer to the staff of the Regional Hospital Officer. Sixteen hospitals containing 4,842 total beds, of which 3,603 were casualty beds, remaining in the portion of Sector I which was in the Metropolitan Police District, and the four hospitals in the 'Brentwood Island', with 1,314 total beds and 945 casualty beds, were taken over by Sector II. The headquarters staff of Sector I and its casualty bureau were dispensed with. There was no change in the civil defence services as these did not concern the Sector organisation.

Region 3. In October, 1941, the High Peak District of Derbyshire containing the hospitals in Buxton, Glossop and Chapel-le-Frith, and the civil defence services in this area was taken over from Region 10 by Region 3 in order that the county authority need only deal with one Region for all E.M.S. purposes. This small enclave had previously been included in Region 10 owing to its proximity to and greater accessibility from Manchester, for whose hospitals it had provided beds for the evacuation of casualties. It was found that the small number of beds available was not required for this purpose. The number of hospitals involved was seven, containing 678 total beds and 375 casualty beds.

These changes, like those previously carried out in Regions 6, 7 and 12, led to smoother administration and to economy in staff.

Alteration of Titles of Hospital and Group Officers in the London Region. As mentioned in Chapter 4, the duties of the Sector Group Officers in the London Region, as far as the administration of the hospitals was concerned, were similar to those of the Regional Hospital Officers, but their titles and that of the Hospital Officer, London Region had not been changed. It had long been felt that these titles were misnomers. In April 1942, therefore, the title of the Hospital Officer, London Region was changed to Casualty Services Officer, his duties being wholly concerned with these services, and Air Marshal Sir Victor Richardson, K.B.E., C.B., formerly Director-General of the Medical Branch of the Royal Air Force, was appointed to the post. The Sector Group Officers were given the title of Sector Hospital Officers.[1]

COURSES OF LECTURES ON SPECIAL SUBJECTS

In order to ensure up-to-date knowledge of advances in the treatment of casualties since the outbreak of the war, a series of lectures by specialists was instituted in each Region in October 1941. These lectures were given at intervals throughout this and succeeding winters at centres so situated as to permit of as large an attendance of medical officers as possible in each of the Regional areas. They were well attended and were found very useful, many matters of interest being brought up and discussed.

INSTITUTION OF SPECIAL CENTRES FOR THE TREATMENT OF FRACTURES

As an addition to the special orthopaedic centres which had been set up in all Regions and in the London Sectors, it was decided in June 1941, that a number of other hospitals should be selected and equipped to ensure that all fractures treated under the E.M.S. Scheme might be placed as soon as possible under the care of surgeons experienced in such cases and in hospitals well equipped to deal with them. Three new classes of fracture treatment centres were formed:

1. Fracture departments 'A' of 100 to 150 beds, for cases requiring treatment for a considerable time, in hospitals suitable from their situation for long-stay cases. These would provide for the proper segregation of patients, facilities for massage, electro-therapy, remedial exercises and occupational therapy.

2. Fracture departments 'B' in certain hospitals, which from their situation were not suitable for long-stay cases, but had the staff, experience and equipment for the segregation and treatment of fractures. These hospitals were suitable for the treatment of ambulant and short-stay cases, i.e. those not requiring more than a week's in-patient treatment.

3. Fracture departments 'C' where civilian patients on discharge from hospital could receive suitable out-patient treatment near their homes when orthopaedic or fracture A and B departments were not suitably placed for this purpose. Certain suitably equipped clinics were also included in this category.

Fracture departments 'A' were established in 56 hospitals fracture departments 'B' in 200 hospitals, together with a further number with fracture departments having 'C' facilities.

Hospital Officers were instructed to ensure the transfer at the earliest possible stage of all fracture cases to these hospitals from those not specially designated for the treatment of such cases.[2]

In some Regions arrangements were also made by which certain of the Joint War Organisation's auxiliary hospitals near hospitals with fracture departments 'A' would receive suitable cases for limited periods after the fractures had been set up in plaster, in order to free beds in the fracture departments for new cases as, in spite of the number of hospitals in which these fracture departments had been started, the demand on their beds was so great that many of them were constantly full. Arrangements were made by which the surgeons and staffs of the fracture departments could visit these auxiliary hospitals and supervise treatment.

SUPPLY OF ARTIFICIAL LIMBS

Amputation Sites. In December 1939, in an E.M.S. Memorandum, Dr. Hebb, then Director-General, had issued to all hospitals valuable notes on the selection of amputation sites, based on the experience of the Ministry of Pensions in dealing with cases from the last war, so as to create the most favourable conditions in amputation stumps for the subsequent fitting of artificial limbs.[3]

Limb-fitting Centres. In July 1940, arrangements for the provision of surgical appliances by the Ministry of Pensions to civilian casualties in hospital were extended to provide for the supply of artificial limbs after their discharge,[4] and the Ministry of Pensions provided limb-fitting centres to which such patients were sent at the appropriate time.

In August 1941, the previous procedure was revised and instructions were issued that all amputation cases should be transferred from E.M.S. hospitals to Ministry of Pensions hospitals.[5] It was recognised that the patient's prospect of ultimately leading a normal life largely depended on the correct preparation of the stump and the provision and accurate fitting of the most suitable artificial limb. Transfers were to be made, therefore, as early as possible—if practicable before operation—the sole criterion in determining the date being the patient's ability to undertake the journey without detriment.

The Ministry of Pensions, acting on behalf of the Roehampton Hospital Committee, had made provision to supply, for payment, artificial limbs to civilians other than those who, as war pensioners, were entitled to receive them free. These arrangements were greatly extended in 1935, and in November 1942, they were further extended to include those who would be able to take up useful work during the war if they were supplied with an artificial limb and if they were prepared to make a contribution towards the cost. For fuller details of the organisation for the supply of artificial limbs see the Ministry of Pensions contribution in The Civilian Health and Medical Services, Volume II, Part II, Chapter 5.

MOBILE X-RAY VANS

In October 1941, the Joint War Organisation of the British Red Cross and Order of St. John provided a number of mobile X-ray vans for the use of the E.M.S.[6] These vans were stationed at selected hospitals in London and in each of the Regions, to form a reserve available for any hospital in temporary need of their services. They provided their own current and could operate by using a flexible cable, up to 100 yards distance from the vans. A radiographer was deputed for duty to each van and additional staff was supplied when necessary from the hospital at which the van was stationed. These vans were meant to be used in circumstances such as the following:

1. During the temporary breakdown of the X-ray service at any hospital, from enemy attack or from any other cause;

2. For the examination of cases in the wards of hospitals with no mobile X-ray apparatus.

These units were found very useful in many Regions.

E.M.S. SERVICE HOSPITALS

In the spring of 1942, in order that the treatment of Service cases should be carried out by medical officers with knowledge and experience of the needs of the Fighting Services, it was decided to concentrate Service cases at certain selected hospitals to be known as E.M.S. Service Hospitals. This measure also permitted greater concentration of medical and nursing staffs for the treatment of all kinds of acute cases, which was necessary in view of the need to release more practitioners and nurses for the Services. A list of 202 of these hospitals in the Regions and 113 in the Sectors was issued to the Medical Directors-General of the three Services.[7] It did not include the special centres. Urgent cases were of course to be admitted to the nearest suitable hospital as before and afterwards transferred as soon as possible to a Service hospital or special centre. Amendments and additions to the list were made from time to time.

NATIONAL WAR FORMULARY

In the autumn of 1941, owing to the increasing scarcity of certain drugs previously obtained from sources no longer available, the Minister of Health appointed a committee to prepare a formulary in order to provide information on the selection of medicines to meet the ordinary requirements of therapeutics, to retain as far as possible more valuable preparations for special use and to eliminate non-essential drugs. Alternatives for certain commonly used drugs that had become scarce were included in this formulary. The formulary was prepared and was ready for use early in January 1942,[8] and amendments to it were issued from time to time as required by fluctuations in supplies.

CO-ORDINATION OF THE CIVIL AND MILITARY MEDICAL SERVICES DURING INVASION

RÔLE OF E.M.S. HOSPITALS AND CIVIL DEFENCE SERVICES

Discussions with the Services during the autumn of 1940 and the spring of 1941 had produced a distinct understanding of the part which both the civilian and military hospitals and the medical services would play in the event of invasion. Clearly the E.M.S. hospitals would have to deal with most of the Service, as well as civilian casualties. It was agreed that they would continue functioning as casualty hospitals even if in the frontal area of military activity, would continue to be operated by the civilian personnel of the E.M.S., and would deal with Service casualties at all stages after the field ambulance and advance dressing station stage. To make this possible, all hospitals in the zones affected were to be cleared of all patients, and Regional Hospital Officers and Commands were to work in close liaison, interchanging medical supplies and pooling all ambulance resources. The staffs of all hospitals in E.M.S. were informed that, unless specially ordered by the competent military authority to evacuate the hospital, they were to remain at their posts.

In each Region provisional plans were worked out and tested frequently by large and small scale combined exercises. One useful lesson was learnt from these exercises, namely, that in an invasion by the enemy from the sea, combined with air-borne troops, the evacuation of patients from the E.M.S. hospitals in the forward areas would be practically impossible, as the available roads might in many cases be in the enemy's hands, or in full use for the movement of our own troops and supplies. Plans were therefore made by which hospitals could hold large numbers of patients for several days in order to meet a situation of this kind. Plans were also made for mobilising all civilian doctors in areas considered likely to be the scene of military operations. These would normally only be required to take duty in the area in which they practised, but they might be required for duty at fixed or mobile aid posts or at a hospital a few miles away. Any doctors raising objections to be mobilised for these duties were informed that a formal 'direction' under the Defence Regulations might be served on them. Instructions laying down the obligations of these doctors in the circumstances referred to above were issued in June 1941.

Another difficulty met during exercises was the difference between the Army pattern stretchers and the stretchers in use in the Emergency Medical Services, which could not be interchanged. To mitigate this, in November 1941, all hospitals and first-aid posts in the invasion zones were supplied with a number of Army pattern stretchers in addition to the civilian pattern already in use.

Defended Areas. In the invasion areas complete plans for the provision of first-aid posts and upgraded first-aid points and the necessary personnel at places at first called 'nodal points', but afterwards 'defended areas', were worked out. When instructed to do so, part of the staffs of certain hospitals outside these 'defended areas' were to move into these areas, the remainder of the staff staying with their patients at their hospitals.

Village Committees. In villages or towns outside the scheduled 'defended areas' local committees were formed, the duties of the inhabitants laid down, and allocated, and supplies of food, drugs and dressings sufficient for seven days arranged for, so that each village could be self-supporting during the periods it was expected they would be isolated by active hostilities in the area. All inhabitants were ordered to make no attempt to evacuate their homes and thus impede the military operations by clogging the roads as the inhabitants of the villages in France and Belgium did when those countries were invaded in May 1940. If any village became a target the inhabitants were advised to take refuge in the surrounding woods and fields.

Administration of Morphia. As in the event of invasion village communities might be altogether cut off from medical aid, a relaxation of the rules under the Dangerous Drugs Act was permitted during invasion. Medical officers of health were instructed to select suitable persons in the villages to administer morphia when urgently necessary. For this purpose the Ministry of Health issued hypodermic syringes and morphia solution to all first-aid points in the invasion areas.

Ministry of Health's Invasion Instructions. In February 1942, the Ministry of Health prepared secret instructions laying down the action which was to be taken at the various stages by all concerned on the issue of warning messages. These were to be three in number—'Preliminary Warning', 'Stand to' and 'Action Stations'. These warnings would be issued to the Ministry of Health by the Home Defence Executive, and in Regions the Senior Regional Officers of the Ministry would be informed by the Regional Commissioners.

The chief action to be taken in the Emergency Medical Services on receipt of instructions to do so, may be summarised as follows:

1. Put in force the pre-arranged plans for clearing the 'Coastal' and 'Green Belt' Hospitals.

2. Evacuate individual hospitals for military reasons when required.

3. Supplement the available hospital beds as required by bringing into use the reserve beds in hospitals, opening reserve hospitals and discharge patients able to leave hospital; this procedure included the auxiliary hospitals.

4. Augment the inter-hospital ambulance service by recalling vehicles previously released but for which the necessary fitments had been stored for this contingency.

5. Re-open first-aid posts which were on a care and maintenance basis.

6. Review the gas cleansing arrangements at hospitals and first-aid posts.

7. Review the arrangements for the casualty services at nodal points and vulnerable defiles.

8. Review the arrangements for retaining in the scheduled towns in the Coastal Belt doctors, dentists, etc., previously designated for this purpose.

9. Review the staffing arrangements at hospitals and put in force the pre-arranged plans for non-resident staff to come into residence. Also review the arrangements for augmenting the medical and nursing staffs of certain hospitals.

10. Remove dangerous mental patients from mental hospitals in the Coastal Belt (Board of Control).

Chain of Command in the E.M.S. during Invasion. After a country-wide exercise held in the spring of 1942, during which the plans for the co-ordination of the E.M.S. with the military Medical Services drawn up and approved in 1940–1 were fully tested, the D.G.A.M.S. expressed the view that the Emergency Medical Services did not yet fit satisfactorily into the military medical scheme to meet possible invasion for the following reasons:

1. (*a*) As several Civil Defence Regions were as a rule represented in one Army Command, the E.M.S. had no representative at the medical headquarters of the Army Commands who could give information and advice to the D.Ds.M.S. of the Commands, and who could issue urgent and authoritative instructions to the E.M.S. organisations in the area during an invasion.

If the military authorities took over control of an area threatened with invasion or actually invaded, their instructions as regards the hospital services, casualty services and the movement of patients and medical personnel, would have to be carried out. It was therefore considered essential that a senior officer of the E.M.S. with full authority to implement the orders of the D.Ds.M.S. rendered necessary by the military situation should be attached to each Command for this purpose.

(b) The delegation of responsibility and executive powers among E.M.S. officers differed considerably between Regions and even in different parts of some Regions; this created difficulties in co-ordinating the work of the two medical services at the lower levels in the chain of responsibility.

(c) There was no code of discipline in the E.M.S. and therefore orders were not easily enforced.

(d) No uniforms were worn by E.M.S. officers, making it difficult for military officers transferred from one area to another to know with whom they were dealing.

(e) This lack of close liaison with the military authorities was also evident in the lower levels of the military medical organisation, such as corps and area headquarters and at hospitals and in local areas as regards the civil defence services.

2. (a) The D.G.A.M.S. therefore proposed that a senior E.M.S. officer should be appointed to each Army Command, to be responsible for the E.M.S. in that Command during active operations and with whom the D.Ds.M.S. would deal direct in preparing plans to meet the changing requirements of the military situation.

(b) To place all E.M.S. officers in uniform with corresponding rank in the military Medical Services so that they would bear the same relation to the Army Medical Services as the Home Guard did to the Army in general.

(c) Other recommendations regarding the appointing of E.M.S. officers of suitable status and rank to corps, district and area headquarters, etc.

LIAISON ORGANISATION

Senior Hospital Officers. As a result of the War Office communication, many conferences and discussions were held and an invasion plan was drawn up and eventually issued to the E.M.S. with a copy to the D.G.A.M.S. for information. The plan consisted in the appointment of five officers to be called Senior Hospital Officers, one to each of the five military Commands in England and Wales, to advise the D.Ds.M.S. on all matters concerning the E.M.S., and with full authority to issue instructions to the Regional Hospital Officers of the Civil Defence Regions when required to do so by the military authorities. A sixth senior officer was proposed for the London District.

Assistant Hospital Officers in each Region were 'designated' to join corps, district and area headquarters in the invasion area when the instructions to 'stand to' were issued, with authority to control the E.M.S. when cut off from communication with the Regional Hospital Officers.

Medical officers of health of counties and county boroughs were requested to carry out the instructions given to them by the Senior Hospital Officers, Regional Hospital Officers and Assistant Hospital Officers as regards the hospitals and Civil Defence Services in their areas.

Medical officers in charge of first-aid posts, officers in charge of civil defence ambulances and medical superintendents, or medical officers in charge of hospitals, were to receive their instructions from medical officers of health. Individual medical officers and nurses would also take their instructions as to action from the medical officers of health.

In London, orders for hospitals would be transmitted through the Sector Hospital Officers, and orders for first-aid posts, ambulances, etc., through the casualty services organisation.

The scheme as issued met with the partial approval of the War Office. They considered that their requirements had to a great extent been met by these provisions, but that the Ministry of Health had not gone far enough to meet their proposals for a complete and uniform arrangement such as they considered essential for a complete integration of the two medical services during active operations in any area. But the Ministry of Health did not see their way to go any farther, chiefly on account of the difficulties which would arise in endeavouring to bring into the military medical scheme a completely civil organisation, which had to deal not only with military casualties, but also civilian casualties and the ordinary civilian sick in its area.

Some of the proposals of the War Office would also conflict with the powers already conferred on Regional Commissioners as regards the casualty services in the face of active operations, and with the responsibilities of the Regional Commissioners when cut off from communication with the central Government.

The proposals regarding uniforms for the E.M.S. were also strongly objected to by the Minister of Health as placing E.M.S. medical officers in the uniform of, and granting them commissions in the Home Guard would bring them under the control of the Home Guard authorities even before they were mustered. He therefore considered that it was essential for them to retain their position as officials, administering both the Emergency Hospital Scheme for which he was responsible and which was essentially a civil organisation, and also the medical side of the Civil Defence Services which were under the control of the Regional Commissioners.

These views were conveyed to the Under Secretary of State for War, and no further action appears to have been taken and, as the organisation which the Ministry of Health had constituted was never put to the test, no opinion can be expressed as to whether the full demands of the War Office were really necessary or not.

Plans for pooling of resources during invasion were revised and expanded. Procedure was laid down by which medical personnel, such as surgical and resuscitation teams, from either the military or the civil services could be made available to both, and arrangements were made for the interchange of ambulances. Detailed instructions regarding action to be taken at various stages of an invasion were issued to all civil and Service officers concerned. As an example of the medical arrangements made in the chief invasion areas, an extract from those of Region 4 (East Anglia) is given in Appendix V.

As many consultants were called up for service with the Forces, some of the smaller hospitals found it difficult to obtain consultant advice, and in 1943 it was agreed that Service consultants could be called upon by any hospital when necessary. Reciprocal arrangements were made between E.M.S. consultants and the Services.

Service Medical Officers. Great help was given by the Services—in particular by the Army—to E.M.S. hospitals by their supplying, whenever the exigencies of the Service permitted, surgeons, physicians, radiologists, anaesthetists, etc., as locums to E.M.S. hospitals for cases of sickness, or in order to permit of well-earned leave. Such help was warmly appreciated: without it few of the staffs of E.M.S. hospitals would have been able to take a holiday.

Armed Forces of the United States. When the U.S.A. Army arrived in this country, contact was made with their medical headquarters and arrangements made for mutual assistance. Reciprocal plans for assistance as regards surgical teams, ambulances, etc., were drawn up, and the Hospital Officers made contact with the officers in charge of the U.S.A. hospitals offering all possible assistance when required and explaining civil defence arrangements. Contact was made by the medical officers of health of the scheme-making authorities with the medical officers in charge of U.S.A. aerodromes and arrangements for mutual assistance, including the admission to the nearest E.M.S. hospital, of casualties requiring urgent treatment, were drawn up similar to those made with British aerodromes. (See Chapter 6.)

Home Guard. When the Home Guard was first formed no special medical arrangements were made. Later, the suggestion was made that the Home Guard should set up its own medical service. This was considered by the War Office and the Ministry of Health who, however, agreed that except in cases where a battalion would be sent out of its own district, its medical officer would, on 'stand to', revert to his civil duties and that before 'stand to' his duties would be confined to teaching stretcher drill and first aid to the Home Guard. It was decided that each battalion would establish a collection point to which its casualties would be brought and that from that point they would be taken care of by the Civil Defence Services. Where possible the collecting-point would be a civil first-aid post or point. If there were no first-aid post or point within reach, representations could be made by the Zone Medical Adviser to the D.D.M.S. or A.D.M.S. District, who would discuss the matter with the medical officer of health of the scheme-making authority. As a result of these discussions, a certain number of additional first-aid posts and points was established.

TREATMENT OF GAS CASUALTIES

LUNG IRRITANT GASES

The possibility of lung irritant gases such as phosgene being used in large quantities by the enemy made necessary a review of the provisions for a defence against gas attacks. The respirators issued to the public were, of course, a completely efficient protection if worn, but the extreme rapidity of action of these gases, especially of phosgene in sufficient concentration, might well cause considerable numbers of casualties amongst the civilian population exposed to their effects. As two and a half years had elapsed since the outbreak of hostilities without gas being used, people had naturally become careless; very few habitually carried their respirators, others had failed to maintain them in serviceable order and some had lost them. The Ministry of Health therefore considered it necessary for E.M.S. hospitals to be prepared to treat considerable numbers of casualties from lung irritant gases.

OXYGEN SUPPLIES

Hospitals had already been supplied with the necessary oxygen inhalation apparatus—(B.L.B. masks)—although there were not enough at any hospital to deal with a large number of casualties. The methods of using this apparatus had been fully explained in E.M.S. Memorandum No. 5 issued in 1940. The shortage of apparatus made it impracticable to increase the supplies at each hospital. Arrangements were therefore made for additional supplies of apparatus to be held at depots throughout the country, to be available to hospitals at very short notice, and for hospitals to come to each other's aid as much as possible.

A small number of 'Arcus' units, by which five cases could be served with oxygen from one cylinder, was also made available at some of the depots for certain hospitals. In addition improvised aids in the administration of oxygen were advised, such as the use of bicycle valve tubing connected by glass Y tubes to the cylinders through a bottle to act as an indicator.

As it was estimated that if phosgene gas were used, 25 per cent. of the patients admitted might need continuous oxygen treatment, each hospital might have to provide oxygen equipment, standard or improvised, for at least 25 per cent. of the beds likely to be available for the reception of gassed cases.[9]

Another difficulty was that of ensuring a sufficient supply of oxygen. The normal supplies to hospitals would be quite inadequate and it was out of the question to keep idle in all hospitals large numbers of cylinders of oxygen which might never be used. Reserve stores of oxygen cylinders were therefore stocked at the depots to be supplied at very short notice. A review was made of the amount of industrial oxygen held by local authorities and by large industrial undertakings; and it was arranged that these stocks of oxygen would also be available in a grave emergency.

It was expected that these provisions would be sufficient to meet even heavy casualties from an initial attack; the need for large quantities of oxygen was not considered likely in subsequent attacks since the great majority of people would again habitually carry their respirators after the warning of the first attack.

DECONTAMINATION UNITS

In October 1942, the Ministry of Health issued instructions simplifying the lay out of these units by the removal of certain of the air locks and gas proof curtains originally provided but now considered unnecessary.[10] Instead of air locks, blanket curtains between the undressing rooms and the rest of the decontamination units were substituted, the risk of gas being disseminated from other than splashed outer clothing being regarded as negligible.

REHABILITATION*

NECESSITY FOR RAPID REHABILITATION IN THE
    FIGHTING SERVICES

In the Armed Forces the primary duty of every medical officer is to maintain the health of all personnel in order that the highest possible percentage may be fit for duty. They must apply the principles of hygiene for the prevention of disease, the highest standards of treatment during illness and the most suitable measures for reconditioning patients after illness, to ensure their return to duty in the shortest possible time. This is the chief reason why civilian practitioners when recruited to the Services, unless as specialists, cannot immediately become adequate substitutes for trained military medical officers, but require special instruction to enable them fully to apply the above basic principles.

POLICY IN THE E.M.S. HOSPITALS

In the E.M.S. hospitals the civilian medical staffs required to treat Service patients were slow to realise the importance of these principles, with the result that in many hospitals Service patients were often retained as in-patients for unnecessarily prolonged periods. (See Army

---

*See also Chapter 13 and Army Medical Services, Volume I, Chapter 2.

Medical Services, Volume I, Chapter 2.) Even after the issue of instructions to accelerate as far as possible the return of patients to duty, either direct or via auxiliary convalescent hospitals and the military convalescent depots, Hospital Officers, Assistant Hospital Officers, Group Officers and Consultant Advisers during inspections found considerable numbers of Service patients retained in hospital for quite insufficient reasons, thus also prolonging the period required for 'hardening' in order to make them fit for duty after the patients had left hospital. Reluctance was also found in the medical staffs of some hospitals in parting with patients obviously requiring specialist treatment at one or other of the special centres.

EQUIPMENT IN E. M. S. HOSPITALS

As the war went on, the demand for man and woman-power gradually increased, which necessitated every effort also being made to fit most categories of civilian as well as military patients to return to work as soon as possible to further the war effort. The Director-General of the E.M.S., on the advice of his Consultant Advisers, took steps to supply every Class IA hospital with the necessary equipment, such as physiotherapy apparatus, apparatus for exercising muscles, etc., to prevent as far as possible the physical deterioration of all patients. The orthopaedic centres had already been supplied with all such special apparatus and also with material for occupational therapy, and provision had been made for organised physical exercises and games under special medical and lay instructors. The hospitals with fracture departments were also fully equipped in this respect when these departments were opened. In addition, a certain number of selected auxiliary hospitals were specially equipped and staffed and physical training instructors from the Army were detailed for duty at these hospitals in order that 'prehardening' could be carried out.

At certain auxiliary hospitals special arrangements were made for the continued rehabilitation of patients from the special centres, such as the special head injury convalescent centre near Oxford and the special neurological centres.

The hospitals in the E.M.S. may therefore be said to have reached a standard considerably higher than that of all but a few civilian hospitals in peace-time as regards facilities for rehabilitation.

THE MINISTRY OF LABOUR AND NATIONAL
    SERVICE SCHEME

In October 1941, the Ministry of Labour and National Service introduced an interim scheme[11] to link the hospitals with certain of the employment exchange services, which provided for interviewing disabled patients in hospitals before their discharge and for consultation with the hospital authorities on their fitness for employment.

Special attention was drawn to patients suffering from medical as well as surgical disabilities. Experience of this scheme had proved its value sufficiently to warrant its development as an essential feature of any permanent rehabilitation scheme.

In January 1942, arrangements were made by which the Ministry's vocational training centres could refer cases commencing training or under training to certain E.M.S. hospitals near these centres for specialist opinion on their suitability for vocations, having regard to the nature of their disabilities.[12] Trainees requiring treatment could be admitted to these hospitals as out-patients. In November 1942, these arrangements were extended to embrace disabled persons undergoing training at technical colleges under local education authorities, and additional hospitals were designated to deal with such cases.[13]

ARMY EDUCATIONAL PERSONNEL

In February 1942, the Army Council made available a certain number of sergeants from the Army Education Corps to supervise diversional occupation and educational activities among Service cases grouped in E.M.S. hospitals to which military registrars were attached. These Army instructors were chiefly concerned with activities of a diversional and educational nature, other than occupational therapy associated with specific treatment under medical supervision. The special attention of all concerned was subsequently drawn to the importance of utilising the services of the A.E.C. for rehabilitation.[14]

THE 'TOMLINSON' COMMITTEE

The need to make use of all possible man and woman-power resulted in the appointment in December 1941, of an inter-departmental committee, with Mr. G. Tomlinson, M.P., as chairman, and with representatives of all interested departments as members, to report on the rehabilitation and re-settlement of all disabled persons. The main terms of reference of the committee were:

(a) to make proposals for the introduction at the earliest possible date of a scheme for the rehabilitation and training for employment of disabled persons not provided for by the interim scheme;

(b) to consider and make recommendations for the introduction after the war of a comprehensive scheme for the rehabilitation and training of, and satisfactory employment for, persons of all categories.

This committee made an interim report on March 10, and finally reported on November 5, 1942.[15]

As regards medical rehabilitation, i.e. of both surgical and medical cases while still under medical supervision as in-patients or out-patients of hospitals, the committee endorsed the policy adopted in the E.M.S. for developing rehabilitation at orthopaedic centres.

other special centres and fracture departments and advocated that these measures should not only be extended throughout the coutryy to the fullest extent possible under war-time conditions, but should also be applied to patients suffering from general medical and surgical conditions as well as to the tuberculous, the blind, cases of neurosis, psychosis, etc.

The committee quoted as an example of the extent to which disabled persons could be employed in industry, an extract from 'Workmen's Compensation' by the late Sir Arnold Wilson and Professor Hermann Levy, in which it was stated that out of 7,882 kinds of work done in the Ford works in America, 670 could be done by legless men, 2,637 by one-legged men, 715 by one-armed men, 2 by armless men and 10 by blind men. At the time this survey was made there were actually 9,563 physically defective employees (about 10 per cent. of the total employment roll) in the factory including about 1,000 cases of tuberculosis, 253 nearly blind in one eye, 3 totally blind, 234 with one foot or leg amputated, 123 with crippled or amputated arm, fore-arm or hands and 60 epileptics.

The Magnitude of the Problem. Fractures and other forms of physical injury formed one of the largest groups of patients requiring rehabilitation. As an indication of the size of the problem the committee recalled that the Delevingne Committee (1936-9) had found that in 1935 about 200,000 fracture cases were treated in hospitals in this country, of which 65,000 were in-patients and that the total number of accident cases was over one and a quarter millions, of which 30 per cent. were industrial accidents and 15 per cent. road accidents. These were peace-time figures, likely to return in similar proportions after the war, but meanwhile war circumstances had altered both the total and the proportions of the different types of injury.

It was found that at the end of hospital treatment most patients in this group were completely restored to their full working capacity or were sufficiently restored to be able to return to their previous or similar occupations. Of the more serious cases treated in orthopaedic centres about 17 per cent., and of other cases a much smaller percentage, left hospital permanently disabled. Most of these, however, were capable of employment but might require a course of vocational training to enable them to take up a new occupation. A small minority would require a prolonged course of specialised training to fit them for any employment, even under sheltered conditions.

Some Recommendations of the Committee

1. *Fractures.* The committee recommended that every effort should be made, even under the handicap of war-time difficulties, to develop the facilities at hospitals and that they should be used to the fullest extent by the medical profession, employers, work people and the general public.

2. *Other Surgical Conditions and General Group of Medical Cases.* It was estimated that the new in-patients in hospitals in this country amounted to about 1,500,000 in a year and that one-third of this number would require medical rehabilitation. The rehabilitation of such cases might be considered as a new conception, except in a few of the larger hospitals where such measures were already in operation. The committee recommended that at the end of hospital treatment provision should be made for convalescent treatment, followed by a course of reconditioning under strict medical supervision. They also recommended that in amputation cases, special attention should be devoted to the provision of artificial limbs, which would greatly enhance the capacity of patients for full employment.

3. *Cardiac Cases.* These cases would require prolonged convalescence and training for occupations requiring very little physical effort; something like sanatorium life was recommended for this group.

4. *Pulmonary Tuberculosis.* It was estimated that 140,000 adults were suffering from pulmonary tuberculosis and that 70,000 could be classified as being able to return to ordinary employment and 20,000 as unlikely to be able to return. These cases would mostly be under full-time treatment in hospitals or sanatoria. In 50,000 cases the disease was arrested or quiescent and full recovery was probable if special measures of rehabilitation were available.

The committee recommended that, although many patients would not be able to undertake full-time employment for a substantial period, many could undertake and benefit by part-time work. Treatment should begin in the sanatoria. Local Authorities and Health Departments should constantly review and develop these facilities.

5. *Blindness and Deafness.* The use of facilities already in existence for training the blind and deaf, mostly under the direction of voluntary organisations, should be encouraged with the view of placing in employment as many persons as possible suffering from these disabilities.

6. *Neurosis and Psychosis.* Cases of neurosis and psychosis require the provision of psychotherapy, occupational therapy, workshops, physical training, etc., on an extended basis. In the existing institutions it had been found that the majority could return to some form of employment, while the minority remained as problem cases and misfits. The committee considered that a neuro-psychiatric service in post-war planning could be provided on a regional basis.

The committee commended the good work that was being done in detecting and arresting the development of disabilities in the early stages at the War Office Centres at Kingston, Skegness and Dunblane, to which minor disabilities were sent, and at the Manchester Docks centres set up by the Ministry of Labour and National Service. Good work was also being done under the Clyde Basin Scheme in Glasgow. (See Volume II, Part II.)

The committee recorded their opinion that the institution of diplomas in rehabilitation should be considered by examining bodies.

Action by the Ministry of Health. As a result of the recommendation of the 'Tomlinson' Committee the Ministry of Health decided to institute systematic visiting of the larger hospitals, including suspended hospitals, in each Region with the view to considering the most practical means of securing any desirable improvement. The visitation in each Region was to be made by the Hospital Officer or one of his assistants and an E.M.S. Officer selected by the Hospital Officer.

They were to submit a list of hospitals recommended by them for the development of rehabilitation facilities based on the possibilities of:

(*a*) making better use of existing facilities by the education of physicians and surgeons and hospital authorities;

(*b*) increasing the provision of trained lay staff, accommodation and equipment of existing centres;

(*c*) making provision at other hospitals, e.g. in cities, particularly for out-patients where, owing to their vulnerability the long stay of patients in hospital was not desirable;

(*d*) making provision at annexes, convalescent hospitals and auxiliary hospitals.

A standard form of report was drawn up for completion, and comments were required on the adequacy of the existing facilities in the light of what was reasonably practicable in war-time and of the attitude to the proposals of the medical staffs and hospital authorities of each hospital.

A medical officer in charge of rehabilitation was to be recommended for appointment at each selected hospital and the medical staff was to be stimulated to apply the principles of rehabilitation indicated in Supplements 28 and 28(a) of the E.M.S. Instructions Part I. The basic principle laid down was that reconditioning of patients should start at the earliest possible stage of an illness and should not be a separate period after treatment, unless the patient was too ill for general physical treatment until some weeks or months had elapsed.

The appointment of an adequate non-medical staff of masseuses, occupational therapists, physical training instructors, etc., was to proceed as far as possible under war conditions.

A circular was issued by the Ministry to each of the selected hospitals to indicate the policy of Government in this matter, making it clear that the limitations on progress imposed by war conditions were fully recognised, but that everything possible within these limits should be the aim of all concerned.[16]

On receipt of the Hospital Officers' reports, the Ministry reviewed their recommendations, took steps to supply the necessary equipment for the improved hospitals and sanctioned the appointment of the necessary technical staff.

In September 1943, arrangements were made for courses of training in rehabilitation methods for physicians and surgeons attached to the hospitals visited during the rehabilitation survey undertaken on the recommendation of the 'Tomlinson' Committee.

Courses were also instituted for masseuses and other ancillary staff selected for this purpose by the hospitals concerned. These courses were started in October, 1943, and were found very useful. In December 1943, the Ministry of Health issued E.M.S. Memorandum 6,[17] which contained full instructions for the benefit of those organising a hospital rehabilitation department.

Post-Hospital Rehabilitation. Instructions were issued to hospitals to encourage the continued out-patient treatment of patients requiring it after discharge from hospital. From time to time the Director-General issued further instructions to improve the organisation for dealing with this most important matter in all its aspects. The chief difficulties met with in the hospitals were due to the shortage of suitable men and women under war conditions, which made it almost impossible to obtain the highly trained and enthusiastic personnel necessary to the degree of success which it was hoped would be achieved under post-war conditions.

The Ministry of Labour in October started an industrial rehabilitation centre at Egham, Surrey, for persons who had any residual disablement after a period of hospital or other treatment for serious injury or illness. These patients were put through a suitable course of an active nature lasting six to eight weeks on the average, by which their return to full employment was greatly accelerated.

The other recommendations of the 'Tomlinson' Committee for courses of reconditioning, vocational training in new occupations, etc., were the concern of the Ministry of Labour and National Service.

Harold Balme, O.B.E., M.D., F.R.C.S., was appointed medical officer in charge of rehabilitation at the headquarters of the Ministry of Health in May 1943, and in the following November outlined the progress made in providing facilities for active rehabilitation in the E.M.S. hospitals.[18]

By that time 48 hospitals possessed full equipment for dealing with all suitable patients, but 35 of these hospitals were only dealing with selected cases, e.g. traumatic.

In addition 102 hospitals possessed partial equipment—e.g. remedial exercises, but no occupational therapy apparatus.

By the end of 1944, 131 hospitals possessed full and 136 partial facilities, and by 1945, 204 hospitals were fully and 129 partly equipped, so that 333 hospitals in all were employing modern methods of rehabilitation; of these hospitals 93 were in the London Region.

In all these hospitals special rehabilitation medical officers had been appointed, but they varied greatly in professional status and specialist

CONSOLIDATION AND IMPROVEMENT

ability. This weakness was chiefly due to the continued shortage of available medical personnel, although 254 representatives from 172 hospitals had been specially trained in the rehabilitation courses referred to above. Adequate physiotherapy departments existed in most of these hospitals and active methods were being more used especially by the younger graduates from physiotherapy schools.

There was still a shortage of remedial gymnasts, but many ex-P.T. instructors were being trained for this work.

The need to introduce 'vocational purpose' into occupational therapy, in hospitals accommodating patients likely to require change of employment on account of their disabilities, was being increasingly felt; but in the opinion of Dr. Balme there was still a serious gap between hospital rehabilitation and resettlement of disabled persons in suitable employment, despite the efforts made to bridge this gap.[19]

RADIO-THERAPEUTIC CENTRES

In November 1943, two radio-therapeutic centres were opened specially to serve the London Sectors; in Mount Vernon Hospital, Northwood, for the Sectors north of the Thames, and in Warren Road Hospital, Guildford, for those south of the Thames. To these hospitals all cases of cancer suitable for this kind of treatment were admitted whether or not they were patients for whom the E.M.S. were responsible. This provision had been found essential to meet the difficulties of providing treatment for cancer by radiation at centres in inner London.

ENEMY ATTACKS
July 1941—December 1942

Enemy attacks from the air during the last six months of 1941 consisted chiefly of small-scale 'tip and run' raids directed against the south-east and south coasts and they continued intermittently during the whole of this period. These attacks at first were usually delivered in daylight, but as the result of mounting losses, were later replaced by night attacks chiefly on sea-port towns. Casualties in England and Wales during this period were 1,207 killed and 1,424 admitted to hospital; of these only 105 killed and 108 admitted to hospital occurred in the London Region.

The same kind of attacks continued during 1942, but in addition a series of attacks known as the 'Baedeker' raids were made between April 23 and June 27 on the cathedral cities of Exeter, Bath, Norwich, York and Canterbury. The numbers of casualties in these cities were:

	Killed	*Admitted to Hospital*
Exeter	247	207
Bath	400	357

144 THE EMERGENCY MEDICAL SERVICES

	Killed	Admitted to Hospital
Norwich	247	264
York	94	107
Canterbury	48	57

Details of these 'Baedeker' raids will be found in Volume II, Part III.

During the year 1942 the only casualties which occurred in London were 27 killed and 52 admitted to hospital during the months of June, July and August. There were no casualties whatever in London during the other nine months of the year. For the whole of the year 1942 the casualties in England and Wales were 3,195 killed and 4,109 admitted to hospital.

REORGANISATION OF THE CIVIL DEFENCE SERVICES

Advantage was taken of the period of comparative inactivity which followed the heavy raids of 1940–1 to apply the experience gained in these raids to improve the civil defence organisation, both in London and in the provinces. An account of certain changes which were made in 1942–3 will be found in Chapter 7, The Civil Defence Casualty Services.

SERVICE ADMISSIONS TO E.M.S. HOSPITALS

The E.M.S. hospitals were, however, by no means idle during this lull. During the last six months of 1941, 76,214 Army sick and casualties (excluding officers) were admitted to hospital and the figure for the R.A.F. for the whole of the year 1941 was 30,932. In 1942, 176,896 Army sick and casualties (including officers) and 47,329* R.A.F. were admitted, of whom 15,867 and 8,559 respectively were women auxiliaries. Of Navy admissions, the number of which must have been considerable, no authentic record is available. The following figures, however, supplied by Dr. Percy Stocks, Medical Statistician to the Ministry of Health, and based on a one-in-five sample of Ministry of Pensions casualty forms, are probably reasonably accurate:

In 1941, 9,520 (including 220 W.R.N.S.); in 1942, 11,540 (including 845 W.R.N.S.). Figures for the Army are direct admissions only, i.e. they exclude transfers, both from other home hospitals and from overseas.

In addition to the above 4,615 Canadian, 1,070 Belgian, 654 Czech and 1,070 Dutch casualties were treated.

CIVILIAN ADMISSIONS

During 1941 the number of civilian 'enemy action' casualties including, 1,660 civil defence and 810 Merchant Navy personnel, amounted to

---

* Great Britain and Northern Ireland.

22,965, while in 1942 these figures were 635, 255 and 4,530 respectively. (See Appendix VIII.)

The above figures also were calculated by Dr. Stocks from the same source as the figures for the Navy. No returns of the numbers of admissions of other civilian categories for which the Ministry of Health had assumed responsibility were required from the hospitals at this time on account of the grave shortage of clerical personnel, nor were the numbers of ordinary civilians admitted to the E.M.S. hospitals asked for, as the daily bed-state returns contained all the information then considered necessary.

ACCOMMODATION IN HOSPITALS

By the end of 1942 the number of hospitals in the Emergency Hospital Scheme had been reduced to 910 and beds to 278,761, of which 149,622 were occupied. Of these 20,993 were occupied by Service sick and casualties, 625 by civilian casualties, and 128,004 by civilian sick. The reduction in the number of hospitals since July 1941, was chiefly due to some having been handed over to the U.S.A. Forces.

Auxiliary Hospitals. An additional 44 auxiliary hospitals had been opened by the Joint War Organisation of the British Red Cross Society and Order of St. John of Jerusalem, bringing the total in use to 229. Among these an increased number were now reserved for W.R.N.S., A.T.S. and W.A.A.F. personnel and a few others for certain civilian categories engaged in essential war work. The total number of beds in these hospitals in September 1942, was 12,657.

The number of admissions during the year ending September 1, 1942, was:

British Forces		Allied Forces	Civilian Patients		Civil Defence Workers		Total
Male	Female		Male	Female	Male	Female	
87,989	3,308	1,914	1,617	3,119	1,558	522	100,027

In addition, 1,981 male and 19 female British and 160 male Allied patients were admitted to the six* convalescent hospitals for officers, including 646 'other ranks' who came as patients to the special convalescent hospital for head injuries.

ENEMY ATTACKS, 1943

During 1943, there was some increase in the weight of enemy attack from the air, an estimated total of 2,320 tons of bombs having been dropped. Casualties were 2,273 killed and 3,350 admitted to hospital. Of these 542 were killed and 989 admitted to hospital in the London Region, the heaviest attacks in London being on the night of January 17/18 by

---

* Includes one Scottish.

74 aircraft and during daylight on January 20 by 60 aircraft. The casualties in London for the whole month were 198 killed and 308 seriously injured. Other relatively heavy attacks were made in March, October and November, but casualties occurred in every month except August.

In the rest of England and Wales the attacks were fairly widely distributed, chiefly along the East and South Coasts; the heaviest attacks were on Hull on the night of July 13–14 and on Sunderland on the nights of May 15–16 and 23–24. Grimsby had its heaviest attack of the war on the night of July 12–13.

The heaviest number of casualties caused at single incidents were:

(*a*) An elementary school in Lewisham was hit on January 20 in daylight by a 250 kilo. bomb, causing 187 casualties, of which 59 were killed and 67 admitted to hospital; most of the casualties were children;

(*b*) A dance hall in Putney received a direct hit on the night of November 7 by a 500 kilo. bomb, causing 288 casualties, of which 78 were killed and 116 admitted to hospital (see Plate X).

A full account of the exceptional and resourceful work of the Ambulance Service in connexion with this incident will be found in Chapter 8 of this volume.

SERVICE SICK AND CASUALTIES

During this year the number of Service sick and casualties treated in E.M.S. hospitals included the following:

Army (including Women's Services, 21,605)	176,022*
R.A.F. (including W.A.A.F., 18,063)†	85,544†
Canadian Forces	3,664
Allied Forces	2,790

As admissions from the Navy are omitted, and the Army admissions exclude transfers, both from other hospitals and from overseas, the total number of Service admissions was much higher than the sum of the above figures. Dr. Percy Stocks has, however, calculated from a one-in-five sample of Ministry of Pensions forms that there were 14,900 Navy admissions to E.M.S. hospitals (including 1,515 W.R.N.S.) during 1943.

CIVILIAN ADMISSIONS

In addition to the above, the routine admission of civilian categories continued. These categories had gradually been added to and by this time made up a formidable list. In April 1943, the Ministry of Health drew up a codified list of all classes of patients for whom the E.M.S. accepted responsibility, either entirely or subject to a contribution by the patient or to the surrender of a contributory scheme voucher (see Appendix IV), and hospitals were required to make quarterly returns of

---

* Direct admissions only.
† Great Britain and Northern Ireland.

in-patients in these categories on the last day of each quarter. Some idea of the scope of the Emergency Hospital Scheme can be gained from tables based on these returns (see Appendix VI). The admissions of civilian 'enemy action' casualties including 430 civil defence and 135 merchant navy personnel during this year were 3,830. (See Appendix VIII.) In addition, Dr. Stocks has supplied estimates of the numbers of admissions of civilian categories not due to enemy action based on the above-mentioned quarterly returns for the years from July 1, 1943 to July 1, 1945. These figures will be found in Appendix VII, they are based on an estimate of an average stay in hospital of twenty-eight days.

ACCOMMODATION IN HOSPITALS

At the end of 1943 the number of hospitals in the Emergency Hospital Scheme stood at 876 and the bed accommodation at 273,304, including 62,045 reserve and 156,676 occupied beds. Of the latter 16,896 were occupied by Service sick, 5,303 by Service casualties, 466 by civilian air raid casualties and 134,011 by civilian sick.

Auxiliary Hospitals. On September 1, 1943, convalescent homes and auxiliary hospitals totalled 231 and the beds available 13,094, the small number of additional hospitals opened during the year being accounted for by the difficulty of obtaining suitable accommodation.

The number of admissions during the year ending September 1, 1943, were:

British Forces		Allied Forces	Civilian Patients		Civil Defence Workers		Total
Male	Female		Male	Female	Male	Female	
85,865	7,209	2,425	2,895	5,350	1,747	1,032	106,523

In addition, 1,911 male and 93 female British and 233 male and 2 female Allied patients were admitted to the Convalescent Hospitals for Officers, which had been reduced to five.*

Service Hospitals. The number of Service hospitals together with bed accommodation as at May 1, 1943, were as follows:

	Number of Hospitals	Occupied Beds	Vacant Beds	Total Beds
Royal Navy	16	3,397	2,010	5,407
Royal Air Force	25†	4,691	1,935	6,626
Army	70	10,439	7,035	17,474
Canadian Army	14	2,523	4,365	6,888

In the twelve Ministry of Pensions hospitals there were at this date 2,410 occupied beds and 3,563 vacant beds, making a total of 5,973 beds.

---

* Includes one Scottish.
† Includes R.A.F. hospitals in Scotland and Northern Ireland.

REFERENCES

[1] Min. of Health Letter to hospital authorities, sector and regional hospital officers, etc., E.M.S./Gen/350, April 30, 1942.
[2] Min. of Health Circular 2395, and Emergency Medical Services Instruction 298, both of June 4, 1941.
[3] Min. of Health E.M.S./Gen/296, December 6, 1939.
[4] Min. of Health Circular 2088, July 8, 1940.
[5] Min. of Health Circular 2436, and Forms 141 and 142 (revised) August 15, 1941.
[6] Emergency Medical Services Instruction 321, October 3, 1941.
[7] Emergency Medical Services Instruction 364, May 19, 1942.
[8] Emergency Medical Services Instruction 335, January 8, 1942.
[9] Emergency Medical Services Instruction 358, April 8, 1942.
[10] Min. of Health Circular 2714, October 27, 1942.
[11] 'Interim Scheme for the Training and Resettlement of Disabled Persons'. Min. of Labour and National Service Leaflet, PL.93/1941. Min. of Health Circular 2449 (Addendum), October 30, 1941.
[12] Min. of Health Circular 2549, January 6, 1942.
[13] Min. of Health Circular 2549A, November 16, 1942.
[14] Emergency Medical Services Instruction 352, February 26, 1942, and Director-General Letter 271, June 8, 1942.
[15] *Report of Interdepartmental Committee on the Rehabilitation and Resettlement of Disabled Persons.* [Cmd. 6415. H.M.S.O.], 1943.
[16] Emergency Medical Services Director-General Letter 242, March 8, 1943.
[17] *Emergency Medical Services Memorandum 6: The Organisation of a Hospital Rehabilitation Department.* (Circulated under Min. of Health Circular 2895, December 20, 1943).
[18] BALME, H. (1943). 'The Advance of Rehabilitation'. Monthly Bulletin of the Ministry of Health and the Emergency Public Health Laboratory Service, 2, 109.
[19] BALME, H. (1946). 'The Present State of Hospital Rehabilitation'. Monthly Bulletin of the Ministry of Health and the Emergency Public Health Laboratory Service, 5, 124.

CHAPTER 6
PERIOD OF ACTIVE OPERATIONS
January 1944 to End of Hostilities

IN the previous chapter the work of the Emergency Medical Services from July 1941 to December 1943, has been recorded. It was a period of comparative quiet, which afforded an opportunity for reorganisation in the light of experience. Facilities for treatment of E.M.S. patients were improved and expanded in order to ensure the highest possible mental and physical capacity for their civil or military duties on discharge from hospital. But much still remained to do, and in 1944, under less restful conditions, further improvements were made notwithstanding increasing difficulties caused by the continued shortage of medical, nursing and lay personnel.

It proved to be an eventful year, in which the Services had to prepare for the treatment of large numbers of battle casualties from oversea while dealing with a considerable increase in air raid casualties, especially in the London area. In this chapter, which covers the period from the beginning of 1944 to the end of hostilities, events are dealt with as in former chapters, not chronologically, but under the separate headings of advances and improvements in the Emergency Medical Services, the preparation for and the reception of battle casualties, and enemy attacks from the air.

ADVANCES AND IMPROVEMENTS IN THE EMERGENCY HOSPITAL SERVICES

RECUPERATIVE TREATMENT FOR INDUSTRIAL WORKERS

With the intensification of the war effort, the demands of the Fighting Services for man-power rapidly increased, while in the industries chiefly concerned in supplying the munitions of war, shortage of labour of all kinds was acute. In Chapter 5 the extensive arrangements made by the Ministries of Health and of Labour to ensure the rapid rehabilitation of disabled persons and their return to employment have been recorded. In furtherance of these objects, these Ministries prepared a scheme, which was brought into operation in May 1944, to provide convalescent treatment for ailing industrial workers. It applied only to factories and certain other industrial establishments, such as coal-mining undertakings, where there was medical supervision by whole-time or part-time medical officers.[1]

Under this scheme, which provided for liaison between the industrial medical officers and the Regional and Sector Hospital Officers, workers recommended for treatment were medically examined at Emergency Medical Services hospitals near their homes, and accommodation was provided in specially selected convalescent homes affiliated to the hospitals. Thirteen homes for men and thirteen for women, containing a total of 973 beds, were opened in the chief industrial areas. The stay of each worker in these homes was normally limited to a fortnight, but in exceptional circumstances a longer stay was permitted. Active convalescent treatment included physical exercises, indoor and outdoor occupations, organised games and rest periods, and convalescents were expected to share in the ordinary domestic duties of the homes. If a worker required hospital treatment while in a convalescent home, he or she was transferred to the affiliated E.M.S. hospital as an E.M.S. patient. This scheme produced fairly satisfactory results, as the majority of patients responded to treatment and were able to return to full or partial employment sooner than they would have done otherwise.

RESETTLEMENT OF PSYCHONEUROTIC AND PSYCHOTIC PERSONS

It had been reported by the Ministry of Labour and National Service that the employment exchanges were having difficulty in dealing with a number of persons who suffered from some form of psychoneurosis or psychosis. These persons were liable to break down in the various posts found for them and it was often a problem to find work which they could usefully do. Breakdowns were also occurring among persons under treatment at the training centres.[2]

Arrangements were therefore made to examine and treat such cases at neurosis centres or clinics, and for reports on their suitability or otherwise for employment, with the result that many persons who had previously been unsuitably employed, were found useful employment appropriate to their condition and capabilities.

The circulars announcing these arrangements (which subsequently were extended to cover members of the Merchant Navy), and laying down the action to be taken, were sent to upwards of 100 selected hospitals containing neurosis clinics.[3]

ADDITIONAL SPECIAL CENTRES

Tropical Diseases. Owing to the increasing numbers of Service patients from oversea, the provisions previously made by the E.M.S. for the reception, investigation and treatment of tropical cases were, by the summer of 1944, proving to be inadequate. Two additional centres for tropical diseases were therefore established in the Emergency Hospital Scheme—at Queen Mary's Hospital, Roehampton and at Smithdown Road Hospital, Liverpool—to which both Service and civilian cases were admitted. R.A.F. personnel, however, continued to be treated for such diseases in their own special hospitals at Halton and Cosford.[4]

Peripheral Nerve Injuries. For similar reasons the accommodation for cases of peripheral nerve injury, already provided at three special centres, was no longer sufficient. Additional accommodation, therefore, was provided as required for such cases at thirteen hospitals with orthopaedic centres and at seven other hospitals.[5]

Injuries of the Spinal Cord and Cauda Equina. It was also found necessary to increase the number of centres for treating injuries of the spinal cord and cauda equina from three to eleven.[6]

PHYSICAL TRAINING

Towards the end of the year 1944, Brigadier T. H. Wand-Tetley, who had retired from the appointment of Director of Physical Training in the Army, joined the staff of the Ministry of Health in order to supervise physical training in all E.M.S. hospitals to which physical training instructors had been appointed. He was specially concerned with relating the work of these instructors to the treatment prescribed by the medical officers in charge of the patients.[7]

PHYSIOTHERAPY

In view of the increasing number of rehabilitation departments which had been established in E.M.S. hospitals throughout the country, the Ministry came to an agreement with the Chartered Society of Physiotherapy for the appointment of four paid part-time liaison officers nominated by the Society, who worked in selected Regions and Sectors under the general direction of the Regional or Sector Hospital Officers.[8]

MEDICAL ARRANGEMENTS FOR THE INVASION OF THE CONTINENT OF EUROPE

PLAN FOR THE RECEPTION OF CASUALTIES

The first indication to the Ministry of Health that an invasion of the Continent of Europe was contemplated in the near future was a notification by the War Office in July 1943, that, unless certain military hospitals in England could be handed over to the Ministry, they might have to be closed, because of the need to provide an efficient medical service for forces oversea. Because of the grave shortage of staff already existing in E.M.S. hospitals, the Ministry doubted the possibility of taking over these military hospitals, but assured the War Office that they would either do so or, alternatively, would arrange to transfer their patients to suitable E.M.S. hospitals. Regional Hospital Officers were requested to discuss the matter with the D.Ds.M.S. of Commands and to arrange accordingly.[9]

In February 1944, the Ministry of Health were authorised to issue a confidential circular to all Class IA hospitals in the E.M.S. Scheme indicating the possibility of having to provide for the treatment of large numbers of casualties during the current year and asking the hospital authorities to be prepared to restrict the admission of civilian patients to those in need of immediate treatment or requiring not more than a few days' stay in hospital, the restriction to begin on a date to be notified by the Regional or Sector Hospital Officers. The object of the Ministry was thus gradually to reduce bed occupancy in all Class IA hospitals to 50 per cent. of accommodation, or probably less in special cases. The reduction was to be maintained for an indefinite period.

The Ministry also indicated that if Service casualties were received in large numbers, hospitals where heavy acute work was being done might require reinforcement at the expense of others doing less urgent work.

Hospital authorities were therefore asked to perfect the necessary advance arrangements for the temporary movement of medical, nursing and lay staffs.

The task of preparing and controlling the scheme for the reception of casualties in this country was entrusted to Sir Claude Frankau, Director, Emergency Medical Services, London and Home Counties, and in April he issued a confidential letter[10] containing full detailed instructions for carrying out the arrangements which had been agreed upon after consultation with the Naval, Military and Air Force authorities. This laid down the procedure to be followed in dealing with all kinds of Service casualties, Mercantile Marine and other civilian casualties at all stages from disembarkation to home base hospitals. It also contained instructions for the accurate recording of casualties and for medical documentation.

Special instructions for dealing with neurosis cases were also drawn up.[11] These were to be labelled 'exhaustion' cases in order to avoid any suggestion of serious illness to the man concerned, and a procedure was laid down by which each type of case would receive the treatment most appropriate to secure early return to suitable duty.

The following summary of the arrangements made for the reception and treatment of casualties is contributed by Sir Claude Frankau:

PRELIMINARY ARRANGEMENTS

After the discussions with the War Office, about the middle of 1943, it was agreed that the treatment of all British casualties in this country from the Second Front should be dealt with by the E.M.S.

SEABORNE CASUALTIES

Some months later certain ports of entry were indicated and active preparations were put in hand to receive and distribute seaborne casualties.

The main ports of entry from 'D' day till October were Southampton, Portsmouth, and, to a lesser extent, Gosport, which were also the embarkation ports for the Expeditionary Forces. Originally Dover and Tilbury had also been selected and equipped; but Dover was never used and Tilbury first came into use in October. By this time the campaign on the Continent had moved forward to the Rhine and casualties were no longer being sent back to base hospitals in Normandy. It entailed a much shorter journey to evacuate them from the Belgian ports to Tilbury.

The hospitals scheduled to receive casualties were divided into three categories:

(*a*) 'Coastal' (or 'Port') hospitals for reception of cases unfit for further travel. These hospitals were all at or close to the ports of disembarkation.

(*b*) 'Transit' hospitals, reached from the ports by road or short rail journey and roughly corresponding to casualty clearing stations.

(*c*) 'Home Base' hospitals, in which patients were to be retained and treated to conclusion.

For purposes of security, the preparations and investigations in regard to coastal and transit hospitals covered a wide area, from King's Lynn to Lyme Regis. It was important not to give any clear indication of the ports of entry as these would serve also as ports of embarkation for the expeditionary force. Considerable heart-burning resulted from the need to delude a number of hospitals; but the fact that the Southampton and Portsmouth areas were the main ports chosen for casualty reception was a decision which had to be concealed from all but a very few until 'D' day.

THE COASTAL AND TRANSIT AREA

Many points had to be considered in making the preliminary investigations, the principal need being to find out the following facts for each hospital:

1. Total available beds;
2. Number of operating theatres;
3. Number of operating tables which could be set up in the existing and improvised theatres;
4. Number of surgical teams available;
5. Resuscitation facilities;
6. Capacity of nursing and domestic staff to work under continual strain;
7. Fuel, food and medical supplies.

It was early agreed to take into account only those beds which were normally staffed and equipped and to keep as a reserve the beds classed as Reserve A and Reserve B; these latter were in fact never used.

All operating theatres were examined and where an extra table could be accommodated, its supply with the necessary equipment was arranged. Extra lighting and other facilities were provided in the improvised operating theatres.

None of the hospitals concerned had an adequate number of surgical teams—based on an allocation of six teams for four tables for a twenty-four hour service—and it was arranged to cover the deficiency by moving teams from London.

Similarly transfer of nurses from London was provided to strengthen the nursing side. Reinforcement of the domestic staffs presented many difficulties but they were eventually solved by calling in the assistance of the British Red Cross Society and Order of St. John, the Women's Voluntary Services and the Army, the last providing a number of R.A.M.C. cooks and clerks and also all the stretcher bearers for work in hospitals and at railheads.

In addition arrangements were made with the Deans of Teaching Schools to obtain the services of a number of medical students in their final year.

THE SOUTHAMPTON, GOSPORT, PORTSMOUTH TRANSIT AND
    COASTAL HOSPITAL SCHEME

For this area, through which all seaborne casualties passed during the first four months, the following is a brief outline of the arrangements:

COASTAL OR PORT HOSPITALS

Available Beds
- 150 St. Mary's Hospital, Portsmouth, serving Portsmouth.
- 50 St. James's Hospital, Portsmouth, serving Portsmouth.
- 400 Haslar R.N. Hospital, serving Gosport.
- 50 Alverstoke Emergency Hospital, serving Gosport.
- 450 Queen Alexandra's Hospital, Cosham, serving Gosport and Portsmouth.
- 50 Borough General Hospital, Southampton, serving Southampton.
- 75 Royal South Hants Hospital, serving Southampton.

TRANSIT HOSPITALS REACHED BY ROAD TRANSPORT

Available Beds
- 450 Queen Alexandra's Hospital, Cosham. (This hospital served a double function as a transit and a coastal hospital.)
- 250 Royal Hants County Hospital, Winchester.
- 100 Winchester Emergency Hospital.

TRANSIT HOSPITALS REACHED BY RAIL TRANSPORT

Available Beds
- 800 Park Prewett Hospital, Basingstoke.
- 600 No. 8 Canadian General Hospital, Aldershot.
- 1,200 No. 2 Canadian General Hospital, Bramshott.
- 600 No. 17 Canadian General Hospital, Pinewood.
- 1,900 Horton, Leatherhead and Sutton Emergency Hospitals (acting as a group).

300 Royal Surrey County and Warren Road Hospitals, Guildford (acting as a group).
700 Botley's Park Hospital, Chertsey.
450 Royal West Sussex, St. Richard's and Summersdale Hospitals, Chichester (acting as a group).

The aggregate number of beds available in the coastal and transit hospitals was therefore approximately 8,000; this would have been just adequate if the general staff estimate of casualties had been reached and if there had been extensive bombing of the marshalling areas, etc. Fortunately, there was no such bombing and the casualty figures were considerably below the estimate. The greatest number of casualties held on any one night in the coastal and transit system was about 4,000. It was soon evident that the beds in transit hospitals were in excess of the number required and those at Chichester and Guildford were withdrawn from the scheme on June 28. On the same day Sutton Emergency Hospital was closed owing to damage from a flying bomb. Shortly afterwards Horton and Leatherhead hospitals were also withdrawn because of danger from flying bombs. Other coastal and transit hospitals were subsequently withdrawn at various dates so that by the beginning of October, Southampton was the sole port of entry. The only hospitals remaining in the scheme were Royal South Hants, Royal Hants County, Park Prewett, Botley's Park and Horton, which had been re-opened on September 14, after the danger from flying bombs had passed.

REINFORCEMENTS TO COASTAL AND TRANSIT HOSPITALS

To provide an adequate surgical and nursing service 48 surgical teams, 29 general duty medical officers, 31 radiographers, 120 medical students and 727 nurses—1,051 persons in all—were moved from London on June 5; but the Army in addition provided 12 surgical teams during the early weeks of the fighting. For security reasons none of the personnel moved knew his destination till he had actually started on his journey. The original intention was to make the movements on 'D' day, but as this was postponed at very short notice from June 5 to June 6 and all the orders had been issued, the moves were made on D-1. For the move 66 buses or other vehicles were used, picking up personnel from over 80 different points.

The coastal hospitals, into which patients unfit to travel were admitted, were more heavily reinforced than the transit hospitals as they were likely to and did in fact deal with the more severe cases. In addition, neurosurgical teams were posted at the Royal South Hants Hospital, Southampton, and at Queen Alexandra's Hospital, Cosham, to deal with injuries of the head and spine, and at a later date a thoracic team was posted at Cosham. A specialist dental surgeon with a roving commission was posted to Alverstoke Hospital to deal with jaw injuries in the area.

RECEPTION AND DISTRIBUTION OF CASUALTIES

The unloading of Landing Ship Tanks (L.S.T.) carriers and other vessels carrying casualties was an Army responsibility, as was the provision of all the road transport; the E.M.S. responsibility began as soon as the patient reached either the ambulance trains or hospitals.

Selection of cases at the ports, a matter of vital importance, was carried out by Army surgical specialists from the 21st Army Group, Lt. Colonel R. K. Debenham, O.B.E., F.R.C.S., R.A.M.C., afterwards Brigadier and Consulting Surgeon to the 2nd (British) Army, and Lt. Colonel A. B. Kerr, T.D., F.R.C.S.Ed. Both these officers were at that time in charge of surgical divisions of military hospitals in the 2nd (British) Army. Their work at the ports and the methods they employed are described in an article 'Triage of Battle Casualties', in the *Journal of the Royal Army Medical Corps*, March 1945.[12]

The chief classes of casualties sent direct to the port hospitals for immediate treatment were acute haemorrhage, gas infections, interference with the circulation of a limb, penetrating wounds of the eye, penetrating wounds of joints not immobilised, compound fractures of the femur not immobilised, paraplegia requiring suprapubic cystotomy, complicated penetrating wounds of the chest, penetrating wounds of the abdomen unless convalescent, extensive burns and severe toxaemia or collapse from whatever cause.

Other cases requiring treatment by neurosurgeons and maxillofacial specialists were sent direct to the Park Prewett transit hospital by road, one hour's drive from the port. All other cases were sent by ambulance train. In the original estimates it was thought that 10 per cent. of the cases arriving would be unfit for a train journey, and would have to be admitted to hospitals at the ports. The actual percentage received into these hospitals was 8·3 during the busy period and the figure was very much lower when more active surgery was being done overseas. The selection was excellent—bad selection would have meant swamping the hospitals at the ports.

Eight civil ambulance trains (casualty evacuation trains) were berthed near the ports of disembarkation for use in transporting cases from the ports to the transit hospitals. The staff of each of these was reinforced by extra nurses and also by two medical students. The trains were provided with penicillin and the necessary equipment so that the treatment of patients with this drug, which was given on the landing ship tanks and hospital carriers, could be continuous.

In order to equalise the load on the hospitals a predetermined schedule of destinations for these trains was drawn up. This schedule was based on the estimated number of casualties and, if this estimate had been correct, would have entailed the larger hospitals receiving three trains each on the first day and the smaller hospitals one, or in some cases, two trains; actually, during the period in which all the transit hospitals were functioning, none of the larger hospitals ever received more than two trains a day and each train-load approximated 200 rather than its full capacity of 300.

In order to provide a quick turn round for the trains at the transit hospital railheads, not less than fifty bearers were always available for unloading and special arrangements were made at all hospitals for the speedy reception and distribution of patients as they came in.

Details of the work of these trains will be found in Chapter 8 (The Ambulance Services).

It was originally thought that the pressure would be so great that only the most urgent cases could be dealt with in the transit hospitals and that all others would have to go on to home base hospitals after examination and re-dressing. But in fact, except for the first two or three days, when a considerable number of patients had perforce to be sent on, practically all cases had any definitive wound treatment required in the transit hospitals. All cases fit to be sent on to home base hospitals were evacuated as soon as possible and only once was the bed accommodation in a transit hospital taxed to the full. At a later stage certain hospitals were able to retain special cases, e.g. fractured femurs and joint wounds, to the great benefit of the patients.

A predetermined schedule of railheads in England and Scotland allowed for a wide and equal distribution of cases and aimed at preventing any particular hospital area becoming overloaded. Like the trains from ports to transit hospitals, the trains used for evacuating the latter were reinforced with extra personnel and were provided with penicillin.

On October 23, the main port of disembarkation was changed to Tilbury, a few cases only coming to this country via Southampton, and the system of primary admission of casualties into transit hospitals was abandoned, all patients fit to travel proceeding direct from the ports to home base hospitals. Owing to the general direction of the railroad system in that area, transfers to transit hospitals from Tilbury would have had to be made by road, and the transport service would have been heavily strained. On the date of this change approximately 70,000 patients evacuated to the United Kingdom by sea had passed through the transit hospital system.

From this date until the end of the year a further 10,500 seaborne casualties were received in the E.M.S. hospitals. From January 1, 1945 to August 15, 1945, the day on which hostilities officially ended, a further 5,100 seaborne casualties arrived, making a total of approximately 85,600.

THE RECEPTION AND DISTRIBUTION OF AIRBORNE CASUALTIES

The Air Ministry had devised a scheme whereby three aerodromes in the neighbourhood of Swindon (Down Ampney, Blackhill Farm and

Broadwell), which were to be used for outward goods transport, would also be used for the reception of casualties brought back in the returning transport planes.

It was expected that about 600 cases a day would be brought back by this method and that, although a small number would be brought back from D + 2, the organised evacuation by air could not begin until D + 14 at the earliest. In fact this method of evacuation of casualties began on D + 7, with an average daily intake in fine weather of 300 and a peak on one day of 934.

The general scheme for the reception of patients was similar to that for seaborne casualties. Cases unfit for transport were retained in Stratton St. Margaret's Hospital, near Swindon (350 beds) or Wroughton R.A.F. Hospital (800–1,000 beds), the remainder being transported to home base hospitals direct by train.

In order to minimise the length of the train journey, detraining points were selected which would not involve a journey of more than four to five hours. Adequate arrangements were made for the retention and care of the patients at the airfields if there were any delay before entraining. As an additional precaution the G.W.R. Hospital at Swindon, with an annexe in the Baths Hall, was also made available in case it should become necessary to house a large number of patients overnight.

The selection of cases fit for transport was an R.A.F. responsibility, and the Army undertook the transport of patients to hospitals or trains.

Special arrangements were made for the immediate transfer by road of cases requiring urgent treatment in special centres, head and spine cases going to St. Hugh's Military Hospital, Oxford, to the Royal United Hospital, Bath, where a special unit had been established for this purpose, and to the Canadian Neurological Hospital, Hackwood Park, Basingstoke; chest cases going to Kewstoke; burns and maxillo-facial cases going to Rooksdown House, Park Prewett or the Canadian Centre at Hackwood Park.

From D-day to October 23, 1944 (after which date Tilbury was the sole port of entry for seaborne casualties), 39,838 casualties transported by air were received into E.M.S. hospitals. Subsequent to this date at least four-fifths of all casualties arrived by air, 10,851 being received by the end of the year and a further 35,770 from January 1, 1945 to August 15, 1945; the total of airborne casualties dealt with was therefore 86,459.

HOME BASE AREA

The home base hospitals were situated in the part of the country north and west of a line from the Wash to Lyme Regis. There were 97 of these hospitals staffed and equipped to do the bulk of the work, with a total accommodation of 50,000 beds, of which 23,000 were vacant on D-day.

Casualties arrived by ambulance train at twenty-three selected railheads, each serving a group of home base hospitals. The railheads were used in rotation to avoid overloading any particular group of hospitals. In order to ensure a quick return of trains to the transit area, the railheads in the Midlands and South Wales were used for the first four days.

From these railheads the patients were distributed to home base hospitals by road transport. Those requiring special treatment were transferred without delay to the appropriate special centres. As soon as the condition and the stage of treatment of the patients permitted, they were transferred from home base hospitals and special centres to 'secondary' accommodation.

The number of beds in 'secondary' hospitals was 58,000, of which 13,500 were vacant and available. 'Secondary' hospitals were of two types which might be called 'reinforcement' and 'decant' hospitals. The former released staff who were transferred to home base hospitals; the latter retained their full staff and to them patients were transferred from special centres and home base hospitals.

In addition to the above accommodation there were 13,000 reserve beds in home base and secondary hospitals which could have been used in emergency. The total number of beds was therefore 121,000 of which 49,500 were vacant. When a suitable stage of recovery was reached patients were transferred to British Red Cross auxiliary hospitals or convalescent depots.

Additional special centres were established as follows:

Neurosurgery	Leicester Royal Infirmary and Cardiff Royal Infirmary
Plastic and Jaw Injury	St. James's Hospital, Leeds
Thoracic Surgery	Leicester City Isolation Hospital

Two home base hospitals—Whittingham Emergency Hospital, near Preston, and Oaklands Emergency Hospital, Bishop Auckland—were designated for the reception of ambulant sick and injured prisoners-of-war.

THE WORK OF THE HOSPITALS

As examples of the work of the hospitals the following accounts of the arrangements and working of the chief port and transit hospitals are of special interest:

THE WORKING OF A PORT HOSPITAL

(Based on a contribution by Brigadier Myles L. Formby, F.R.C.S., Surgeon, E.N.T. Dept., University College Hospital)

THE HOSPITAL

This was the Royal South Hants and Southampton Hospital, which provided 160 beds for casualties and which was specially prepared for the reception of casualties evacuated from Normandy, mostly in landing ship tanks, whose condition was such that they could not be sent to 'transit' or special hospitals.

THE STAFF

The medical staff was reinforced by London surgeons, anaesthetists, house surgeons, senior medical students and an R.A.M.C. general duty officer, and in addition by an appropriate number of sisters, nurses, radiographers and a detachment of R.A.M.C. stretcher bearers.

THE PLAN OF WORK

Reception of Cases. The ambulances drew up at the entrance to the out-patients' hall in which the patients were transferred to stretcher trolleys and taken into one of the two reception wards where the stretchers were placed on beds. Each case was at once seen by the resuscitation officer on duty.

There were four resuscitation teams, each consisting of an experienced house surgeon or general duty officer and a senior medical student; a radiographer was always available for duty with each team. The surgical staff was divided into six teams, two local and four from London, each team consisting of a surgeon and an assistant surgeon, an anaesthetist, theatre sister and theatre nursing staff. One was a specialised neurological team, another was orthopaedic, and four were general surgical teams.

Distribution of Patients. After resuscitation, the distribution of cases was dealt with by a co-ordinating officer, who, according to their nature, allotted them to the various surgical teams on duty. It was part of his duty to know the number of cases arriving, their nature and the commitments of each surgical team. There were three operating theatres and the day was divided into three eight-hour shifts, ensuring three surgical teams always on duty. After operation, cases were removed to two post-operative wards where the patients remained in charge of the operating teams, who spent much off-duty time in these wards.

The R.A.M.C. stretcher bearers also worked in eight-hour shifts, unloading ambulances, conveying cases to reception wards and operating theatres and loading cases for evacuation to transit or special hospitals. The sisters and nurses adhered to their customary day and night duties.

Pathological services were available at all times in spite of the increased work entailed by the issue of penicillin and transfusion supplies.

Case sheets containing full information regarding the cases, such as clinical notes, resuscitation treatment, operative treatment and findings, post-operative treatment, pathological reports, X-ray films, etc. were kept and duplicates made.

THE CASUALTIES

These with few exceptions were of the serious type which the hospital was meant to deal with, showing that the sorting at the 'hards' had been done with great skill and sound judgment by two experienced R.A.M.C. officers normally in charge of the surgical divisions of general hospitals. The general condition of the casualties was better than was expected. Most of them were tired and sleepy, some were hungry, a few seriously dehydrated and others more affected by a rough channel crossing than by their wounds. The first batches had had little treatment and so contained a proportion in very poor condition. After the sixth day many of the serious cases had been dealt with by the Paratroop Field Ambulance or Field Service Units and were in remarkably good condition. From the fourteenth day wounds were for the most part less serious, but there was a proportion of cases untreated, except for first field or shell dressings, and these were in poor condition.

Up to D + 16 a total of 282 cases had been admitted, which was approximately a quarter of the number expected. The largest number admitted on one night was 40, on the night of D + 5/6. From D + 17 to D + 26 a further 228 cases were admitted, making a total of 510 in all. These latter cases were on the whole much less serious than the former.

TYPES OF WOUNDS

Multiple injuries were strikingly predominant. Buttock wounds were common, chest wounds numerous, but burns infrequent. Severe head wounds, spinal and maxillo-facial injuries were in larger proportion than was expected, probably because the officers at the 'hards' were aware that specialists in these branches of surgery were available at this hospital.

Excluding closed head injuries, penetrating wounds of the brain and simple rupture of the tympanic membrane, there were 60 cases with wounds of the head and neck, with which an E.N.T. surgeon could usefully assist, and as several of these had eye injuries as well, the inclusion of a whole-time ophthalmic surgeon in the team would have been an advantage. There were only 3 cases of gas gangrene and none of tetanus.

MISSILES PRODUCING CASUALTIES

Mortar bombs were responsible for a high proportion of the casualties; bullet wounds were seldom seen.

DEATHS

Of the 510 admissions, 17 died; of these 6 were moribund on admission and in 4 others the prognosis was hopeless from the first.

VISITS BY CONSULTANTS

Numerous and welcome visits were made by consultants, whose practical assistance in maxillo-facial cases and helpful advice in general surgery, in chest cases and in neuro-surgery were of the greatest value.

X-RAY WORK

The value of the work of the radiographers cannot be too strongly emphasised. Their aid was an essential accessory to early diagnosis and correct treatment.

PENICILLIN

Practically every case arriving had received penicillin with varying regularity. Brigadier Formby remarked that 'there is a limit to what the well-disciplined British soldier will stand' and thought that being 'jabbed' by a needle regularly every three hours might be too much for even his patience under treatment, especially when it was frequently supplemented by irregular and often larger 'jabs' for transfusion, A.T.S., A.G.G.S., morphia, etc. Those few who complained were informed that these repeated injections were unavoidable and for their own protection.

RESUSCITATION

The effects of resuscitation—which varied from natural sleep, warmth, drinks, food, morphia, etc., to the transfusion of several pints of plasma or whole blood—were described by Brigadier Formby as amazing.

PORT CASES IN TRANSIT HOSPITALS

There was naturally a laudable anxiety among the surgeons concerning the wounded whom they had treated and passed on to the transit hospitals, and an early visit to one of these hospitals proved instructive and brought out the following points:

(i) A defective ambulance took more out of the patients in a nine-mile journey than the cross-channel voyage. One such ambulance was forthwith discarded.

(ii) The chief complaint in the transit hospital was that little or no surgical treatment was required for the cases coming from the port hospital.

GENERAL COMMENTS

Subsequent visits to the hospital confirmed the impressions recorded by Brigadier Formby in his account of the work during the first twenty-six days after invasion day.

It would appear that the functions of a port hospital were carried out efficiently and expeditiously, which must have been a prime factor in saving lives and in shortening the period of hospital occupancy by the patients passing through it.

Administrative Arrangements at Park Prewett Hospital while acting as a Transit Hospital

(Contributed by Mr. A. Innes, F.R.C.S., Surgical Director of the Hospital)

Instructions had been received before 'D' day that when the Western invasion commenced, this hospital would cease to function as a general hospital and would operate as a transit hospital.

Steps had been taken in advance to reduce the number of occupied beds and on June 6, 1944, the bedstate was as follows:

Equipped beds for the reception of battle casualties	1,301
Occupied beds	244
Vacant beds	1,057

STAFF

(a) *Medical:* The normal hospital establishment was:

Surgeons, whole-time	5
,, part-time	3
House surgeons	7
Physicians	2
House physicians	4

To supplement these on June 5, 1944, there reported for duty at the hospital:

Surgical teams, civilian	3
,, ,, Army	1
House surgeons	6
Medical students	24

The services of a qualified R.A.M.C. Ophthalmic Surgeon was also available during the transit phase.

On August 8, 1944, the surgical teams were withdrawn.

On August 14, 1944, the number of medical students was reduced to 12.

(b) *Nursing:* 102 additional nurses reported from London on June 5, 1944.

(c) *Orderlies:* 58 R.A.M.C. orderlies and bearers were allotted to the hospital during the transit period to supplement the 40 civilian nursing orderlies and stretcher bearers.

DETRAINING FROM AMBULANCE TRAINS

This was carried out at the Southern Railway siding, Basingstoke, under the supervision of the hospital military registrar with the help of forty-eight R.A.M.C. bearers detailed for this purpose. An adequate supply of transport for stretcher and sitting cases was placed under the orders of the medical superintendent for conveyance of casualties from the train to the hospital.

AMBULANCE TRAINS

Seventy-one trains were received from the ports.

Sixty-one trains were used to evacuate cases fit for transfer to base hospitals in the Midlands and North.

ADMISSION OF CASES TO HOSPITAL

All admissions were passed through a central reception room, where a brief clinical examination of every case was made. Three cases could be dealt with simultaneously, three teams (each consisting of a senior surgeon, a sister and a nurse) being on duty.

The surgeons on duty, after examining the patients and the details on his field medical card, placed the case in one of the following categories, indicated by affixing a coloured gummed slip on to the outside of the field medical card envelope:

(*a*) Severe shock requiring resuscitation—violet slip.

(*b*) Urgent operation priority—red slip.

(*c*) Operation—but not immediate—green slip

(*d*) For observation—white slip

(*e*) Not requiring operation, fit for evacuation—yellow slip

(*f*) Severe burns and/or maxillo-facial cases—white with black 'P' slip

(*g*) Medical case—blue slip.

ALLOCATION TO WARDS

At the exit of the reception room a card was handed to each patient indicating the ward to which he was allotted. The total number of cards available for each ward corresponded to the empty bed-state of that ward, and the official in charge of allocation of patients to wards was thus in possession of a minute-to-minute picture of the number of empty beds in each ward.

A and D particulars of each patient were taken in triplicate at one of a series of 'clerking points' *en route* to the wards and thence the patient was conveyed to the appropriate ward as indicated by the card given him on leaving the reception room, where one of the copies of the A and D forms was handed to the ward sister. Of the remaining two copies, one was passed to the military registrar and the other filed in the hospital E.M.S. records.

The stretcher bearers then returned to await further ambulances.

The time taken for examination, categorisation and admission was reasonably short, the average rate of admission of a convoy being 3·2 cases a minute, i.e. a convoy of 250 cases would take approximately one and a half hours to clear.

EVACUATION

(*a*) On receipt of information from the Hospital Officer, Region 6, Reading, as to the time of arrival of evacuation ambulance trains at Basingstoke, their capacity and destination, an allotment was made to each ward of the number of stretcher and walking cases to be entrained, and the reverse process from detraining was put into action.

(*b*) Canadian patients were evacuated to Canadian general hospitals by motor ambulances under arrangements made by the Canadian military authorities.

(*c*) American patients were evacuated to American general hospitals through similar channels.

It should be noted that, apart from the large convoys of 200–250 cases sent by train from the coast ports, this hospital also admitted cases direct to the plastic and orthopaedic units.

There was a later modification when AIRVAC came into operation and the severest types of orthopaedic, spinal, burns, or maxillo-facial cases were transferred by road from the airport concerned direct to the appropriate unit in the hospital without passing through the mechanism used for the reception of the larger convoys.

NUMBER OF CASES ADMITTED

By convoy	13,911
By direct transfer	1,650
Total number of cases admitted from June 6, 1944, to November 1, 1944	15,561

This total was made up of:

Allied casualties	13,080
Prisoners-of-war	2,481
	15,561

NUMBER OF CASES EVACUATED

Canadians		2,639
British, American and other Allied Forces		
Officers	440	
Other ranks	8,928	
		9,368
Prisoners-of-war		2,430
Civilians		9
		14,446
Other transfers		327
		14,773

TREATMENT WHILE IN HOSPITAL

Arrangements had been made, using the augmented personnel, to run a complete twenty-four hour ward and operating theatre service for as long as was necessary.

The cases admitted to the wards were again examined there, and a check made of the admitting surgeons' categorisation.

The graph which follows gives an idea of the number of operations performed for each convoy from D-day to D + 96. The operation rate per convoy varied slightly and dropped as more holding hospitals were established on the far shore.

It is of interest to note that although a ward of twenty beds had been set aside for resuscitation purposes, on only seven occasions was a case admitted to that ward for resuscitation from a convoy. Minor cases requiring blood and/or plasma were treated by mobile 'shock' teams, which were available day or night.

A ward of fifty beds was also set aside for the treatment of severely wounded cases with penicillin, a penicillin unit comprising a registrar and four dressers being made available by the M.R.C. for this purpose. To assist with this work the massage personnel—twelve in all—were trained in the administration of the drug by continuous drip and intermittent methods.

MORTALITY

The deaths among the casualties were extremely low and during the transit period amounted to:

Allied mortality	23
Prisoner-of-war mortality	10
Total	33

This total included the deaths among the special centre cases—i.e. burns, severe facial, orthopaedic and spinal injuries, which formed a very high proportion of the whole. Mortality rates were thus:

Allied	0·17 per cent.
Prisoners-of-war	0·40 per cent.
Combined	0·21 per cent.

RELAXATION OF THE RESTRICTIONS ON ADMISSION OF CIVILIAN PATIENTS

In September 1944, when it became possible to estimate more accurately what was required in E.M.S. hospitals for casualties from oversea, it was decided to relax the restriction on the admission of civilian patients in order to meet the great and increasing demand for hospital accommodation. Regional and Sector Hospital Officers were

PERIOD OF ACTIVE OPERATIONS

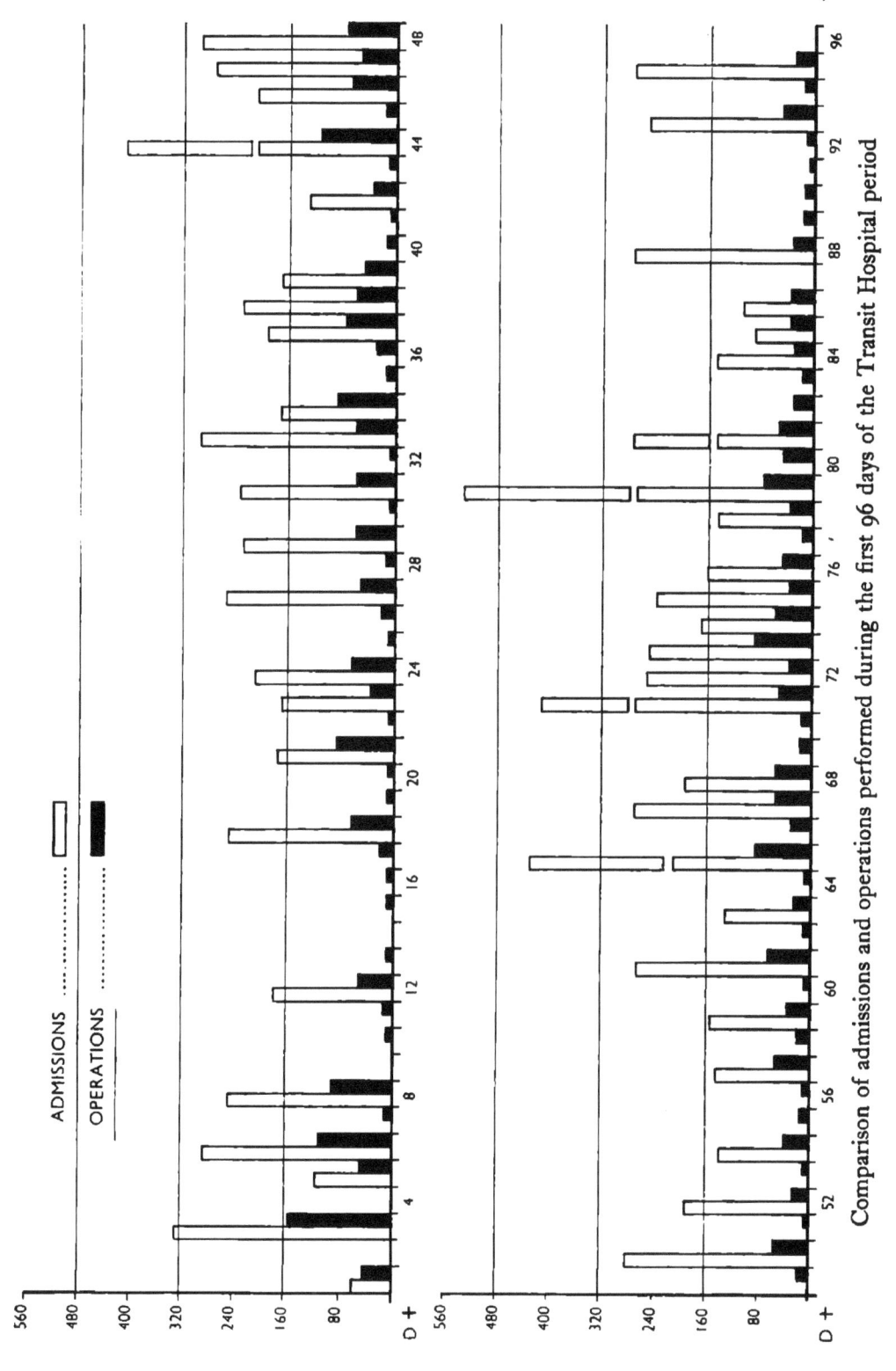

Comparison of admissions and operations performed during the first 96 days of the Transit Hospital period

therefore asked to review the position in their areas and to determine how far beds might be freed for civilian sick while keeping an adequate number of beds fully staffed for the reception of Service casualties.[13]

In hospitals in which no casualties had been received or were likely to be received and from which no staff had been transferred to other hospitals, complete or almost complete relaxation of restrictions was effected at once, and in other hospitals various degrees of relaxation were carried out. In London Sectors, where the demand for acute beds was increasing and was expected proportionately to increase with the return of evacuees from the provinces, the practicability of reducing E.M.S. bed reservation was considered and reductions were effected in accordance with the circumstances in each case.

As the result of further experience, it was decided in October, that all the restrictions laid down in February 1944, could be withdrawn except for their retention in modified form in one or two areas where the demand for accommodation of battle casualties was still high, and that except in Regions 4, 5 and 12 there was no need to reserve any beds for air raid casualties.[14]

In December 1944, it was agreed that E.M.S. arrangements must be based solely on operational considerations and that all hospital beds not likely to be required for E.M.S. purposes should be released. For this purpose the following decisions were made:[15]

(i) Numbers of beds likely to be required by the E.M.S. were to be specified for hospitals, and hospitals in which no beds were required were to be suspended or withdrawn from the scheme.

(ii) The reservation was to be based entirely on operational needs except for the holding of a few beds in smaller hospitals so as to continue the policy of transferring cases to hospitals near their homes.

(iii) Where hutted wards had been provided, the reservation was normally to be not less than the number of beds in the unit, excluding any units released to the owning authorities for non-E.M.S. purposes.

(iv) Where 'annexes' had been attached to hospitals, but were no longer required for the E.M.S., their future use was to be settled after discussion with the hospital authorities. They were either to be released or retained for E.M.S. patients on a 'suspended' basis.

(v) The fixed reservations were to hold good for six months, after which the position would again be reviewed.

No action as regards local authority hospitals was to be taken until the receipt of further instructions; those instructions were issued in February 1945.[16]

SIR GIRLING BALL

The E.M.S. suffered a great loss through the death of Sir Girling Ball, F.R.C.S., on July 16, 1945. Sir Girling was Dean of St. Bartholomew's

Hospital Medical School, and when war threatened was an energetic member of the various committees on whose advice the E.H.S. and E.M.S. were planned. He was largely responsible for the shaping of the Sector scheme for London and was in charge of Sector III from its formation till the end of hostilities in Europe. The important part taken by the medical schools of London in staffing and equipping the upgraded and expanded hospitals in the Sectors was to a great extent due to his guidance and help. He was chairman of the London Sector Hospital Officers and of the Services Committee of the Central Medical War Committee.

Throughout the war Sir Girling was a source of strength to the headquarters staff of the E.M.S. in Whitehall, and by his example, leadership and efficiency contributed in no small degree to the magnificent service rendered by E.M.S. hospitals to the people of London during the years of heavy enemy attack from the air. He gave all his strength and impaired his health to help win the war.

ENEMY ATTACKS, 1944-5

PILOTED AIRCRAFT

In the year 1944 E.M.S. hospitals were affected less by the results of piloted air attacks than by casualties and damage inflicted by the robot 'flying bomb', first used in June of that year, and by the long-range rocket which followed three months later.

The early days of the year, however, were not entirely uneventful, they were marked by a slight increase in the enemy's air activity against this country by night—intended, presumably, to be regarded in Germany as comparable with the massive attacks then being carried out by the Air Forces of the Allies. But these enemy raids were of little consequence until the night of January 21-22, when a fairly heavy attack was made on south-eastern England and the southern part of East Anglia, during which 27 aircraft penetrated the London area. Fatal and seriously injured casualties were 29 and 104 respectively, of which 4 fatal and 74 injured occurred in the London area. This was followed a week later (January 29-30) by a heavier raid in which over 160 aircraft were in operation, including about 100 long-range bombers. The area attacked was again south-eastern England and part of East Anglia, with a few planes penetrating as far as Hampshire and Oxfordshire. Civilian casualties were 51 killed and 124 seriously injured, mostly in the London area.

Light raids continued intermittently until there occurred between February 18 and 25, a series of five brief concentrated attacks on London, the heaviest since May 1941, in which some 600 civilians were killed and 1,300 seriously injured. In these raids over 1,800 fires were caused, 94 per cent. of them in London, and 17 hospitals were damaged.

170 THE EMERGENCY MEDICAL SERVICES

Amongst the major incidents was one in Kings Road, Chelsea, on the night of February 23–24, when a block of flats received a direct hit and 72 persons killed, 111 seriously injured and 40 missing were reported. On the same night 3,000 houses were destroyed or rendered uninhabitable in Battersea, and 1,200 people were made homeless in Fulham.

Thereafter raids were few and scattered, and casualties light. London casualties by the end of April totalled 1,249 fatal and 2,541 seriously injured. A few further casualties occurred in May (68 killed; 75 seriously injured), all outside London, bringing the totals up to 1,563 killed and 2,916 seriously injured, of which 79·9 per cent. and 87·1 per cent. respectively were in London.

FLYING BOMBS (V.1)

On Tuesday, June 13, 1944, aerial attacks took a new but not wholly unexpected form with the launching from the French Coast of high-speed flying bombs against London and south-east England. Each contained an explosive charge of rather less than one metric ton, the weight varying according to the kind of filling used.

The first casualties in this novel, disturbing and destructive form of attack occurred in the London area in the early hours of June 13, when a railway bridge at Bethnal Green was hit and demolished and severe damage to surrounding property was caused by blast. Six civilians were killed and 12 seriously injured. Other incidents occurred in Kent and Sussex and the day's casualties were 9 killed and 23 seriously injured.

Attacks rapidly gained momentum. Within a week of the first incident 776 flying bombs had been reported in operation and casualties had mounted to 723 civilians killed and 2,610 seriously injured. By the last week of August flying bombs had taken a toll of approximately 5,500 killed, 16,000 seriously injured and 30,000 slightly injured. Over 93 per cent. of these casualties occurred in the London area, which was throughout the primary target, and by the seventh week of the attacks every one of the ninety-six Greater London local authorities had been involved. Kent, Sussex, Surrey and Essex were the counties most affected outside the London area.

Casualties from these flying bomb incidents up to September 1, are given in the following table, the figures in brackets being casualties per projectile:

	Flying bomb strikes	Killed	Seriously injured	Slightly injured	Total casualties
London region	2,334	5,126 (2·2)	14,712 (6·3)	25,983 (11·1)	45,821 (19·6)
Other regions	2,789	350 (0·1)	1,206 (0·4)	3,829 (1·4)	5,383 (1·9)
	5,123	5,476 (1·1)	15,918 (3·1)	29,812 (5·8)	51,206 (10·0)

During the daylight attacks of the Battle of Britain in the summer of 1940, casualties per estimated ton of bombs despatched against the United Kingdom were: 0·15 killed and 0·19 seriously injured. Compared with these, the rates of killed (0·68) and seriously injured (1·99) per flying bomb launched were respectively four and a half and ten times greater.

For the night raids of September 1940, to May 1941, casualties per ton despatched were: killed 0·92, seriously injured 1·07. Casualties per flying bomb launched were approximately one-fourth less than these in killed but nearly double in seriously injured.

As from September 1, 1941, the Bomb Census covered the whole country, and weights of bombs dropped were recorded. For the nine months to May 1942, the casualties per metric ton dropped were: killed 0·83, seriously injured 0·93. Flying bomb casualties per incident were: killed (1·1) one-third greater, and seriously injured (3·1) three and a third times greater.

These comparisons, however, while sufficient to indicate that the flying bomb was a potent offensive weapon, leave certain factors out of account. In the daylight raids of the Battle of Britain, for instance, the main objects of attack were not the densely populated residential areas which bore the brunt of the flying bomb offensive, and in the night raids which followed a large proportion of the population was protected by shelters. Flying bombs were in operation both day and night and many major incidents occurred during the busiest hours when streets and shops were full.

During the early period of the attacks, useful field work, directed by Professor S. Zuckerman, C.B., F.R.S., was undertaken by the Oxford Extra Mural Unit under the Ministry of Home Security Research and Experiments Department. A considerable number of London incidents were investigated and, from these, standardised casualty (killed and hospitalised) rates were worked out giving the average number of casualties to be expected per flying bomb strike in a neighbourhood with a population density of one person per 1,000 sq. ft. These standardised casualty rates were of the order of 10 by night and 20 by day, indicating that an area of the above relatively high population density could expect 100 fatal and hospitalised casualties per ten flying bomb incidents by night and some 200 by day. Of these at least 25 per cent. were likely to be fatal casualties, the remainder being hospital cases. Some critics regarded these estimates as more theoretical than practical.

The population density varied considerably but was generally well below one per 1,000 sq. ft., and the rate of killed and seriously injured (day and night incidents) up to September 1 proved to be 8·5 per incident, of which 25·8 per cent. were fatal casualties.

Casualties were similar in type to those caused by the parachute bomb in earlier raids and included a large number of lacerations and eye injuries, due to splintered glass and flying debris, especially in the earlier days of the attacks before the importance of taking cover was fully appreciated. Later, the habit of taking cover was accompanied by an increase in injuries from masonry, many who escaped death in the open being buried—some with fatal results, others with varying degrees of trauma—by collapsing buildings. It was recorded by one small E.M.S. hospital that of 259 flying bomb casualties admitted (of whom 18 died), 52 (of whom 9 died) were injured by masonry. In these cases injuries tended to be severe and included 23 fractures of limbs and pelvis (3 deaths) and 7 fractured skulls (6 deaths). Whereas some 20 per cent. of admissions and 50 per cent. of deaths of flying bomb victims in this hospital were due to falling masonry, over 40 per cent. of admissions were injured by glass, but only one death occurred among these. That there was not amongst the admissions a single case of crush syndrome with oedema of the injured part, anuria and uraemia was regarded by the Resident Surgical Officer as 'probably due in great measure to the increased speed of the A.R.P. rescue service, and possibly to a lessening in the enthusiasm for intravenous plasma therapy'.[17]

The following comparisons are based on an analysis of injured among surviving casualties from 122 flying bomb incidents and a series of 119 hospitalised casualties caused by parachute mines, and indicate a general similarity in types of injury caused by the respective weapons:

	Fractures Compound	Fractures Simple	Eye Injuries	Lacerations	Others
	per cent.	per cent.	per cent.	per cent.	per cent.
Parachute mines	8	33	14	29	16
Flying bombs	15	30	19	26	10

	Glass	Other flying debris	Other causes
Parachute mines	25	13	62
Flying bombs	30	20	50

At no time during the flying bomb attacks were the casualty services fully extended and no strain was imposed on E.M.S. hospitals by the number of injured admitted for treatment. Indeed, hospitals were affected more by material damage to their premises and by the consequent loss of beds.

Damage to Hospitals. The regularity with which hospitals suffered throughout the flying bomb ordeal was remarkable. They had been among the earliest victims of the attacks, as many as seven being damaged in one night. Several were hit in the first week, including St. Mary Abbot's L.C.C. Hospital, Kensington, at 4.30 a.m. on June 17, when 5 members of the staff and 13 patients were killed and 18 staff and 10 patients injured. The children's isolation block, night nurses' home and central block of the nurses' home were completely demolished; four ward blocks were partly demolished. The hospital was evacuated and closed, involving the loss of 832 beds, of which 346 were eventually brought into use again. Another L.C.C. hospital—St. Olave's, Bermondsey—after being severely damaged, without casualties, on June 23, was again hit on August 13, when the pathological laboratory was demolished and further extensive damage was caused. Fortunately injuries to patients and staff were few and slight; but the hospital was evacuated and temporarily closed, with the loss of 570 beds, of which the majority were subsequently restored.

London County Council hospitals in the E.M.S. Scheme, of which there were 41 in the London Region, were involved in no less than 60 incidents, of which 15 were major incidents. Staff casualties amounted to 13 killed and 67 injured. The numbers of patients killed (26) and injured (24) were surprisingly low; but 1,271 beds were permanently and 4,528 temporarily lost.

The Royal Free Hospital, Gray's Inn Road, was another early victim. Damage was extensive and 140 patients had to be evacuated. Considering that the building had a direct hit, it was astonishing that only 5 persons were killed—a nurse, a kitchen maid, 2 men patients and a woman patient. Many more hospital incidents were to follow and by the end of October not less than 100 hospitals had been damaged. In the London Sectors alone 76 were damaged involving the permanent loss of some 2,600 beds, the temporary loss of over 6,000 beds and the evacuation of approximately 8,000 civilian patients to other Regions. Casualties among staff and patients were fortunately low. Of the staffs, only 24 were killed and 146 injured. Patients killed and injured numbered 138 and 1,155 respectively (see Plates XI to XV).

Blast Damage to Property. Severe damage was caused by blast. Over 700 'Key Point' incidents were recorded and in the London Region alone there were more than a million housing casualties. Over 25,500 houses were destroyed or damaged beyond repair and more than 52,000 were rendered uninhabitable; 77,000 were seriously damaged but habitable, and 873,000 less seriously damaged.[18]

Progress of the Attacks. Combined fighter, gun and balloon defences, which had brought down about one-third of the flying bombs launched during the first week of the bombardment, became so efficient that on one day, August 28, out of 101 bombs which approached the English Coast, 97 were destroyed and only 4 got through to London. By the end of August the main fight against this form of attack was practically won. With the Allied advance through France and into the Low Countries the attacks rapidly diminished in number and frequency. A few incidents occurred in East Anglia and Kent during the first week of September, but no V.1 bomb fell on London between August 31 and September 15, when the offensive was resumed on a small scale by night and London again came under fire. But it was not until 8 a.m. on Tuesday,

October 31, that London was again attacked by daylight, and 3 fatal and 15 seriously injured casualties resulted at West Ham.

Having lost their launching sites, the Germans were now adapting Heinkel aircraft as carriers for flying bombs, which were launched from over the North Sea in many subsequent attacks, several of which appeared to be directed against Norwich, until the range was again extended to London and the Thames Estuary.

These attacks, mostly by night, continued throughout the month of November, in which 264 flying bombs were plotted in operation, resulting in 101 incidents of which only 10 occurred in London. In December, attacks were on a smaller scale and by the middle of January 1945, they seemed to have come to an end. For six weeks not a single flying bomb struck. It was generally supposed by the public that this weapon had been finally abandoned in favour of the long-range rocket from which South-east England, and especially London, had been under attack for four and a half months. But early in March, flying bomb attacks were resumed, apparently with a new type of increased range, launched from land bases in Holland. They were short-lived and of little effect; 160 further bombs in operation succeeded in causing only 58 incidents —less than one-fourth of which occurred in London. Casualties were 26 fatal and 106 seriously injured, of which all but 4 fatal and 23 seriously injured were inflicted on London. The last attack was made on Thursday, March 29, 1945, when eleven bombs were plotted in operation and there were three incidents in Essex, one in Hertfordshire and one in Kent, all without casualties.

Over 9,000 flying bombs had been plotted, nearly 6,000 of them overland, and 5,609 incidents had resulted, of which 2,416 occurred in London and 3,193 in other Regions. Casualties amounted to 5,837 killed, 16,762 seriously injured and approximately 24,000 slightly injured; 92 per cent. of the fatal casualties, 91 per cent. of the seriously injured and 83 per cent. of the slightly injured occurred in the London Region.

Evacuation. The flying bombs' toll in killed and injured would undoubtedly have been higher but for the resumption of officially arranged evacuation. Some 818,000 people left the London area, including 228,000 mothers and expectant mothers, 537,000 children and 53,000 old, invalid and blind persons.[19]

Evacuation of Hospital Patients. The extensive damage which was being caused to hospitals and the consequent temporary or permanent loss of beds made it expedient in the interests of the patients to carry out a partial evacuation of the London hospitals especially those in the areas receiving the greatest punishment from these missiles.

Consequently, organised evacuation began on August 3, 1944, and continued till August 30, during which period over 13,000 patients were transferred in ambulance trains from hospitals in the danger areas, chiefly to hospitals in the North, West and Midlands, and some to Scotland. Full details of the distribution of the patients sent to Scotland will be found in the Scottish E.M.S. History (Volume II, Part I, Chapter 6).

As in previous evacuations many complaints were made by friends and relatives of the patients, but the great majority realised that these moves were necessary. Arrangements made to keep relatives informed of patients' location and progress were generally satisfactory, although difficulties arose here and there owing to errors in the nominal rolls. The chief cause of complaint was that—except in special cases, such as patients on the dangerously ill list—relatives could not obtain free travel vouchers for visiting, this concession being considered inexpedient by the Ministry because the distances involved were long and the railways were already overcrowded.

In September, after consultation with the hospital authorities in the London area, the Ministry instructed the Regional Hospital Officers[20] to make arrangements for the gradual return to London of evacuated patients, priority to be given to:

(*a*) Patients occupying beds in acute hospitals required for battle casualties or to meet the needs of the local civilian sick;
(*b*) Children's units;
(*c*) Tuberculous patients and groups of chronic sick who had been evacuated with staff.

These groups of patients were to be moved back as ambulance trains were available.

This gradual movement was accelerated after the end of hostilities in Europe, when instructions were issued[21] to return all hospital patients, including those evacuated in 1939-40, to the areas of origin responsible for their maintenance.

'BOMB ALLEY'

Although London was the main objective of the flying bomb attacks, the counties of Kent and Essex, especially the former, necessarily suffered severely from being in the direct line of approach of the majority of these missiles. Large numbers fell short of their objective through defects in their mechanism, but many more were shot down by fighters and A.A. batteries.

The following story of the effect of these defensive activities in Region 12 is of interest:

Although the remarkable success of the defences saved many citizens from wounds or death and much property from damage or destruction in the London Region, a price had unavoidably to be paid by other Regions in which flying bombs were intercepted and exploded in the air or brought down before reaching the target area, but where the same amount of explosive caused less human and material damage.

Especially was this the case in the South-eastern (No. 12) Region (comprising Kent, Sussex and Surrey, less portions of Kent and Surrey in the London (No. 5) Region), which contained the thirty-mile wide 'bomb alley' running north-west from the Beachy Head, Dungeness and Folkestone coastline right up to the target of London from Dartford in the east, round to Walton and Weybridge in the west. This Region was involved from the beginning of the attacks on June 13, 1944. The first four weeks, with a rising casualty rate and a daily average of 60 was the phase of the fighter plane, the inland gun battery and balloon barrage. The second four weeks, with the daily casualty average falling to 51, saw the policy of evacuating the main flying bomb 'lanes', coupled with the use of table shelters for those remaining, and the transfer of the gun batteries to the coastline, beginning to tell. In the third four weeks the fuller effect of these tactics was shown in the reduction of the daily casualty rate to 27. With the military capture of the European launching sites the daily rate fell to one for another month, after which casualties were few and intermittent until the attacks ceased.

The number of flying bombs recorded by this Region during the twelve weeks of the main attack was 3,576. Of these 1,011 (28·3 per cent.) were brought down in the sea and 1,942 (54·3 per cent.) fell on land without causing casualties. Many of them had been exploded in the air. The remaining 623 (17·3 per cent) inflicted casualties in the Region, but fortunately approximately 77 per cent. of these casualty incidents occurred in rural districts, in which the casualty rate per 1,000 acres was only 1·2 compared with 4·1 in urban districts, 6·0 in municipal boroughs, 5·6 in county boroughs and 1·8 in the Region as a whole.

The Region's casualties for this period were:

Killed	326 (0·1 per land strike	0·5 per casualty producing strike)
Seriously injured	955 (0·4 ,, ,,	,, 1·5 ,, ,, ,, ,,)
Slightly injured	2,599 (1·0 ,, ,,	,, 4·2 ,, ,, ,, ,,)
Total casualties	3,880 (1·5 ,, ,,	,, 6·2 ,, ,, ,, ,,)

Of the casualties 58·8 per cent. occurred in rural districts and of these 9 per cent. were killed, 26 per cent. seriously injured, and 65 per cent. slightly injured.

During the twelve weeks of the main attacks the Region experienced from 7 to 8 casualty incidents per 24 hours. Casualties averaged approximately 6 per casualty-producing flying bomb, 4 slightly injured and 2 seriously injured, 1 of these was killed for every 2 incidents. In the first four weeks most of the casualties occurred at night, but in the second and third phases an increasing majority of flying bombs fell during working hours. The decentralisation of rescue and first-aid resources, that was necessary for scattered incidents, was widely achieved by the principle of the 'flying squad on limited patrol', which, with the Light

Medical Unit, made the ideal team. The rescue and ambulance teams that dealt with an incident were often the first to locate it. To quote from a report by one of the Region's Casualty Service Officers, Dr. H. N. Garrus:

'Often early information would reach Control or depot of the general direction of an incident—i.e. whether this was near built-up property—although in rural areas the precise location and the number of casualties necessarily took longer to come in. During this period the flying bomb squad nearest the known direction mobilised and patrolled in an agreed area, keeping Control informed. Such decentralisation in an extensively built-up area subject to the multiple incidents of bombing raids would quickly spell disaster; with single-casualty incidents from missiles whose undeviating course is visible at all hours, in areas almost wholly manned by part-time staff, it is the only effective and economical method.'

Rescue work in rural areas was largely confined to removing surface debris and casualties, often from isolated and lightly built dwellings:

'The light rescue work involved largely obviated the need for sodium bicarbonate and morphia, or for full first aid, except for the few who had to be sent a long journey to hospital. There never was any shortage of medical equipment, although it was necessary to issue liq. adrenalin to upgraded first-aid points as a few A.T.S. urticarial reactions were reported on the second injection.

Surprisingly little use was made of the veritable network of all types of first-aid points, both official and unofficial. It was quicker to deal with casualties near the incident with the Light Medical Unit and Rescue, taking the rest direct by ambulance or sitting case car to first-aid post or hospital. Every general practitioner is a potential L.M.U. and if kept in the picture is one of the key men.'

For illustrations of the work of the Civil Defence services in dealing with the casualties caused by pilotless planes see Plates XVI to XXIV.

THE LONG-RANGE ROCKET (V.2)

The lull in aerial attacks that followed the remarkable success of the defences against flying bombs towards the end of the summer, was disturbed on Friday, September 8, by the fall—at Chiswick—of the first long-range rocket to be used against London and South-east England. In this new weapon, weighing 12 tons and containing an explosive warhead of about 2,000 lb., yet attaining an altitude of 60–70 miles and having a range of over 200 miles, the Germans had produced a projectile which could not be intercepted in action and of whose approach, at a speed much greater than that of sound, no warning could be given.

Against attacks with such a weapon there could be little defence other than the destruction or capture of launching sites and the throttling of supplies by dislocating communications. Neither active fighter plane nor passive balloon could check the rocket's flight. A.A. guns were silent, the siren alarm no longer sounded; nothing was heard of the hurtling projectile before its impact and explosion. Deep shelters were used to some extent as a precaution against night attacks, but taking cover on a large scale by day was not practicable. This was an important factor in producing higher casualty rates per rocket strike than those of the flying bombs.

But the absence of warning was to some extent compensated by the fact that the public accepted the position, and in general, the daily round was broken only at the time and in the immediate neighbourhood of an incident. The fall of several rockets at short intervals in the same area would naturally cause local alarm, but in general, there was less interruption of work, less preoccupation and apprehension than when flying bombs were known to be, or were actually heard and seen, on their way.

London appeared to be the target of V.2, as of V.1. Within a fortnight of the first strike, of some 50 rockets launched, 24 had fallen on land—16 in Greater London, 7 in Essex and 1 in Sussex. These early attacks provided pointers, but hardly sufficient evidence upon which accurately to assess the potentialities of this weapon. In one incident it had pierced a concrete-surfaced road and made a crater 20 ft. deep and 40 ft. in diameter and thus showed great penetrating power. Blast seemed to be forced upwards, causing less extensive damage than the flying bomb, although considerable damage to houses was caused by ground vibration. All the fatal casualties (61) and all but four of the seriously injured (183) within the first two weeks of the attacks occurred in the London area. Here it appeared that not less than 4 fatal and 11 seriously injured casualties per rocket strike must be expected—approximately double the casualty rates from flying bombs—and this was borne out by subsequent events. By the time the 500th long-range rocket had struck, four months later, casualties in Greater London had mounted to 1,241 killed (5·2 per strike), and 2,943 seriously injured (12·5). Although more than half (264) of the rockets had fallen outside the London Region the casualties in other Regions were few in comparison, amounting to only 102 killed (0·4 per strike) and 276 seriously injured (1·0). Combined fatal and seriously injured casualties for the 500 incidents amounted to 4,562, i.e. 9·1 per strike.

Up to this time the proportions of V.2 (rocket) incidents and casualties occurring in the London area were remarkably similar to those of the previous V.1 (flying bomb) attacks. As the following table shows London experienced less than 50 per cent. of the incidents but suffered over 90 per cent. of the casualties in each case:

	Incidents		*Killed*		*Seriously injured*	
	London per cent.	Elsewhere per cent.	London per cent.	Elsewhere per cent.	London per cent.	Elsewhere per cent.
V.1	45.6	54·4	93·6	6·4	92·4	7·6
V.2	47·2	52·8	92·4	7·6	91·4	8·6

Casualties were sometimes surprisingly few in comparison with the extent of damage to small, densely populated property. In Poplar, for instance, a rocket on the night of Friday, November 24, demolished over 40 dwellings and damaged over 1,000 others; but the casualties were only 18 fatal and 53 seriously injured. Over 1,500 houses were damaged in East Ham on Sunday, January 28; the fatal and seriously injured civilian casualties were respectively 13 and 30. From Whitstable, Kent, only 1 fatal and 4 seriously injured casualties were reported when 300–350 houses were seriously damaged and 1,000 slightly damaged on Monday, January 15.

These incidents are mentioned as showing that casualties were sometimes very much lighter than might have been expected; but there were, of course, many other rocket strikes of far more serious consequence. The worst incident occurred on Saturday, November 25, at New Cross, when shortly after 12.30 p.m. a Woolworth's store received a direct hit. The store was crowded, mostly with women and children—160 persons were killed and 108 seriously injured. The next heaviest casualty list amounted to 110 killed and 123 seriously injured, when at 11.10 a.m. on Thursday, March 8, 1945, a rocket struck Farringdon Market Buildings, Finsbury, and penetrated to the L.N.E.R. depot below (see Plate XXV). The last morning of the attacks, March 27, was marked by a serious incident at Stepney, when two five-storey blocks of flats were destroyed, one block partly destroyed, and a hospital seriously damaged. There were 134 fatal casualties and 49 seriously injured. On the afternoon of that day the last rocket fell, at Orpington, Kent, killing 1 person and injuring 23. Plate XXVI gives an excellent impression of the damage caused by a typical V.2 strike in a built-up area.

Including a certain number which burst in the air too high to cause casualties, 1,102 long-range rocket projectiles (L.R.R.P.) which reached this country had inflicted a combined total of 9,415 fatal and seriously injured casualties as shown below:

	Number of L.R.R.P.	Killed	Seriously injured	Slightly injured	Total casualties
London region	516	2,503 (4·9)	6,050 (11·7)	13,219 (25·6)	21,772 (42·2)
Other regions	586	221 (0·38)	641 (1·1)	1,891 (3·2)	2,753 (4·7)
Total	1,102	2,724 (2·5)	6,691 (6·1)	15,110 (13·7)	24,525 (22·3)

(Figures in brackets are casualties per L.R.R.P.)

Casualties sent to hospital spread over the twenty-nine weeks of the attacks, averaged only 231 per week.

In London 20 E.M.S. hospitals had been damaged, resulting in 633 beds being put out of use temporarily and 260 permanently—including

100 non-E.M.S. beds for chronic sick—and necessitating the transfer of 386 patients to other hospitals. Except for a few slightly injured, there were no casualties amongst hospital patients.

Hospital staffs suffered only 3 fatal, 2 seriously injured and 11 slightly injured casualties.

CROSS-CHANNEL SHELLING

No story of Britain under fire would be complete without reference to the ordeal of the inhabitants of Dover, Deal, Folkestone, Ramsgate and neighbouring villages under cross-channel shelling.

The first shell in the bombardment burst near Dover on August 12, 1940. By September 30, 1944, when it was officially announced that all long-range guns on the other side of the Channel had been captured, 2,226 shells had been recorded in Dover, 120 in Deal and 219 in Folkestone. Ramsgate was shelled seven times. Thanks to the alertness of observers and the efficiency of their warning, and still more to the safe shelter afforded by caves, casualties were not heavy. Although over 2,500 shells were recorded, excluding Ramsgate's unknown number, and nearly 6,000 properties were damaged, casualties amounted to only some 150 killed, 250 seriously injured and 400 slightly injured. Of these by far the greatest numbers (approximately 100 killed, 200 seriously injured and 220 slightly injured) occurred in Dover, which bore the brunt of the attacks. Here it appears that less than 25 per cent. of the shells were effective in producing casualties, i.e. it took approximately twenty shells to kill 1 person and injure 4, of whom 2 were seriously and 2 slightly injured. Thus the casualties from cross-channel shelling, compared with those inflicted by bombs, were few and, spread over a period of four years, clearly imposed no tax on E.M.S. resources within the area concerned. But the strain and stress borne by those who experienced the shelling over a long period were, of course, considerable and the fact that the area came to be known as 'Hellfire Corner' vividly suggests the far heavier losses which would have resulted had the population not been reduced by evacuation, and adequate shelter had not been available to those that remained.

TOTAL CASUALTIES IN UNITED KINGDOM

The first and second chapters of this History of the Emergency Medical Services are largely concerned with speculations and estimates regarding the numbers of air raid casualties to be expected in the event of war with Germany, and with the initial steps taken to provide for their accommodation and treatment. The development of aerial warfare and its application in Abyssinia and Spain had forced the conclusion that casualties would be extremely heavy. The possibility of a million seriously injured within a month of the outbreak of hostilities was admitted, and pre-war hospital accommodation was seen to be woefully

PERIOD OF ACTIVE OPERATIONS

inadequate for an influx of cases at the envisaged rate of 30,000 a day. This estimate was no wild guess but was based on the known strength of the Luftwaffe. That it was not unreasonable to anticipate such numbers became evident later, when casualties on a still heavier scale were inflicted by the Air Forces of the Allies in some of their concentrated attacks on certain German cities.

But the enemy failed to strike immediately after the declaration of war, when our cities were most vulnerable, and by the time their heavy air raids developed the Luftwaffe had lost much of its initial advantage. Thus, in contrast to those early fears of devastation, death and mutilation, the numbers in the following table of civilian casualties that actually occurred are seen to be mercifully light:

The table shows that there were 146,777 civilian casualties due to enemy action in the United Kingdom. Of these 60,595 were killed or missing, believed killed, and 86,182 were injured and detained in hospital. 49·3 per cent. of the fatal, 58·6 per cent. of the seriously injured and 54·8 per cent. of the total casualties occurred in the London Region. Of casualties amongst Civil Defence workers, on the other hand, the majority occurred outside London, 59·3 per cent. of the killed and 51·8 per cent. of the seriously injured being in other Regions. Of the 6,838 Civil Defence casualties 6,220 were men and 618 women.[22]

It will be noted that the table does not include slightly injured casualties, of whom 150,832 were recorded: 145,481 in England and Wales, 3,558 in Scotland and 1,793 in Northern Ireland. In addition, unrecorded numbers of civilians are known to have had their slight superficial injuries attended to in chemists' shops and by their own doctors without passing through the first-aid posts, etc., of the casualty services; but any estimate of these would be pure guess work (see Army Medical Services, Volume I, Chapter 6.)

The above figures reveal that hospitalised air raid casualties for the whole period of the war were fewer than the number which would have required admission in a single week had the pre-war estimates been realised.

The comparatively light demands made on its resources by air raid casualties enabled the E.M.S. to provide adequate medical and surgical care for civilian sick and various categories of war workers, and to fulfil what became its main function, viz. the treatment and restoration to health of Service casualties from overseas.

ACCOMMODATION IN HOSPITALS, 1944

E.M.S. Hospitals. By the end of 1944 the number of live hospitals in the E.M.S. had been reduced to 819—57 less than at the end of 1943—with a bed accommodation, including 42,208 reserves, of 249,137. Of these beds 153,228 were occupied: 16,383 by Service sick; 22,619 by Service casualties; 1,178 by civilian air raid casualties and 113,048 by

Air Raid Casualties in Great Britain and Northern Ireland
September 3, 1939 to May 31, 1945
(Excluding Casualties in the Armed Forces)

	KILLED					SERIOUSLY INJURED			
	Men	Women	Children	Uncl.	Totals	Men	Women	Children	Totals
London Region
Civil Defence General Services (while on duty)	506	61			567	1,024	125		1,149
Police (while on duty)	106	1			107	261	1		262
National Fire Service (while on duty)	285	9			294	720	19		739
Other civilians	12,063	13,516	3,326	17	28,922	20,342	23,757	4,258	48,357
	12,960	13,587	3,326	17	29,890	22,347	23,902	4,258	50,507
Other Regions
Civil Defence General Services (while on duty)	639	149			788	1,084	220		1,304
Police (while on duty)	183				183	302			302
National Fire Service (while on duty)	429	11			440	681	22		703
Other civilians	12,712	11,652	4,410	520	29,294	16,324	13,678	3,364	33,366
	13,963	11,812	4,410	520	30,705	18,391	13,920	3,364	35,675
Great Britain & Northern Ireland	26,923	25,399	7,736	537	60,595	40,738	37,822	7,622	86,182

civilian sick, both those for whose treatment the Ministry had from time to time accepted financial responsibility and others. Roughly two-thirds of this reduction had been effected during the last quarter of the year.

Auxiliary Hospitals and Convalescent Homes: Convalescent Hospitals. On September 1, 1944, the War Organisation of the British Red Cross Society and Order of St. John of Jerusalem was controlling 234 auxiliary hospitals and convalescent homes, equipped with 14,334 beds, 10,256 of which were occupied, a considerable increase in bed accommodation over the previous year, mainly accounted for by the provision of emergency beds at existing convalescent homes following 'D' day. In addition, provision had been made for a further 600 beds required to complete the 15,000 beds finally asked for by the Ministry of Health. Beds in the five* convalescent hospitals for officers totalled 237, with an additional 91 for 'other ranks'. Owing to increased pressure on accommodation it was hoped to open a further convalescent hospital in the South of England.

Service Hospitals. At the end of April the numbers of Service hospitals—with bedstates—were as follows:

	Number of Hospitals	Occupied Beds	Vacant Beds	Total Beds
Royal Navy	18	3,566	2,424	5,990
Army	59	10,613	4,252	14,865
Royal Air Force	26†	5,142	2,523	7,665
Canadian Army	16	5,965	3,789	9,754

The twelve Ministry of Pensions hospitals were in all equipped with 5,781 beds, of which 3,286 were occupied and 2,495 vacant.

CIVILIAN ADMISSIONS, 1944

As in the case of the previous war-years only the figures given in Appendix VIII for 'Enemy Action' casualties are available and these including 540 Civil Defence and 115 Merchant Navy Personnel amounted to 19,065 during the year.‡

The estimate of admissions of the other civilian categories for 1944 will be found in Appendix VII.

During 1944, Service casualty and sickness cases admitted to E.M.S. hospitals included the following:

Royal Navy (including W.R.N.S. 1,175)	18,265‡
Army (including Women's Services, 15,559)	128,443§
Royal Air Force (including W.A.A.F., 12,053‖)	56,200‖
Canadian Army	9,351

---

* Includes one Scottish.
† Includes R.A.F. hospitals in Scotland and Northern Ireland.
‡ Calculated from one-in-five sample, as in previous chapter.
§ Direct admissions only.
‖ Great Britain and Northern Ireland.

A relatively small number of Allied Service patients were also treated in E.M.S. hospitals.

The admissions to convalescent homes and auxiliary hospitals in the year ending September 2, 1944, were as follows:

British Service		Allied Forces	Civilians		Civil Defence Workers		Total
Male	Female	Male	Male	Female	Male	Female	
104,519	8,323	2,386	3,664	5,336	1,103	811	126,142

Convalescent hospitals treated 2,754 patients, including 102 from Allied forces.

ACCOMMODATION IN HOSPITALS, 1945

E.M.S. Hospitals. Although the reduction of hospitals had naturally been considerable during the year 1945, particularly in the period March 2 to June 1—when numbers dropped from 810 to 538—there still remained in the E.M.S. 458 live hospitals at the close of the year. The total bed accommodation in these hospitals was 152,240, including 19,325 reserves, with a bed occupancy of 11,962 Service sick; 7,618 Service casualties; 92 civilian air raid casualties and 75,975 civilian sick: 95,647 occupied beds in all. Bed accommodation represents 61 per cent. of that at the end of the previous year, and Service and civilian patients respectively 50 per cent. and 67 per cent. of the corresponding figures for 1944.

Auxiliary Hospitals and Convalescent Homes: Convalescent Hospitals. On September 1, 1945, only 139 auxiliary hospitals and convalescent homes, with a bed occupation of 5,699, were still fully functioning as compared with 234 a year previously. One further convalescent hospital for officers had been added to the five* already in commission, and until August all remained open. During August and September three were closed. Beds in the remaining three numbered 135.

Service Hospitals. (a) At the end of April 1945, the numbers of Service hospitals—with bedstates—were as follows:

	Number of Hospitals	Occupied beds	Vacant beds	Total beds
Royal Navy	19	4,654	2,005	6,659
Army	51	8,171	4,510	12,681
Royal Air Force	23†	2,925	5,758	8,683
Canadian Army	15	8,080	2,604	10,684

In Ministry of Pensions hospitals—still twelve strong—bed accommodation was as follows: 3,431 occupied beds, 1,706 vacant beds: 5,137 in all.

---

* Includes one Scottish.
† Includes R.A.F. hospitals in Scotland and Northern Ireland.

PERIOD OF ACTIVE OPERATIONS

(b) A comparison of the above figures with the statement below, indicating the position at the close of 1945, shows the gradual decline in British Service hospital accommodation and the rapid drop in that of the Canadian Military Medical Services:

	Number of Hospitals	Occupied beds	Vacant beds	Total beds
Royal Navy	17	3,525	2,817	6,342
Army	42	7,533	4,314	11,847
Royal Air Force	21*	3,877	3,296	7,173
Canadian Army	4	2,166	1,278	3,444

Bed accommodation in the eleven existing Ministry of Pensions hospitals totalled 5,035 beds, of which 2,301 were occupied and 2,734 vacant.

The table overleaf summarises the bedstates in E.M.S. hospitals at various dates throughout the war, omitting figures at dates for which returns are not available:

CIVILIAN ADMISSIONS, 1945

The admissions of 'Enemy Action' civilian casualties (see Appendix VIII) including 20 Civil Defence and 45 Merchant Navy personnel amounted to 3,370 during the year.†

For the estimated admissions of other civilian categories, see Appendix VII.

The 1945 admissions to E.M.S. hospitals included the following Service casualty and sickness cases:

Royal Navy (including W.R.N.S. 820)	10,325†
Army (including Women's Services, 11,795)	122,544‡
Royal Air Force (includes W.A.A.F., 6,215§)	36,858§
Canadian Army	1,928

No figures for 1945 admissions of Allied Service patients to E.M.S. hospitals are available.

Auxiliary hospitals and convalescent homes in the year ending September 2, 1945, admitted:

British Service		Allied Forces	Civilians		Civil Defence Workers		Total
Male	Female	Male	Male	Female	Male	Female	
92,977	6,012	2,966	1,837	2,828	136	204	106,960

Convalescent hospitals treated 1,562 patients, including 233 officers from Allied forces.

---

* Includes R.A.F. hospitals in Scotland and Northern Ireland.
† Calculated from one-in-five sample, as in previous chapter.
‡ Direct admissions only.
§ Great Britain and Northern Ireland.

The Bedstates in Emergency Medical Service Hospitals at Various Dates

(1) Date	(2) Live Hospitals in the Emergency Medical Service	(3) Occupied beds	(4) Vacant beds	(5) Reserve A beds*	(6) Reserve B beds†	(7) Total beds including Reserves	(8) E.M.S. beds (inc. in Column 7)	(9) 'Category' Patients‡ (inc. in Column 3)	(10) Other Patients (Civilian sick) (inc. in Column 3)
Outbreak of war	2,370	—	163,500	—	—	—	—		
End of 1940	1,104	162,577	78,913	23,582	31,683	296,755	197,678		
" " 1941	991	153,580	79,223	22,433	32,966	288,202	185,969		
" " 1942	910	149,622	65,612	26,881	36,646	278,761	107,307		
" " 1943	876	156,676	54,583	25,368	36,677	273,304	106,157	40,049	116,627
" " 1944	819	153,228	53,701	18,312	23,896	249,137	108,418	55,614	97,614
" " 1945	458	95,647	37,268	19,325		152,240	62,197	29,806	66,841

* Immediately available beds for which no additional staff would be required.

† Stored beds for use of which additional staff would be required.

‡ Classes of patients for whose treatment the Ministry of Health from time to time accepted financial responsibility. (See Form 227 (Revised) —Appendix IV).

UNITED STATES MILITARY HOSPITALS IN THE UNITED KINGDOM*

The reciprocal arrangements which had previously been made with the combatant services of the United Kingdom and Canada for pooling medical resources and hospital accommodation when expedient or necessary in grave emergencies were extended to include the Forces from the United States early in the year 1942. (See Chapter 4.)

The Historical Division of the Office of the Surgeon-General, United States Army (as the result of agreements entered into at the meeting of the Commonwealth Medical Histories Liaison Committee held in Ottawa in September, 1947, at which the Medical Historians of the U.S. Army and Navy were present as observers), supplied full information as to the number of hospitals and bed accommodation available in the United Kingdom throughout the war.

This permits of the inclusion in the E.M.S. History of a comprehensive picture of the total accommodation available in U.S.A. hospitals from time to time for the treatment of war casualties of all kinds in addition to U.S.A. casualties.

U.S. HOSPITALS AND BED ACCOMMODATION

The total number of military hospitals established by the United States authorities in the United Kingdom was 122 with a normal bed capacity of 107,551, and an expanded bed capacity of 148,609. Of these, 109 were in England and Wales with a normal capacity of 102,306, and an expanded capacity of 143,022; including five tented hospitals with 4,480 beds and seven convalescent hospitals with 17,575 beds. The rate of expansion in numbers of these hospitals and beds throughout the United Kingdom, shown in the table below, was mainly due to the foresight and enterprise of Major General Paul R. Hawley, Chief Surgeon, European Theatre of Operations, at whose instigation hutted hospitals taken over by the U.S.A. were greatly extended:

Date	Number of Hospitals	Total beds	Occupied beds	Vacant beds
April 30, 1942	1	350	310	40
April 30, 1943	20	12,191	3,524	8,667
April 30, 1944	74	55,782	29,356	26,426
April 30, 1945	95	95,800	69,298	26,502

(*Note*.—The peak period of U.S.A. hospital accommodation in the United Kingdom was in February 1945, when 99 general hospitals and 5 large convalescent hospitals provided a total of 138,160 beds and the peak patient census was attained on February 8, 1945, when 129,289 patients were under treatment.)

---

* See Army Medical Services, Volume I, Chapter 2.

During the war six E.M.S. hospitals containing 3,300 beds were taken over by the U.S.A. The bed accommodation in these hospitals was permanently expanded in hutted additions by 3,122 and by 2,852 emergency beds in tents making a total of 9,274 beds. Two other hospitals containing 1,904 beds were taken over from the R.A.M.C. who had previously taken them over from the E.M.S.

THE TREATMENT OF U.S.A. MILITARY PERSONNEL IN E.M.S. HOSPITALS

United States Army provision of hospitals in Great Britain lagged considerably behind the flow of U.S. troops into the country. A 250-bed station hospital accompanied the first contingent which landed at Belfast on January 26, 1942, but did not become operational until March 9, 1942, at Londonderry. The first U.S. general hospital to function in the United Kingdom opened in Belfast in the latter part of May. Two more general hospitals opened in July, at Oxford and Mansfield in England, and by the end of 1942 some 4,900 fixed hospital beds were available for the United States troop strength of approximately 135,000.

Throughout the whole of 1942, U.S. Army medical authorities were cognisant of the inadequacy of their own fixed hospitals fully to care for the American force being assembled in Great Britain, particularly in view of the wide dispersion of that force. Accordingly, early arrangements were made to admit U.S. troops to Emergency Medical Service and British and Canadian Army, Navy and Air Force hospitals. No charges were made for this service, which also included out-patient and necessary dental treatment. In return, British and Canadian Army, Navy, and Air Force personnel were accorded similar medical service in U.S. military hospitals, as they became available, to the furthest possible extent.

Unfortunately, available records are not sufficient to show the total number of U.S. military personnel treated in Emergency Medical Service hospitals located in Great Britain over any given period. Accurate patient accounting was not begun until the autumn of 1942 and the available statistics covering only a one-year period, are sketchy at best. They do not show a distinction between E.M.S. hospitals in England, Wales, Scotland, and Northern Ireland, and, in some instances, are believed to include U.S. patients in hospitals not belonging to the E.M.S.

The available figures are as follows: In mid-August of 1942, 172 U.S. patients were reported in E.M.S. hospitals throughout the United Kingdom. On September 4 this census was reported as 158, and on October 9, it had increased to 590. After the latter date the records show only the total admissions from November 12, 1942, to October 15, 1943, as 2,056.

This eleven-month tabulation of admissions to E.M.S. hospitals, plus the three separate census figures previously cited, produces a total of 2,976 U.S. troops known to have received treatment at Emergency Medical Service hospitals over a fourteen-month period. It is reasonably certain that a fairly large number was also admitted to E.M.S. facilities in the six and a half months when U.S. troops were in Great Britain before mid-August, 1942, and a smaller group in late 1943 and in 1944. But no clues, either to total numbers or areas of treatment, are available in the records.

THE TREATMENT OF BRITISH CIVILIAN AIR RAID CASUALTIES IN U.S.A. MILITARY HOSPITALS

It is reasonably certain that only a very small number of British civilian air raid casualties received treatment in United States Army hospitals in Great Britain. No mention of such treatment is made in the headquarters reports submitted by Army medical authorities in the United Kingdom and a search of the unit records of hospitals serving in metropolitan areas and in the South of England failed to disclose any specific numbers.

The records of one U.S. hospital, the 16th Station Hospital, which operated in the Vincent Square Infants' Hospital in London, show the admission and emergency treatment of an unspecified number of British civilian air raid victims on three separate occasions in 1944. The first was the six-day period, February 19–25, a period marked by the renewal of the Luftwaffe attacks on London, and the second and third came on the nights of March 15 and July 3. The total civilian admissions were less than 75 for the three dates.

This brief citation is the only mention of the treatment of civilian air raid casualties in U.S. hospitals contained in the records. It is believed that had such treatment been at all extensive, it would have been recorded in the annual historical accounts submitted by the U.S. hospital units. It must be assumed that other instances, if they did occur, were infrequent.

BRITISH ASSISTANCE IN AMBULANCE TRANSPORT

The U.S. War Department had no record of the number of United States Army personnel carried in ambulance transport of the British Emergency Medical Services, but assumed it to be correct that 47,319 U.S. Service personnel were carried in E.M.S. ambulance trains. (See Chapter 8.)

Several British organisations helped the U.S. evacuation services by transporting patients within the United Kingdom. The Emergency Medical Services placed one of their trains at the disposal of the U.S.

Army Medical Department in the middle of 1944. In addition, the entire evacuation of U.S. Air Force crash landings and forced landings in the British Southampton Command was jointly conducted by the E.M.S. and the Royal Army Medical Corps.

THE MEDICAL SERVICES OF OTHER ALLIED FORCES IN GREAT BRITAIN

The withdrawal of the Allied military forces from the Continent in 1940 was followed by the establishment of war-time National Administrations by our Allies in Great Britain. These administrative services were concerned on the one hand with the continued share in the conflict by those naval, military and air forces which remained available or later became available to them as the war progressed, and, on the other hand, with the arrangements for the medical care of their nationals, both military and civil.

At first Allied sick and wounded were largely cared for in British hospitals, but gradually, as medical and nursing personnel became of sufficient strength to deal with the problem, separate hospitals, sanatoria and convalescent homes were set aside for their use, in some cases with the collaboration of the British Authorities and sometimes also with the help of voluntary societies, including the British Red Cross.

Information on the working of the Allied Medical Services is far from complete. At the time when such data as are necessary to present an adequate account of their activities could best have been given, i.e. at the end of the war, the Allied nationals were hastening to return to their own countries. The Free French Naval Forces, Belgium, Norway and Poland did however supply such information, which is now briefly summarised. The medical work carried out in this country by the National Administrations of the Netherlands, Czechoslovakia, and Yugoslavia was on similar though less extensive lines.

BELGIUM

The Belgian Army Medical Service in Great Britain was established in May 1940, with the arrival in England of 350 Belgian sick and wounded soldiers evacuated from the Continent. The medical staff at first was small, but grew as additional medical and nursing staff arrived. At first all the sick and wounded were found beds in British hospitals. Later some hospital facilities were established in Carmarthen with a Belgian staff of 3 medical officers, 3 N.C.O.s, 3 medical students, a qualified nurse and 4 nursing sisters. A hospital, with 30 beds was afterwards established at Buttlers Marston. Nevertheless, the majority of Belgian sick and wounded were treated in British hospitals in agreement with the British and Belgian Authorities. The number of Belgians treated in British hospitals increased during the war as will be shown by the following table of bed occupancy:

1940	5·460 bed days
1941	14·100 ,, ,,
1942	24·740 ,, ,,
1943	37·600 ,, ,,
1944	36·765 ,, ,.
1945 (first quarter)	16·349 ,, ,,

A rehabilitation centre was set up at Wimbledon in 1941, which subsequently became a surgical unit with modern equipment given by the British Red Cross.

The Belgian Authorities also established a pharmaceutical service specially adapted to the needs of their medical staff and more in conformity with the Belgian pharmacopoeia.

The arrangements carried out by the Belgian Authorities, either in conjunction with British hospitals or in their own institutions, had to cover a growing number of civilian as well as Service sick and wounded owing to the varying influx of refugees during the war.

THE FREE FRENCH NAVAL FORCES

It was in June 1940, that all Frenchmen able to do so were called upon to unite in continuing the struggle. The headquarters of the Free French Forces in London, set up immediately afterwards, had at first so small a staff that there was only one medical department for all three branches of the Fighting Services. Subsequently, a naval headquarters was set up with a Medical Directorate. But there were few medical officers, no medical establishments and only one sick bay in one warship. Consequently, from July 1940 to July 1941, all naval sick and wounded were treated in British naval hospitals. This diffusion of French wounded with consequent language difficulties, was resolved to a certain extent by the opening of a medical centre for Free French Forces at St. John's Wood, London, the premises of which had been generously offered by the Duchess of Hamilton. This medical centre functioned as a 'sorting office', where patients were examined by a French medical officer, who decided whether the patient should be treated by French doctors or whether he should be admitted to a British hospital.

The medical centre had 35 beds and a special wing for cases of venereal disease. It also included dental and pharmaceutical services. The Centre later became known as the 'Albert Calmette Medical Centre'.

Between November 1940, and April 1943, the four following convalescent homes were established:

For convalescents requiring medical supervision
- *In England*
  'Pasteur-Lister Naval Convalescent Home', 'Butlers Court', Beaconsfield.
- *In Scotland*
  Knockderry Castle Auxiliary Hospital, Cove, Helensburgh, Dumbartonshire.

For convalescents not requiring supervision
- *In England*
  'Steep House', Petersfield, Hants.
- *In Scotland*
  Quothquhan Lodge, Biggar, Lanarkshire.

The distribution between England and Scotland of these provisions for medical care saved much time. Patients for instance from corvettes and submarines operating in Northern waters could be treated without sending them long distances to Southern England.

Particular attention was given to cases of pulmonary tuberculosis. During the latter part of 1940 and in 1941 all cases of pulmonary tuberculosis among Free French sailors were treated in British sanatoria. But the adverse affect of isolation in these institutions, where often they could not make themselves understood, soon became evident; morale suffered and the therapeutic value of treatment was lessened.

British sanatoria also were increasingly overburdened as the war progressed and the provision of a sanatorium for the Free French Naval Forces became urgent. Property was acquired at Beaconsfield, adjoining the Pasteur-Lister Convalescent Home, and was equipped with modern appliances. The first patients were received in February 1942. Though the sanatorium, 'Highfield', accommodated 40 patients, it was soon found to be too small, and adjoining property was subsequently acquired and equipped with 40 beds, this annexe being reserved for cases under observation and for non-infectious cases.

Some 7,500 French sailors served under the Cross of Lorraine during the war. The arrangements for their medical care, described above, together with the provision of well-equipped base sick quarters in London, Clapham Common, Smethwick, Cowes, Greenock and Dundee, proved very satisfactory and liaison with the British Naval Authorities and hospital services was most cordial and helpful.

NORWAY

The Norwegian Medical Services in Great Britain comprised:
(a) The Armed Forces Medical Units, and
(b) The Public Health Service.

(a) The Armed Forces Medical Units consisted of 74 medical officers and 70 sisters and nurses. All Norwegian units serving in the Allied

Forces had their own medical personnel. The medical service was organised on the same lines as the British. Indeed, the Norwegian Air Force medical service was incorporated in that of the R.A.F.

There were 3 Norwegian hospitals with 220 beds, and 1 small 'Brigade Hospital' with 50 beds. In addition, there was a general hospital of 160 beds operated in collaboration with the Norwegian Public Health Service. Norwegian sick or wounded were sometimes accommodated in British hospitals. Up to May 1944, the approximate number of Norwegian Service men killed outside Norway was 795, and about 2,000 were wounded. Most of the casualties occurred in the Navy and Air Force.

Apart from casualties, the gravest problems confronting the Norwegian Medical Services were tuberculosis and venereal diseases. About 150 beds were available in Norwegian hospitals for the treatment of tuberculosis.

All expenditure incurred by the Norwegian Forces in Great Britain during the war was met by the Norwegian Government from income derived from the Norwegian Merchant Navy.

(b) The Norwegian Public Health Service in Great Britain was set up to provide health and medical attention for seamen of the Mercantile Marine. The first Medical Department was established in London in June 1940, and there were four others at Newcastle, Glasgow, Liverpool and Cardiff, the ports which had the greatest Norwegian traffic during the war.

A number of small civilian hospitals were established, two in London, one near Edinburgh, one near Glasgow and one near Liverpool. Two convalescent homes were also in operation.

Economically, the medical services were on the lines of those in Norway in peace-time. All seamen and other civilians employed by the Norwegian Government were members of the Government-organised Sickness Insurance Fund. The premiums of the members covered part of the cost, and the Government contributed the remainder.

A number of Norwegian doctors served in British hospitals during the war and were with British units in the Navy, Army and Royal Air Force from Iceland and Spitzbergen to Italy and Africa.

A small number of Norwegian medical students studied at British Universities during the war.

POLAND

Of the Polish medical officers who arrived in Great Britain during the war, some were employed on the Polish War Establishment, others were directed to Polish refugee work in various countries and some eighty-seven were placed at the disposal of the British War Office. Other Polish medical officers were released from the Polish Army and worked with the Polish and Allied Merchant Navies.

One of the main problems was the shortage of female nursing staff which was solved in part by the setting up of the Polish Women's Auxiliary Service.

The British Authorities furnished the equipment of the Polish Army Medical Services and assisted in the setting up of Polish Departments in various British hospitals and convalescent homes.

Among Polish medical establishments in Great Britain were the military hospital of 430 beds at Taymouth Castle, Aberfeldy, Perthshire, a casualty clearing station of 120 beds at Dupplin Castle, Perth, district reception stations and dental centres at Kirkcaldy, Falkirk, North Berwick and Edinburgh, a hospital for disabled soldiers at Auchentroig near Stirling, a hospital for the treatment of tuberculosis at Callowhill, Newcastle, and the Paderewski Hospital of 120 beds in Edinburgh, which was run in connexion with the Polish Medical Faculty in that city.

It is unique for a foreign Faculty of Medicine to exist in any country. Such a unique case, however, was the establishment of a Polish Faculty at the University of Edinburgh during the war. It was formed in 1941 as a result of an agreement signed between the Vice-Chancellor and Principal of the University and the Minister of the Interior of the exiled Polish Government in Great Britain.

The Polish Army, which had escaped from France in 1940, was largely concentrated in Scotland, and arrangements had been made for Polish medical officers to receive instruction in British military medical methods by attending the military hospital at Edinburgh and for certain officers to work in the medical departments of the University. Subsequently, to meet language difficulties, post-graduate courses given by Polish teachers were inaugurated, and this led to the establishment of a Polish School of Medicine. The Polish Faculty was inaugurated in the McEwan Hall on March 22, 1941. The first Dean was Dr. Antoni Jurasz, who was later succeeded by Dr. Tadeusz Rozalski. The staff consisted of 8 professors, 9 senior lecturers, 21 senior assistants, and 8 junior assistants.

The School began with 77 students, 47 of whom were serving in the Forces. About 30 had completed their studies in Poland but had not passed their examinations, and refresher courses were arranged for them. For the second academic year there were 120 students. The first to receive the diploma M.B., B.Ch. was a pilot of the Polish Air Force who then returned to his fighter squadron.

During the war Poles from the battlefields and from the underground Army within occupied Poland, came to Britain to study at their own Medical Faculty. This came to an end when the war was over, but the experiment had proved successful, the number of students in its last year being 241, a third of whom were women. Between March 1941, and July 1949, 226 students graduated MB., Ch.B., and 18 obtained the M.D. degree.

The establishment and work of the Polish Faculty of Medicine at Edinburgh during the stress of war represents a fine example of international co-operation in medicine.

DEMOBILISATION

HOSPITALS

Demobilisation in the E.M.S. and the release of hospital beds for civilian use cannot be said to have had any parallel in the Fighting Services, in which little demobilisation, if any, could be effected until the end of hostilities in Europe.

The policy in the E.M.S. was to release hospital beds and medical and nursing staffs to meet the urgent requirements of the civilian population as soon as it was reasonably certain that this could safely be done, while still retaining adequate accommodation for the treatment of Service personnel and for the estimated numbers of casualties. Such was the flexibility of the organisation that this policy could be put into force and also reversed at very short notice as the operational situation indicated.

In these circumstances it was possible to introduce measures for partial demobilisation as early as September 1944, when in certain areas all restrictions on the use of hospitals by the civilian population were almost completely relaxed.[23]

In October all beds reserved for air raid casualties in the voluntary hospitals were released in every Region except Regions 4, 5 and 12, and in December many voluntary hospitals were suspended or withdrawn from the Emergency Hospital Scheme as quite unlikely to be used again, many hospital annexes were given up and in many hospitals the additional beds supplied were taken down and stored. In hospitals where beds were still reserved, the arrangements were to be reviewed in six months' time.

In February 1945, similar releases of beds were put into effect in the local authority hospitals.

With the end of hostilities in Europe, the release of beds and hospitals continued and when Japan surrendered in August, the pace of release was considerably increased.

The table below shows the numbers of hospitals and beds retained for E.M.S. cases in the years 1944–5:

Date	Live hospitals in E.M.S.	E.M.S. beds in Live E.M.S. hospitals
June, 1944	863	108,081
December, 1944	819	108,418
June, 1945	538	80,026
December, 1945	458	62,197

DEMOBILISATION OF THE CIVIL DEFENCE SERVICES

The principles referred to above did not apply to the same extent to the demobilisation of civil defence staff. It was possible, however, greatly to reduce the civil defence establishments in certain areas which, it was reasonable to assume, would not again be subjected to heavy attacks from the air; in such areas releases on a considerable scale were made before hostilities in Europe ceased, in order to relieve as much as possible the general shortage of man-power. In the autumn of 1944, after the rapid advances of the Army in France and the elimination of the launching sites for flying bombs, the reduction of civil defence establishment was accelerated and it was continued in the spring of 1945 when the attacks by rockets had ceased.

With the end of hostilities in Europe, demobilisation of the Civil Defence Services began and was rapidly completed. (See Chapter 7.)

DEMOBILISATION OF DOCTORS*

As early as the autumn of 1942, the Government had set up a reconstruction secretariat and an inter-departmental committee on the machinery of demobilisation, presided over by Sir Alfred Hurst, K.B.E., C.B., to prepare a general demobilisation scheme.

The Central Medical War Committee in November of that year considered the question of demobilisation as it affected medical personnel. They were supplied by the Ministry of Health with a short outline of the official plan which had been tentatively agreed in order that any recommendations they might make should be kept within the framework of that plan.

After several meetings and conferences in November 1943, they submitted the following recommendations to the Ministry of Health:

(1) That in order to facilitate the demobilisation of medical officers from the Services and pending a general conscription plan applicable to the community, the recruitment of young practitioners, i.e. those within five years of qualification, or who were under the age of 28, should continue for a limited period on the present lines after the cessation of hostilities.

(2) That all practitioners who were serving with the Forces, who were 44 years of age and over on January 1, 1940, should, subject to their consent, constitute a priority group for demobilisation.

(3) That practitioners who were prisoners-of-war, or had been interned, should be given special priority.

(4) That hardship cases should be covered by the appropriate procedure under the general demobilisation plan and dealt with through their commanding officers.

(5) That the primary consideration for the demobilisation of the remaining groups should be age and length of service, and that the table set out in the appendix be submitted to the Ministry of Health.

---

* See Army Medical Services, Volume I, Chapter 9.

(6) That to meet cases which would not be covered by the demobilisation plan, there should be an arrangement in the procedure at present in operation to secure the release of serving officers where this is shown to be necessary on the grounds of civil needs.

(7) That the recommendations 5 and 6 are put forward on the assumption that the Service Departments will give effect to the recommendation of the Central Medical War Committee for the release of individual practitioners on the grounds of civil needs.

The table in the appendix contained a plan for release by points, based on age and length of service, which differed from the plan drawn up by the Government for general demobilisation because as doctors entered the Service at a much later age than the combatant officers and other ranks, a different arrangement of age-groups was considered necessary.

With certain exceptions these recommendations were considered acceptable. The exceptions were departures in matters of detail from the approved procedure for dealing with releases in general. These were not considered justifiable. It was agreed also that the numbers of doctors released in advance of their turn should not at any time be allowed to exceed the numbers of young practitioners recruited, and with reference to Recommendation 7 of the Central Medical War Committee, that the Service Departments must have an overriding right to refuse the release of any individual if for military reasons his services could not be spared. These conclusions of the Inter-departmental Committee were communicated to the Central Medical War Committee for their information and received the acquiescence of that body.

In September 1944, a White Paper[24] on the re-allocation of manpower between the Armed Forces and civilian employment during any interim period between the defeat of Germany and the defeat of Japan was presented to Parliament. The Central Medical War Committee then published a statement on the demobilisation of doctors[25] which gave a general summary of the Government's plan as far as doctors were concerned. In this the profession were informed that the table for age plus length of service releases would be the same for doctors as for all other persons, that there would be no special priority for the release of returned prisoners-of-war or internees, that priority would be given to special cases of compassion and proved hardship and to individuals whose services were specially required to meet the needs of the civil population, but that in no case would these special releases exceed the numbers of young practitioners recruited.

EFFECT OF THE SCHEME ON THE HOSPITALS

Remobilisation. In the immediate post-war period, the application of these principles to the release of the medical staff of the Forces affected primarily these officers as individuals, but it was also of considerable interest to those responsible for the staffing of the civil hospitals. For them it was a period of remobilisation in order to enable them fully to resume their obligations to the civil population, though continuing to treat the gradually diminishing numbers of military and other E.M.S. patients in the hospitals in which beds still had to be retained for this purpose. The demobilised officers might be divided into four classes:

(*a*) General practitioners of various ages who had established practices to return to, their work having been carried on either by partners or by other practitioners under the scheme brought into being by the Ministry for this purpose;

(*b*) Junior officers who had been recruited to the Forces immediately after completing their term of service in the hospitals in 'A' or 'B2' appointments;

(*c*) More senior officers who had done approved service in 'B1' appointments and had been studying for, or had actually obtained, higher qualifications necessary to fit them for specialist or consultant appointments in the future;

(*d*) Officers on the consultant staffs of hospitals who had been recruited direct as specialists to the Services.

Those under head (*a*) were of no concern to hospital authorities, but the other three classes were the material from which the staffs of the hospitals of the future would largely have to be taken.

In the large teaching hospitals and in local authority hospitals, the depleted establishments had to be brought up to full strength and normal arrangements made to replace the many temporary expedients resorted to during the period of hostilities, such as the dispersal of medical staffs to outer zone base hospitals and special hospitals and the temporary arrangements, both part-time and whole-time, for the specialist and ordinary treatment of Service and civilian patients.

The permanent members of the senior staffs of specialist and consultant status referred to under (*d*) above, when released from service, gradually filled up some of the vacancies, but many gaps remained because of the deaths and retirement of medical men who had continued to serve their hospitals beyond the retiring age. To fill these vacancies adequately was an immediate problem of considerable difficulty. These posts would normally have been filled by the highly eligible and experienced men and women referred to under (*c*) above, who at the outbreak of the war had served for considerable periods in hospital appointments as medical and surgical registrars, clinical tutors, etc., and who possessed the necessary higher academic qualifications and experience of general and special hospital practice.

The great majority of them had been called up for the medical branches of the Forces and had been serving for several years. The result was that, although they had gained much new experience and knowledge of military medicine and surgery and of the prevention and treatment of tropical diseases and war disabilities, they lacked the experience they would have gained with the multifarious causes of disability met with in hospital practice among the civil population. The fears of men of this type were from time to time freely expressed in the medical journals, that those who remained in civil life owing to some medical disability or because they were indispensable to the efficiency of the E.M.S. and were therefore retained in its hospitals, would obtain an unfair advantage over those who had volunteered or had been recruited to the Forces.

These fears were commented on in November 1945, by Lord Moran,[26] President of the Royal College of Physicians, London, who emphasised the danger of filling vacancies without giving the claims of Service doctors the consideration they plainly deserved. He said that the Demobilisation Committee of the Royal College of Physicians held that hospital authorities should adopt some system of deferment in filling vacancies until demobilisation was further advanced. There was also the danger that, for economic reasons, many of these men, if they did not obtain suitable hospital appointments, might be forced to take up practice as assistant or junior partners and that their services would therefore in all probability be lost to the hospitals.

For the junior practitioners mentioned under (b) above, many of whom had either obtained higher qualifications or were studying for them it appeared essential to provide suitable appointments of the 'B1' type in order that they might be able to resume their careers.

It was obvious, therefore, that some action on the part of the various hospital authorities and of the Ministry of Health would be necessary, and these difficulties and others connected with medical demobilisation had indeed been considered at the Ministry of Health for some time. A conference on these matters, at which representatives of the universities and other hospital authorities were present, was held in October 1944, with the result that the following scheme, which was embodied in a memorandum[27] by the Ministry of Health, was decided on:

1. *Young practitioners recruited to the Forces within a year or two of qualification:* In accordance with the recommendations of the Central Medical War Committee, young practitioners who were at the termination of service in 'A' or 'B2' posts in the hospitals and who had done no military service, would continue to be recruited to the Forces after the end of hostilities in Europe, and the holders of 'B1' posts would also be so recruited. Vacancies would thus be provided for officers on release from the Forces who were desirous of occupying such appointments, with the object of obtaining a form of postgraduate education.

As some of the E.M.S. hospitals would continue to function for at least one year after 'cease fire' there would also be posts available in the E.M.S. establishment. The Ministry of Health undertook the financial responsibility for the salaries of officers filling posts additional to the normal establishment of hospitals, either directly in the case of E.M.S. hospitals, or if not, by means of grants to the hospitals or universities.

These posts would be of 'B1' status tenable for six months and the salaries would be £350 per annum, plus the usual allowances.

The scheme also provided financial assistance where the courses of training did not involve the holding of hospital appointments, e.g. the D.P.H. course, for those desirous of obtaining Public Health appointments. This scheme enabled demobilised officers wishing to continue their studies in order to qualify as consultants, to take up their careers under the best conditions. Many such extra appointments were created in the large teaching and local authority hospitals by agencies designated for the purpose in London and in the Provinces, and Deans or Directors of postgraduate education were appointed to these agencies to make the necessary administrative arrangements.

2. *Practitioners recruited from General Practice:* For this class the Ministry of Health undertook the financial responsibility for reimbursing suitable hospitals for giving short courses of instruction to practitioners who wished to brush up their work before they returned to practice, or while actually continuing their practices. The Ministry advocated courses covering twenty-two half-days, either consecutively or at intervals, and agreed to pay seven and a half guineas to the hospital authorities instituting such courses and to pay travelling and out-of-pocket expenses to the practitioners who wished to take them. This scheme, of course, did not affect in any way the staffing of the hospitals.

3. *Practitioners who on recruitment were being trained as Specialists or Consultants:* The posts available for this class were existing senior 'B1' posts and similar posts, approved by the universities, which fell vacant by the recruitment of the medical officers holding them, whether in the E.M.S. hospitals or not. Additional posts of this kind that might be required would be provided as part of the general plan for implementing the Goodenough Committee's proposals[28] for staffing the hospitals of the future. The salaries of these posts would be of the order of £550 per annum, plus allowances, and would be met as under Class I above by the Ministry of Health. The Service authorities were informed of these arrangements and the medical press gave publicity to the scheme. Released medical officers who desired to take advantage of the scheme were advised to apply to the hospital authorities or to the Deans or Directors of postgraduate education in London and the Provinces.

Dental Practitioners. Similar arrangements to those for Class II practitioners were made to provide postgraduate education for dental officers but no hospital appointments were provided for them.

These arrangements were obviously of special benefit to both the junior and senior classes of officers who wished eventually to attain consultant status, but they did not altogether solve the difficulty. In 1946 when officers had completed six months' service in these special appointments and had either obtained higher academic qualifications, or were still studying for them, it was found that the number of hospital appointments available on the senior staffs of hospitals was quite insufficient and that many of these officers had no employment suitable to their status and experience.

The new National Health Service Bill had passed through its various stages in Parliament and provided for a large number of appointments for specialists and consultants to carry out the provisions of the Bill, but as the Act was not to come into force until July 1948, a period of eighteen months remained during which these highly qualified and eligible medical officers would have no suitable employment. The Presidents of the three Royal Colleges pointed this out in a letter in July 1946.[29] They proposed that in order to fill this gap practitioners employed in the senior 'B1' posts referred to above should have their term of office extended if they so desired until the Act came into operation, if the postgraduate Deans who selected them were satisfied with their work. For the older group of men who had been qualified for ten years or more and who normally all had consultant qualifications, they suggested that the Ministry of Health should create a number of more senior salaried whole-time appointments and that hospitals should be asked how many posts of this kind they needed, the appointments to be made by a small committee in each Region. They suggested that the period of office in these appointments should end when the new Service came into being. Publication of these proposals led to correspondence in the medical press, warmly supporting the proposals of the Presidents of the Royal Colleges and emphasising the urgency of some administrative action of this kind. One specialist correspondent even expressed his view that in many cases, his own included, the action was too late and he had had to give up his hopes of a consultant career and go into general practice for economic reasons.

In November the Minister of Health, after considering these representations, agreed that appropriate steps should be taken to meet the difficulty both in the interests of the practitioners themselves and to obviate the risk of their loss to the projected specialist service of the National Health Service. He therefore requested all county borough and county councils and certain voluntary hospitals to consider increasing the establishment of their general hospitals by posts to be made available to ex-Service specialists, wherever the volume of specialist work would justify the increase. Proposals for the extra posts at salaries of the order of £1,000 p.a. were to be submitted to him for approval; the costs would be covered by grants made by the Ministry. The duration of the posts was to be limited to the period pending the establishment of the National Health Service.[30]

For specialists not yet qualified to take full responsibility in the higher posts, provision had already been made to extend the tenure of senior 'B1' appointments and the Minister decided that, although the scope for further additions to these posts was limited, in so far as they were practicable they should be made. The enactment of these proposals met with general approval and they were put into practice by the authorities concerned.

E.M.S. BEDS

At the end of the year 1946, by arrangement, 35,132 beds, out of a total of 116,128 in 366 suitably distributed hospitals—of which 344 were Class 1A, 6 Class 1B and 16 Class II—were available for E.M.S. patients. Many of these were long-stay civilian and Service patients for whose accommodation the Ministry of Health continued to be responsible. This arrangement enabled patients to be treated in hospitals near their homes and avoided the need to retain any special E.M.S. medical and nursing personnel. Some of the special centres were, however, retained in certain hospitals pending the establishment of the National Hospital Service in 1948.

CONCLUSION

This chapter concludes Part I of the general narrative of the inception, evolution and work of the Emergency Medical Services in England and Wales.

The story, as unfolded herein, has its beginning as far back as the year 1922 when, less than four years after the 'cease-fire' of the War of 1914–18, the Committee of Imperial Defence were considering the potentialities of the aeroplane as a long-distance offensive weapon. The air arm of warfare, though young, slow and comparatively feeble in the 1914–18 War, was seen to be growing stronger and longer in reach, and would soon be capable of striking swift, smashing, knock-out blows against any unprepared victim. The danger that it might be wielded against this country, though not at that time menacing, was one that could not be ignored. If, as it was apprehended, there was no certainty that such an attack would never be made, and if, when it was made, there was no sure means of meeting and deflecting the sudden blow before it took effect, then, obviously, civilian casualties must be provided for and the Ministry of Health must co-operate with other departments in the early as in the later stages of civil defence. As a precautionary measure, therefore, plans were laid for a civil defence organisation in which the Ministry of Health was to take an early and important part.

The various stages in the formation and development of the main E.M.S. organisation have now been recorded, with particular emphasis on the establishment and work of the Emergency Hospital Service. In planning and building up this Service, bearing in mind the expected sequence of events, provision had to be made on the largest possible scale, first for air raid casualties at home, for whom it had been estimated that a million beds might be required, and later for battle casualties from oversea, and for the great civilian army of war-workers who became officially entitled to medical care and treatment in E.M.S. hospitals. Nor could the continuing needs of the ordinary civilian sick, of the aged and infirm, of the mentally afflicted, of the tuberculous, of maternity and infancy, be ignored.

In Chapter 1 we have seen that, as an essential preliminary to expansion, the extent of existing accommodation was ascertained in 1938 by a hospital survey which revealed in 3,128 hospitals a total of some 403,000 beds, of which nearly 75 per cent. were occupied. On the basis of the 103,000 vacant beds, a programme of classification, crowding, pooling, adaptation and building was gradually worked out which was to give in 2,370 E.M.S. hospitals, nearly half a million potential beds for all purposes (300,000 for casualties) at the outbreak of a war which, it had been estimated, might in its earliest phase produce air raid casualties at the rate of some 52,000 a day, of whom 28,000 daily would require admission to hospital and 22,000 would need to be retained more than 48 hours (Chapter 2). Providentially, the expected onslaught on such a scale was never made, and by the time of the first real test in 1940 (Chapter 4) the organisation, administration and equipment had been reviewed, consolidated and strengthened by the measures recorded in Chapter 3. E.M.S. hospitals, it will be noted, had been reduced in number by the withdrawal or suspension of many that were unlikely to be much used for casualties, but the accommodation, staffing and equipment of the 1,207 that remained had been greatly improved.

For obvious reasons it was essential throughout the war to make the utmost use of available resources, in accommodation, equipment, appliances and drugs, and not least in professional skill and experience. That the best possible use of medical personnel was made was not always admitted by hard-pressed medical practitioners, to whom the Forces at home appeared to have an undue share during their long period of comparative inactivity between Dunkirk and D-day. But just when and where the strains and stresses of war would be most acutely felt could never be predicted with certainty. To the danger of massive air attacks there was added the threat of invasion, for which, as our reconnaissance flights in the autumn of 1940 revealed, the enemy's preparations were well advanced. Under this threat, comprehensive plans were prepared, Coastal and Green Belt schemes were developed, and liaison between civilian and Army and Air Force medical services was established (Chapters 4 and 5).

Adaptability, mobility and flexibility were of cardinal importance and were assisted by a large measure of decentralisation under the Regional scheme. By pooling hospital resources, all classes of patients, Service and civilian, were provided for throughout the country; the treatment given being co-ordinated and enhanced by the work of Consultant

Advisers, Regional Consultants and Group Advisers, and by the establishment of Special Centres in which certain types of disease or injury were concentrated and treated by specialists of outstanding skill and experience in their particular field, and where expert nursing and the application of the principles of physical medicine helped to ensure rapid recovery and rehabilitation, or the minimum degree of permanent disability in those unfortunate enough to be damaged beyond complete repair.

Thus, under the compulsion of war, a great experiment was made in working a hospital system on a national basis, and its success did much to prepare both the medical profession and the general public for a State hospital service, the establishment of which was to be one of the first constructive tasks of peace.

In 1944, the long-awaited invasion of Europe was accomplished, and in Chapter 6 the E.M.S. arrangements for the reception and distribution of overseas casualties have been described. This chapter also records the flying bomb and long-range rocket attacks which inflicted over 27 per cent. of the total number of seriously injured air raid casualties and damaged many E.M.S. hospitals.

The war history of the Navy, Army, and Air Force hospitals, referred to in this narrative, will be found in the Services volumes. In contrast to the position during the 1914–18 War, the number of purely military hospitals functioning in this country was very limited, as from the outset the Ministry of Health undertook the provision of hospital facilities for Service patients, of whom more than 1,250,000 were treated in E.M.S. hospitals during the six years of war.

The construction of the E.M.S. machine has been given in some detail. In operation, it proved adequate to the demands actually made upon it and always held reserve resources against the possibility of a heavier weight of casualties. Fortunately the health of the people was, on the whole, surprisingly good, and the nation was spared the ravages of any epidemic in any way comparable with the pandemic of influenza which took such heavy toll in 1918.

Faced with the challenging demands of a war of destiny, a small civilian army of medical and lay workers of both sexes tackled all problems as they arose and overcame all difficulties in a great and sustained effort of devoted and untiring service which earned the gratitude of millions, and which was in some measure recognised in the following awards to members of the staffs of hospitals in England and Wales:

> O.B.E., 3; M.B.E., 15; George Cross, 1; George Medal, 37; British Empire Medal, 13; Commendation, 63.

Part II, which follows, contains in Chapters 7 to 15, a series of contributions on the work of the ancillary services, describing in greater detail the collection and transport of casualties, the organisation of medical supplies, the work of the pathological and blood-transfusion services, the application of radiology and physiotherapy and the provision of medical and nursing personnel.

The organisation of the Emergency Medical Services in Scotland and Northern Ireland, which differed in some respects from that in England and Wales, is described in the next volume, which also contains the dramatic story of the air raids on London and selected provincial centres in the United Kingdom. These vivid accounts, mostly written by medical officers of health while the scenes which they describe were fresh in their minds, reveal the courage and patience of all classes under the strain of total war, and show afresh the spirit in which the casualty services carried out their humane, arduous and dangerous work. The same spirit permeated the whole of the Emergency Medical Services.

REFERENCES

[1] Min. of Health Circulars A.S. 345 and D.G.L. 345, May 4, 1944.
[2] Min. of Health E.M.S./D.G.L. 337, April 6, 1944.
[3] Min. of Health Circulars 24/44 and 24A/44, April 6, 1944, and 91/44, August 9, 1944.
[4] Min. of Health Emergency Medical Services Instruction 476, June 16, 1944.
[5] Min. of Health Emergency Medical Services Instruction 495, September 15, 1944, and Amendment, November 30, 1944.
[6] Min. of Health Emergency Medical Services Instruction 496, September 19, 1944.
[7] Min. of Health E.M.S./D.G.L. 453, December 7, 1944.
[8] Min. of Health E.M.S./D.G.L. 426, September 21, 1944.
[9] Min. of Health E.M.S./D.G.L. 282, July 20, 1943.
[10] Min. of Health E.M.S./D.G.L. 340, April, 1944.
[11] Min. of Health Emergency Medical Services Instruction 463, May 16, 1944.
[12] DEBENHAM, R. K., and KERR, A. B. (1945). *J. R.A.M.C.*, **84**, 125.
[13] Min. of Health E.M.S./D.G.L. 424, September 14, 1944.
[14] Min. of Health E.M.S./D.G.L. 432, October 17, 1944.
[15] Min. of Health E.M.S./D.G.L. 466, December 30, 1944.
[16] Min. of Health E.M.S./D.G.L. 476, February 14, 1945.
[17] BELL, R. C. (1944), *Brit. med. J.*, **2**, 689.
[18] *Parliamentary Debates, House of Commons, Official Report*, fifth series, Vol. 403, September 28, 1944 (403 H.C. Deb., Cols. 411–12).
[19] *The Times*, September 21, 1944 (Report of Mr. Willink's address to the Rotary Club of London, 20.9.44).
[20] Min. of Health E.M.S./D.G.L. 425, September 14, 1944.
[21] Min. of Health E.M.S./D.G.L. 495, May 15, 1945.
[22] *Strength and Casualties of the Armed Forces and Auxiliary Services of the United Kingdom, 1939 to 1945*, Table XI. [Cmd. 6832], H.M.S.O., June, 1946.
[23] Min. of Health E.M.S./D.G.L. 424, September 14, 1944.
[24] *Re-allocation of manpower between the Armed Forces and civilian employment during any interim period between the defeat of Germany and the defeat of Japan.* [Cmd. 6548], H.M.S.O., 1944.
[25] *Brit. med. J.*, 1944, **2**, 605–6.
[26] *Brit. med. J.*, 1945, **2**, 663–4.
[27] Min. of Health Memo. 'Postgraduate Education for Medical Officers on release from the Forces—Administrative and Financial Arrangements'.
[28] *Report of Inter-departmental Committee on Medical Schools* (1944), London, H.M.S.O.
[29] *Brit. med. J.*, (1946), **2**, 134.
[30] Min. of Health Circular 202/46, November 8, 1946.

APPENDIX I

OFFICIAL PUBLICATIONS ON AIR RAID PRECAUTIONS

Issued by the Home Office (Air Raid Precautions Department)

HANDBOOKS:

No. 1. Personal Protection against Gas. (2nd edition).
No. 2. First Aid and Nursing for Gas Casualties. (3rd edition).
No. 3. Medical Treatment of Gas Casualties (1st edition).
No. 4. Decontamination of Materials (1st edition).
No. 4A. Decontamination of Clothing (including anti-gas clothing and equipment) from persistent gases.
No. 5. Structural Defence (1st edition).
No. 5A. Bomb Resisting Shelters.
No. 6. Air Raid Precautions in Factories and Business Premises (1st edition).
No. 7. Anti-Gas Precautions for Merchant Shipping (2nd edition).
No. 8. The Duties of Air Raid Wardens (2nd edition).
No. 9. Incendiary Bombs and Fire Precautions (1st edition).
No. 10. Training and Work of First-Aid Parties (1st edition).
No. 11. Camouflage of Large Installations (1st edition).
No. 12. Air Raid Precautions for Animals (1st edition).
No. 13. Fire Protection—for the guidance of occupiers of factories and other business premises.
No. 14. The Fire Guards Handbook.

MEMORANDA:

No. 1. Organisation of Air Raid Casualties Services (2nd edition).
No. 2. Rescue Parties and Clearance of Debris (3rd edition).
No. 3. Organisation of Decontamination Services (2nd edition).
No. 4. Organisation of the Air Raid Wardens' Service (1st edition).
No. 5. Anti-Gas Training (2nd edition).
No. 6. Local Communications and Reporting of Air Raid Damage (1st edition).
No. 7. Personnel Requirements for Air Raid General and Fire Precautions Service and the Police Service (1st edition).
No. 8. The Air Raid Warning System (1st edition).
No. 9. Notes on Training and Exercises (1st edition).
No. 10. Provision of Air Raid Shelters in Basements (1st edition).
No. 11. Gas Detection and Identification Service (3rd edition).
No. 12. Protection of Windows in Commercial and Industrial Buildings (1st edition).
No. 13. Inspection and Repair of Respirators and Oilskin Clothing and Decontamination of Respirators (5th edition).

No. 14. Domestic Surface Shelters.
No. 15. Care and Custody of Equipment (4th edition).
No. 16. Emergency Protection in Factories (1st edition).
No. 17. Civil Defence Uniforms.
No. 18. Civil Defence Motor Transport (1st edition). (Joint Publication of the Ministry of Home Security, the Ministry of Health and the Department of Health for Scotland).

APPENDIX II

1. CONSULTANT ADVISERS AT HEADQUARTERS

Subject	Consultant	Date of Appointment
Neurology	Gordon M. Holmes, Esq., C.M.G., C.B.E., M.D., F.R.C.P., F.R.S. (afterwards Sir Gordon Holmes).	Outbreak of war.
Psychiatry	Bernard Hart, Esq., C.B.E., M.D., F.R.C.P.	Outbreak of war.
General Surgery	Sir Cuthbert Wallace, Bart, K.C.M.G., C.B., F.R.C.S.	Outbreak of war. (Died May 1944).
Orthopaedic Surgery	H. A. T. Fairbank, Esq., D.S.O., O.B.E., M.S., F.R.C.S. (afterwards Sir Thomas Fairbank)	Outbreak of war.
Orthopaedic Surgery	Harry Platt, Esq., M.D., M.S., F.R.C.S. (afterwards Sir Harry Platt)	April 1940.
Casualty Services	E. Rock Carling Esq., F.R.C.S., F.R.C.P. (afterwards Sir Ernest Rock Carling).	Outbreak of war.
Plastic and Maxillo-Facial Surgery	Sir Harold Gillies, C.B.E., F.R.C.S.	Outbreak of war.
Thoracic Surgery	A. Tudor Edwards, Esq., M.Ch., F.R.C.S.	November 1939. (Died Aug. 1946).
Head Surgery	Professor Hugh Cairns, D.M., F.R.C.S., (afterwards Sir Hugh Cairns)	Outbreak of war.
Neuro-Surgery	Professor G. Jefferson, C.B.E., F.R.S., M.S., F.R.C.P., F.R.C.S. (afterwards Sir Geoffrey Jefferson)	February 1940.
Gynaecology	Sir William Fletcher Shaw, M.D., F.R.C.P., P.R.C.O.G.	June 1942.
General Medicine	Professor F. R. Fraser, M.D., F.R.C.P., (afterwards Sir Francis Fraser)	Outbreak of war.
General Medicine	The Rt. Hon. The Viscount Dawson of Penn, G.C.V.O., K.C.B., K.C.M.G., M.D., F.R.C.P.	Outbreak of war. (Died March 1945).

Subject	Consultant	Date of Appointment
General Medicine	Professor J. A. Ryle, M.D., F.R.C.P.	May 1941. (Died Feb. 1950).
General Medicine	Sir Charles Wilson, M.C., M.D., F.R.C.P. (afterwards Lord Moran of Manton)	July 1941.
Ear Nose and Throat	W. M. Mollison, Esq., C.B.E., M.Ch., F.R.C.S.	Outbreak of war.
Ophthalmology	C. B. Goulden, Esq., O.B.E., M.Ch., F.R.C.S.	Outbreak of war.
Radiology	A. E. Barclay, Esq., O.B.E., M.D., F.R.C.P.	Outbreak of war. (Died April 1949).
Dental Surgery (with special reference to Jaw Injuries)	W. Kelsey Fry, Esq., C.B.E., M.C., M.R.C.S., L.D.S. (afterwards Sir William Kelsey Fry).	Outbreak of war.
Physical Medicine	Sir Robert Stanton Woods, M.D., F.R.C.P.	Outbreak of war.
Rehabilitation	J. Rhaiadr Jones, Esq., (Honorary)	September 1940.
Peripheral Nerve and Spinal Injuries (Honorary)	Colonel (afterwards) Brigadier G. Riddoch, M.D., F.R.C.P.	January 1942. (Died Oct. 1947).
Anaesthetics	I. W. Magill, Esq., C.V.O., M.B., B.Ch., D.A.	October 1942.

2. SPECIAL CENTRES

Classification	Number
Injuries requiring orthopaedic surgery	22
Peripheral nerve injuries	3
Injuries of the spine and cauda equina	8
Injuries to the chest	13
Head injuries	14
Maxillo-Facial injuries	13
Burns	6
Neurosis	14
Rheumatism	3
Effort syndrome	1
Skin diseases	25
Children's diseases (London Sectors)	18
Amputations (Ministry of Pensions Hospitals)	10
Total	150

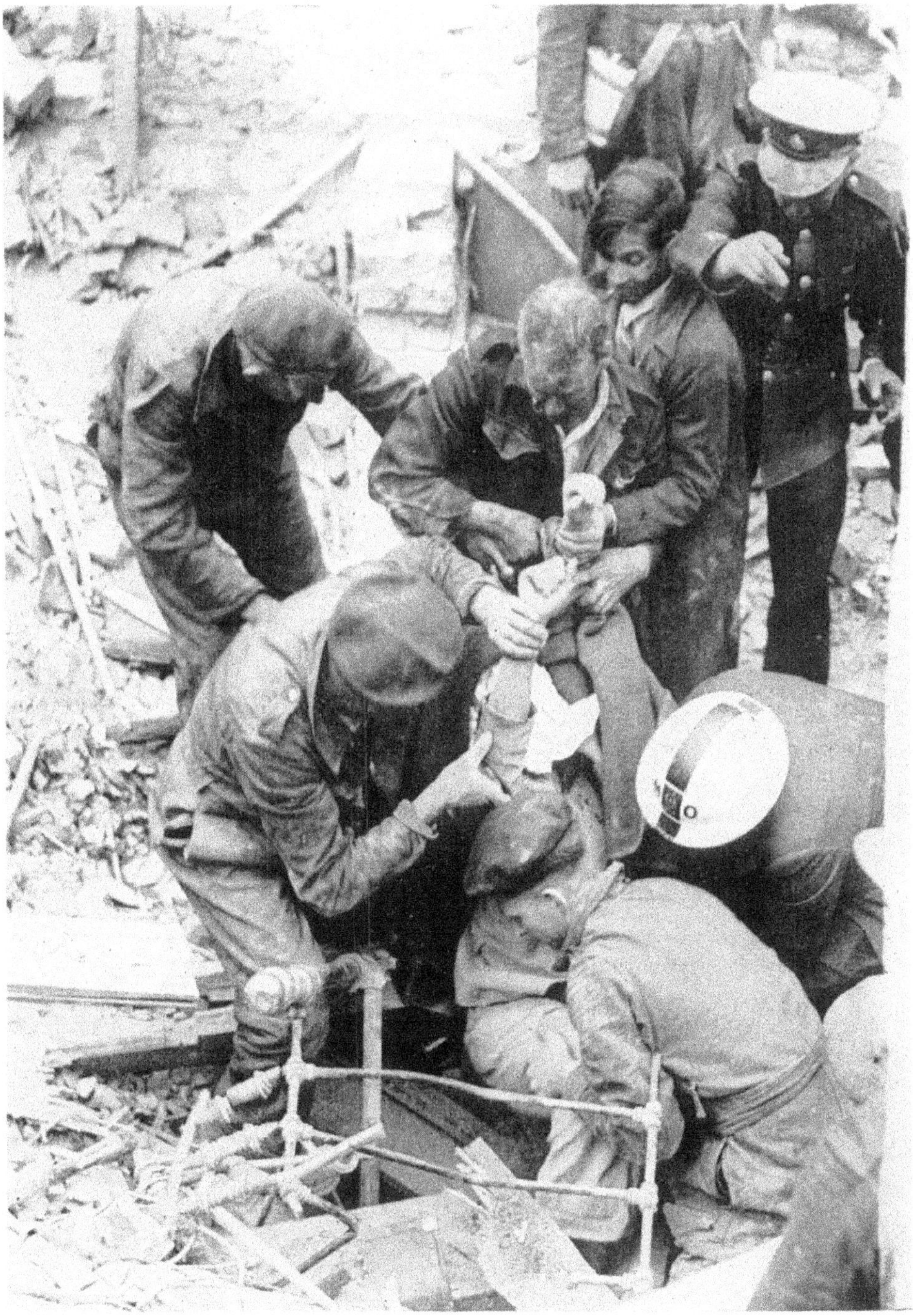

(Imperial War Museum)

PLATE XVII. A man rescued after a pilotless plane strike having been buried $3\frac{1}{2}$ hours. June 24, 1944

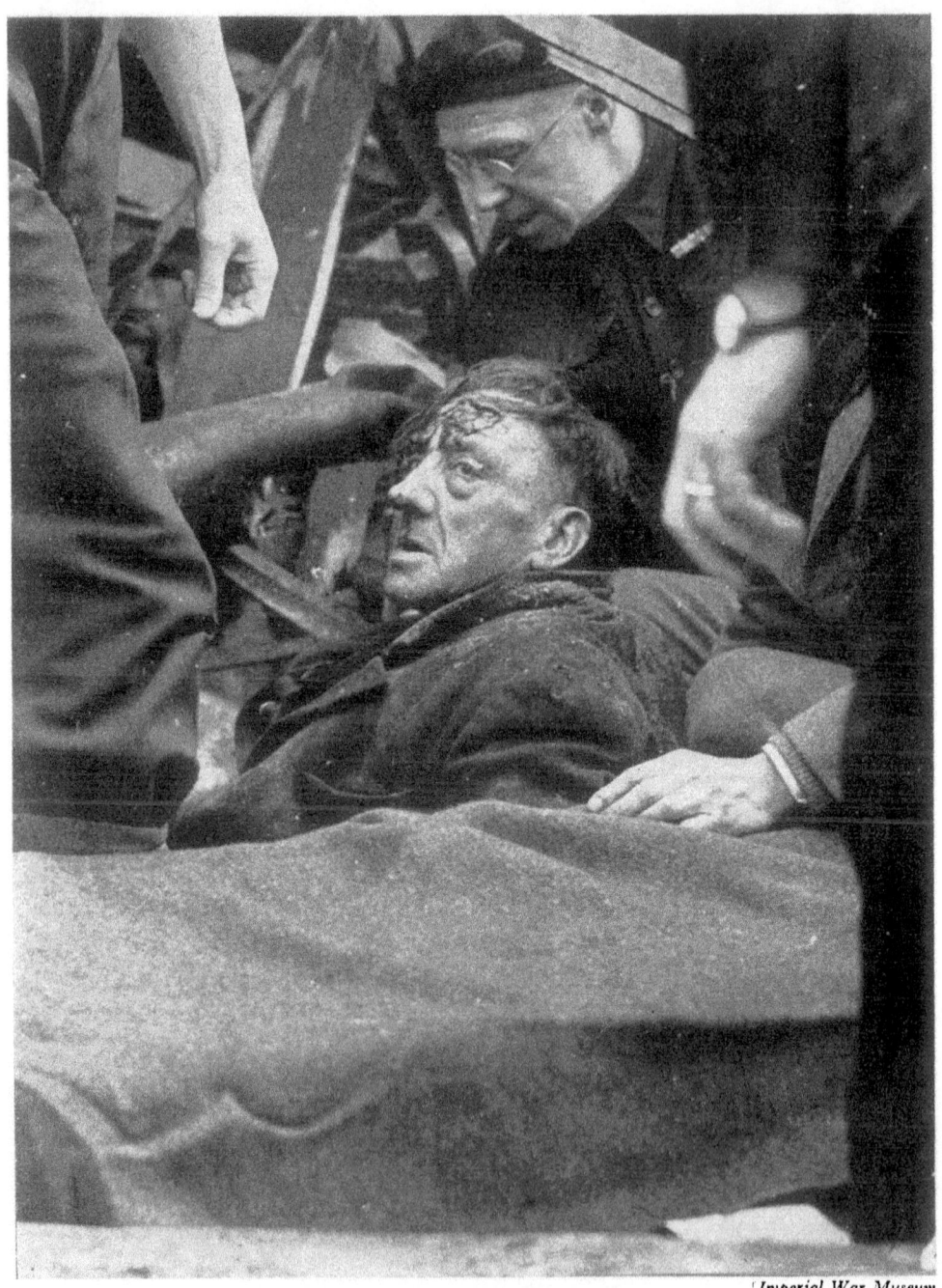

PLATE XVIII. A casualty being rescued from debris after a pilotless plane strike

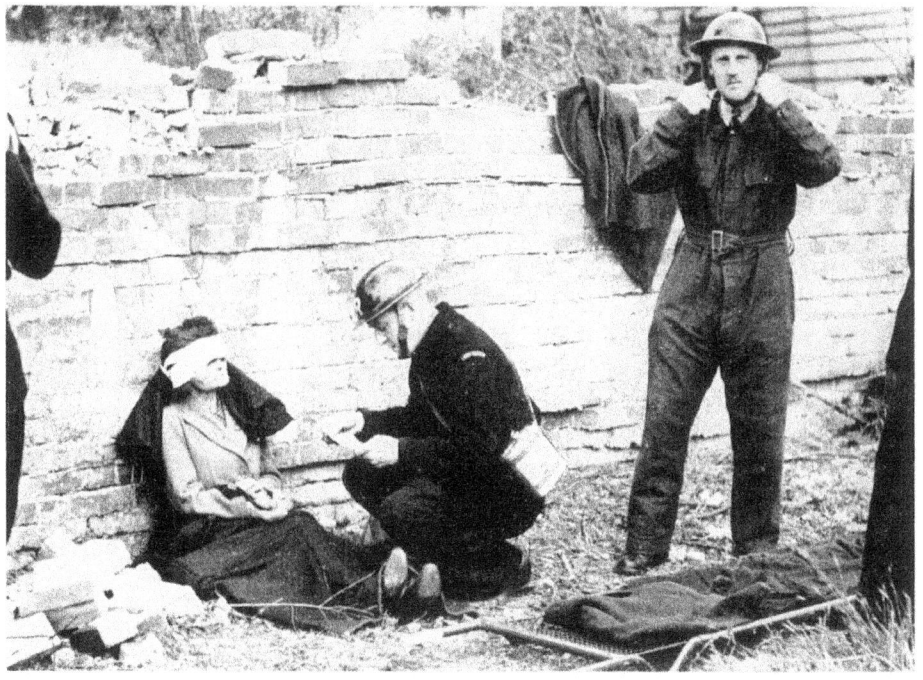

PLATE XIX. Members of the Civil Defence Force attending a casualty after a pilotless plane strike in a London road on July 11, 1944

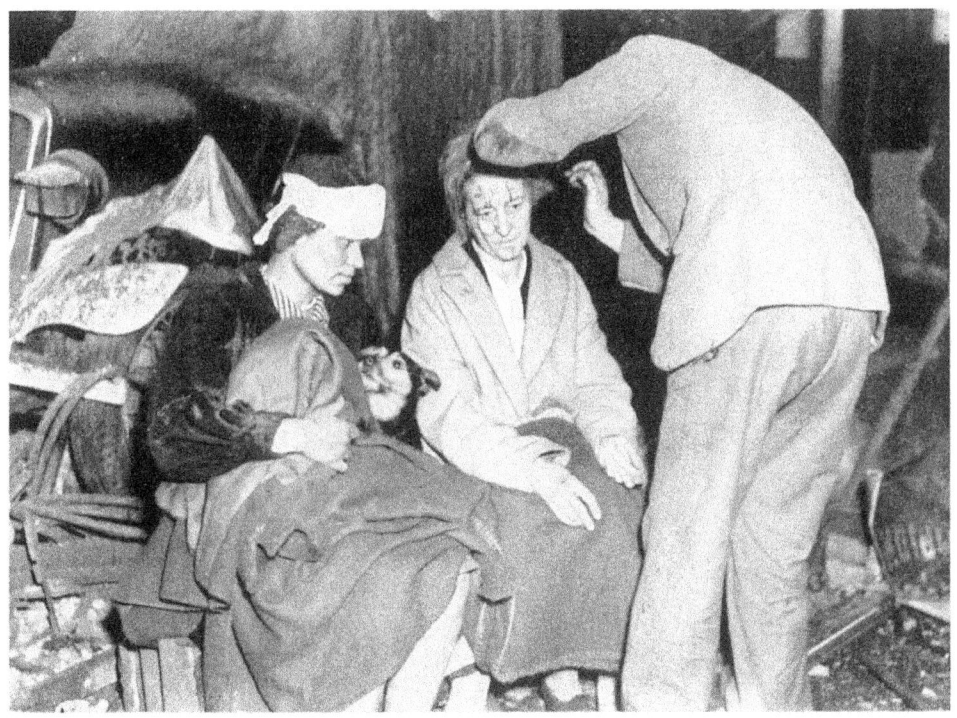

PLATE XX. First aid on the spot after a pilotless plane strike in London.

PLATE XXI. Alsatian dog searching for casualties after a V.1 (pilotless plane) strike

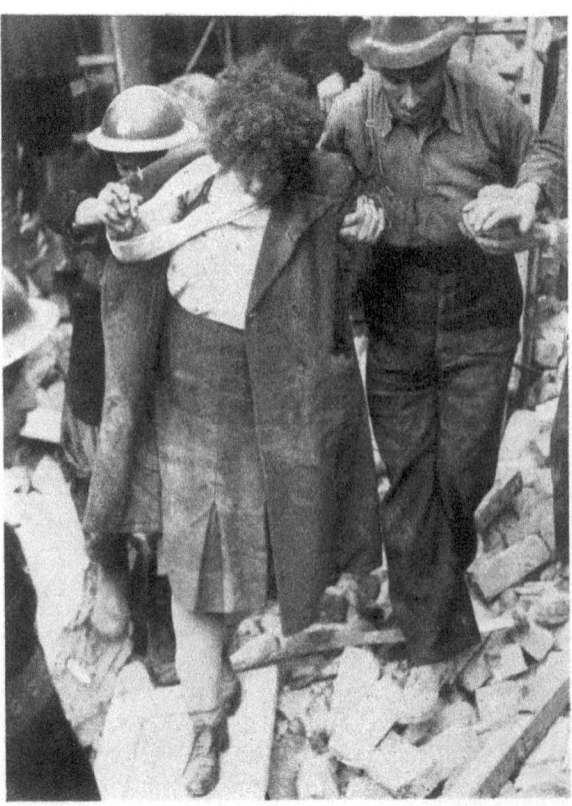

PLATE XXII. A woman after rescue from the roof of a public-house after a pilotless plane strike

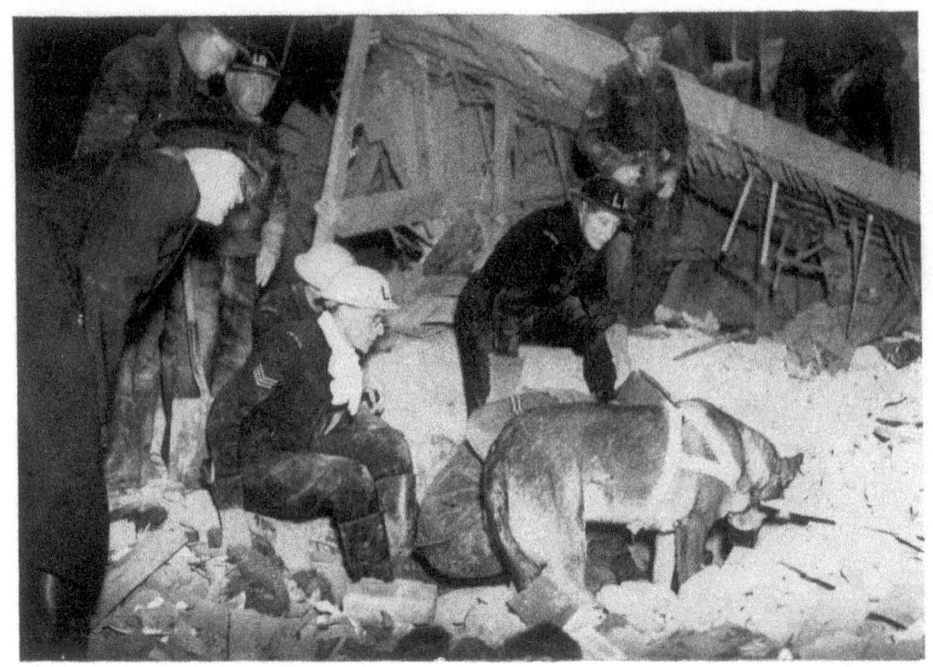

[Imperial War Museum

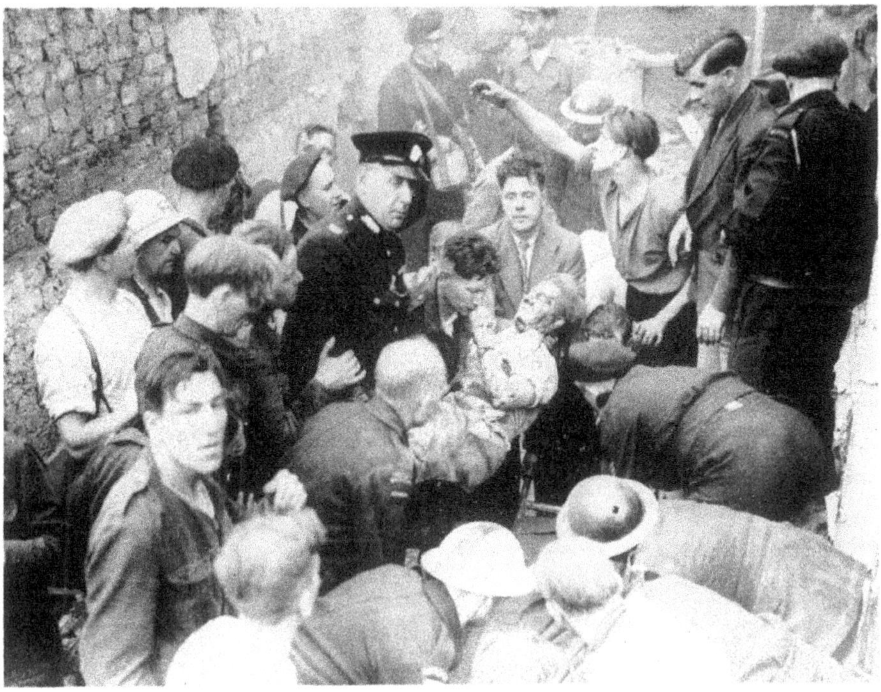

PLATE XXIII. A casualty dug out from under debris after a pilotless plane strike. He was buried for over an hour

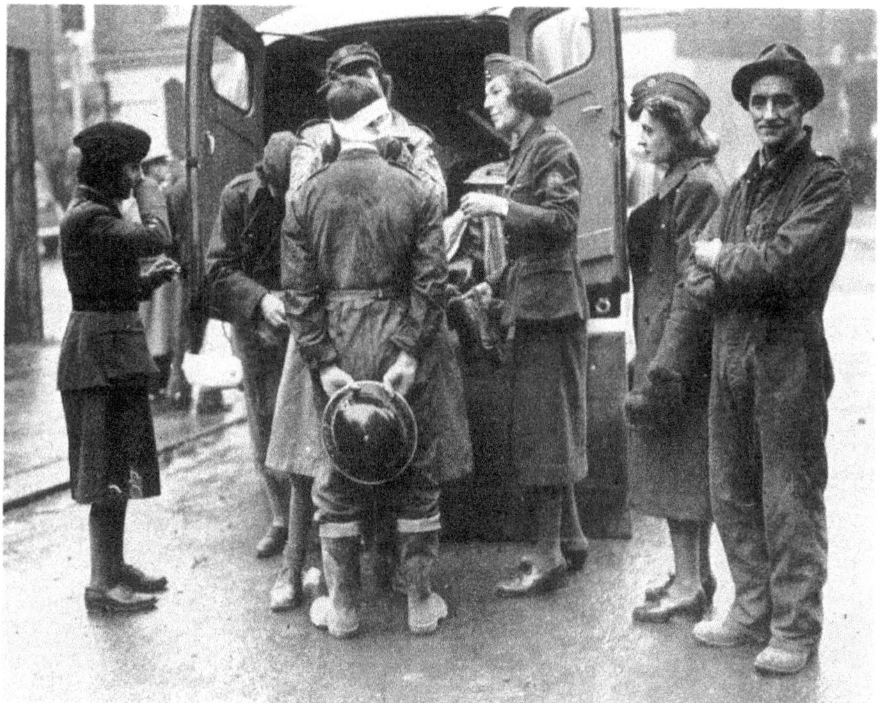

[Imperial War Museum

PLATE XXIV. An Anglo-American ambulance in London after a convent and a block of flats had been hit

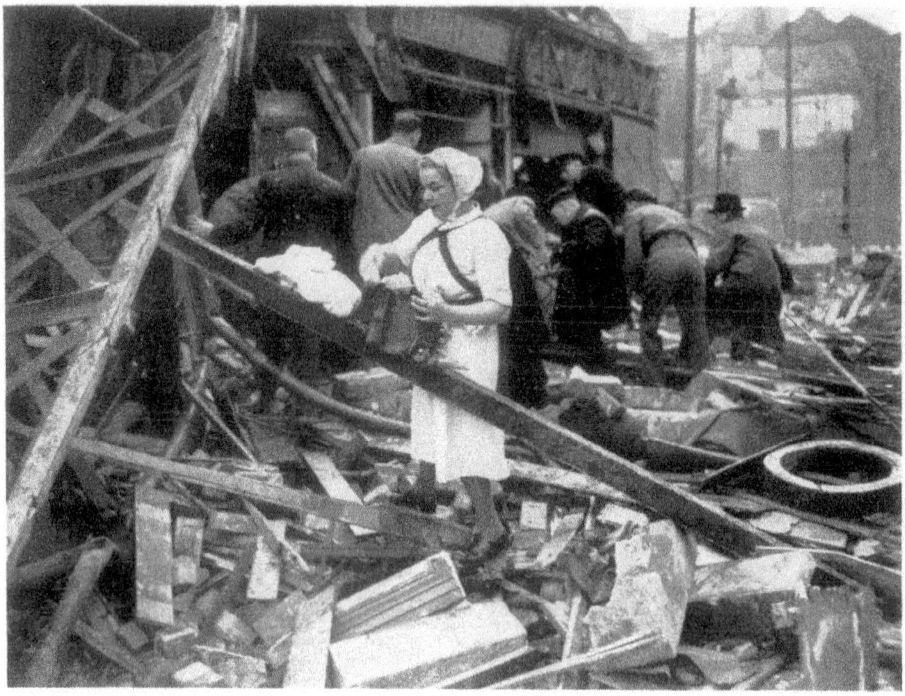

Imperial War Museum

PLATE XXV. Rescuers freeing casualties from debris in Farringdon Street, after the long-range rocket strike on March 8, 1945

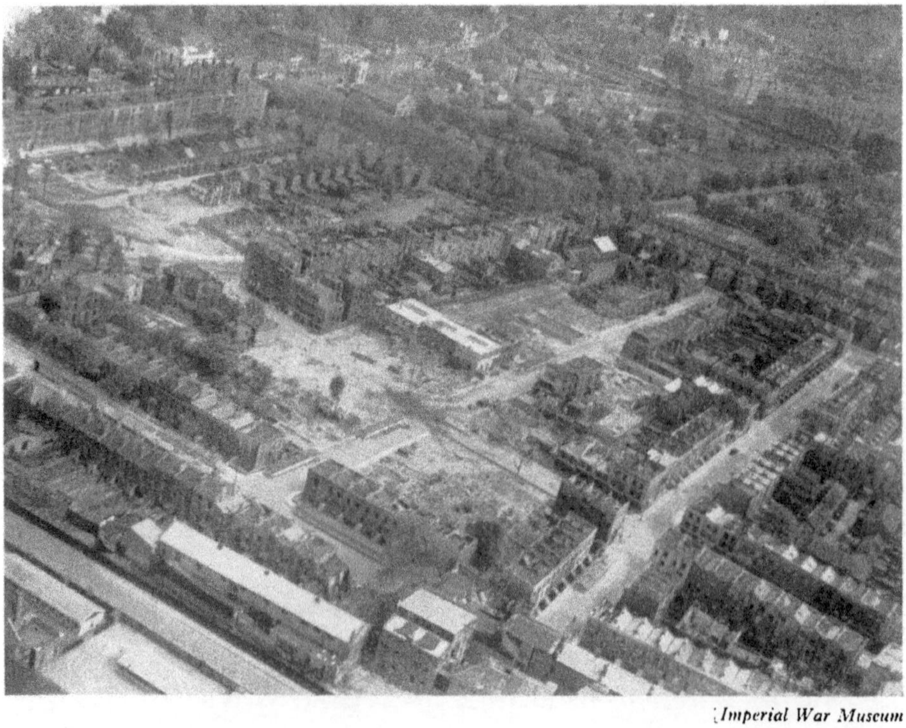

Imperial War Museum

PLATE XXVI. A view of the damage caused by a V.2 (long-range rocket), Islington. The casualties caused were 72 killed, 86 seriously injured and 182 slightly injured

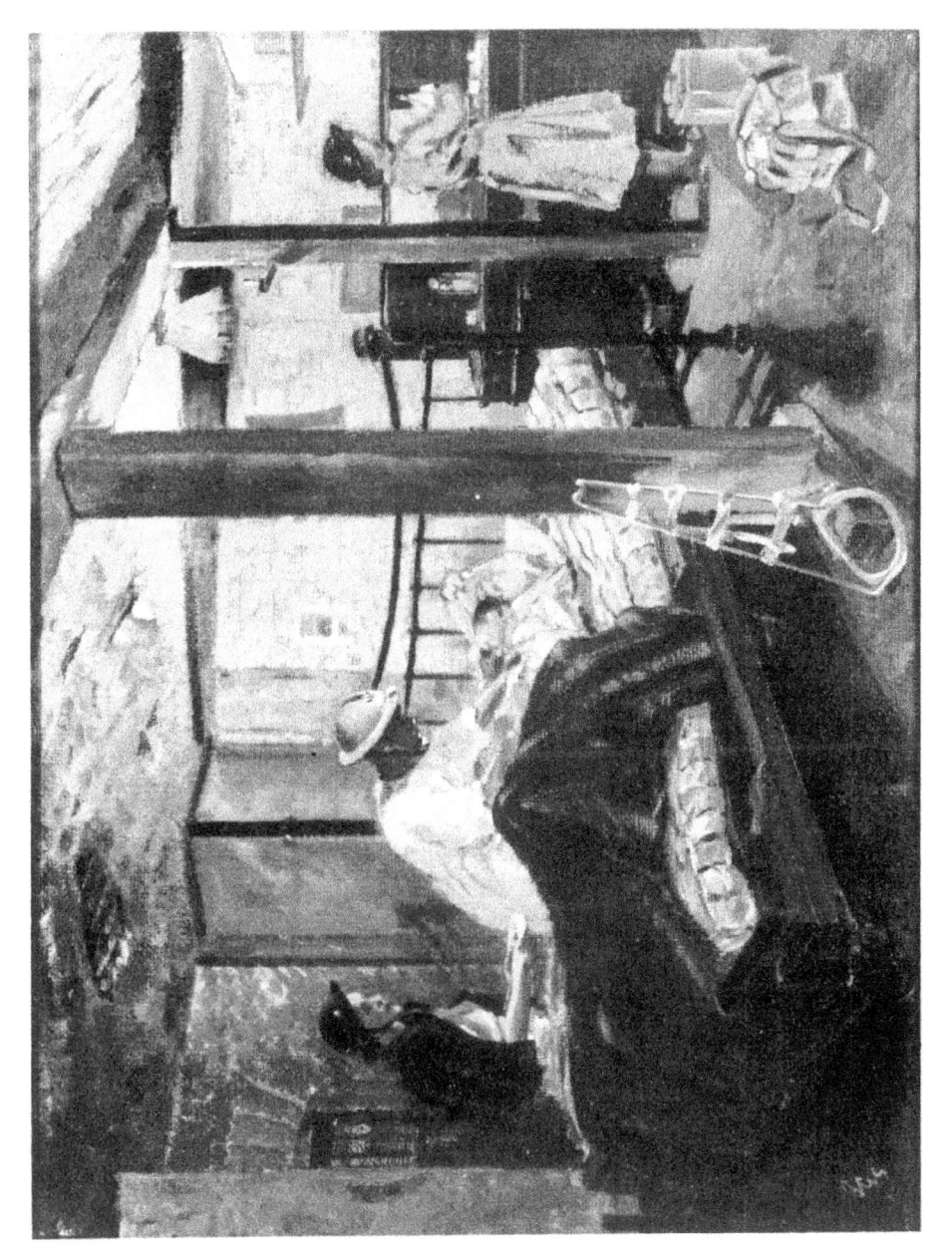

PLATE XXVII. Photograph from official war artists' painting. 'A mobile first-aid unit at work in a basement'

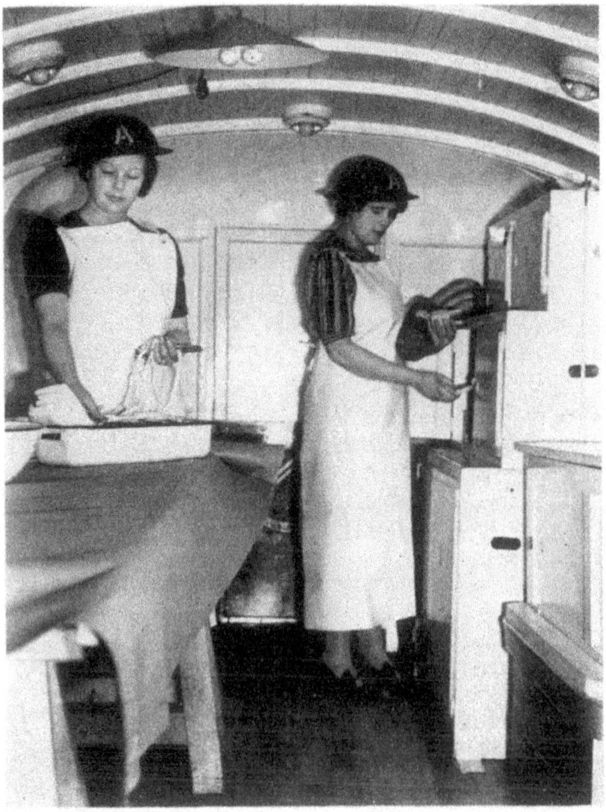

Fox Photos Ltd.

PLATE XXVIII. A mobile operating theatre, Preston

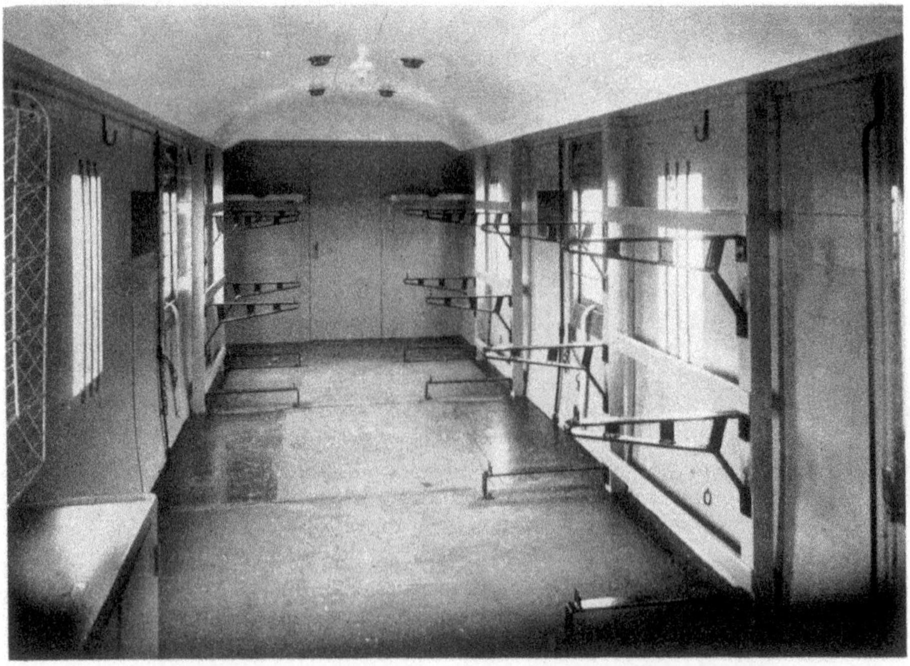

PLATE XXIX. L.M.S. brake van fitted for stretcher cases

APPENDIX III
CIVILIAN TRANSFERRED PATIENTS—FORM E.M.S. 116
January 1, 1940 to December 31, 1945
England and Wales

	1940	1941	1942	1943	1944	1945	Total
Regions	7,943*	21,871*	29,355*	39,279	19,175	10,960	128,583*
London	50,833†	67,734‡	79,404	86,919	54,060	49,474	388,424
Grand total	58,776*†	89,605*‡	108,759*	126,198	73,235	60,434	517,007*

* Approximate figures only in respect of Regions 1 and 9.
† Includes January/April 1941 in respect of Sector VII.
‡ Excludes January/April 1941, in respect of Sector VII.

APPENDIX IV

CLASSES OF E.M.S. PATIENTS

FORM E.M.S. 227 (Revised)

A. Patients entitled to Free Treatment in General Wards (Note (a))—whether admitted at first instance or transferred from another Hospital

Group	Description of class	Relevant circulars, etc.	Documents or evidence establishing title
A.1	*Civilians*, including regular Police [Note (d)]		
	(i) suffering from war injuries;	Cmd. Paper 6061 Circs. 1874*, 1938*, 1938A†, 2246*, 2246A†. Letter dated 31.8.39 to British Hospitals Association.	Cases received from F.A.Ps Stretcher Parties, Police, etc. In case of doubt the local head of the Service in question should be able to certify that the patient is enrolled as a member of that Service.
	(ii) suffering from war service injuries incurred in the course of Civil Defence duties. For full definition see Personal Injuries (Civilians) Scheme, S. R. & O. 226 of 1941 and 563 of 1942. Included among others are Police War Reserve, and Royal Observer Corps. This class also includes National Fire Service personnel, members of the American Ambulance in Great Britain, enrolled Blood Donors, and members of the Home Guard injured on duty and before mustering for active service. (Upon such mustering the Home Guard would be treated as soldiers under A2 below.) [These classes are not entitled to be treated for ordinary sicknesses or for accidents sustained whilst not on duty.]	Circs. 2467 and 2516	
A.2	*Members of the Fighting Services* whether injured or sick [Notes (a), (e), (f), (g), (h), (k).] Besides serving officers and men of the Royal Navy, Army and Royal Air Force, including Women's Auxiliaries, and V.A.D. members actually serving with the Forces, this class includes	As above	Service identity particulars
	(i) dependants of certain Service officers and men, and officers on half pay, when certificates are produced from the appropriate Service authority [Note (m)];	Circ. 1938*, 1938A†	A.F.O. 1668 R.A.F. 3467(W) T. 124X or T. 124T
	(ii) naval men serving on T. 124X or T. 124T agreements;	Circ. 2572	Service identity particulars
	(iii) cadets and University candidates on Service courses (only when on duty, and, in the case of sea cadets, only until fit to be removed home);	Circ. 2467	
	(iv) repatriated prisoners-of-war;		Service identity particulars
	(v) Dominions and Allied Forces, including members of U.S. Army, Navy and Marine Corps, of Air Forces attached to these Corps, of the nursing staffs of these services; officers of the U.S. Public Health Service; U.S. medical and nursing staff attached to E.M.S.; Canadian Firemen and Red Cross personnel;	Circs. 2246*, 2246A†, 2467, 2497, 2690	Service identity particulars
	(vi) officers and men of the Merchant Navy (including foreign seamen) injured on duty or suffering as a result of exposure. (See also B. 3(iv) below). [Note (m).]	Circs. 2346*, 2346A†, 2467 Circs. 2246*, 2246A†	Certificates of discharge or competence Under escort
	(vii) prisoners-of-war and interned enemy aliens;		
	(viii) Ministry of Pensions cases, (a) readmitted casualties and war service injuries; (b) cases defined in Circulars 2516, 2530, 2530A.;	Circ. 2400 Circs. 2516, 2530, 2530A, 2860, 46/44, E.M.S.I. 475	Directions from Hospital Officer
	(ix) Certain members of the National Fire Service; National Fire Service Overseas Contingent.		
A.3	*Special Classes* comprising (i) unaccompanied children (Note (b)) evacuated under the Government Scheme;	Circs. 1938*, 1938A† 2157 2246*, 2246A† Letter 99047/676/101	Billeting forms
	(ii) mothers and children admitted for 48 hours' rest and shelter; (iii) sick civilians removed from shelters, rest and feeding centres and houses in target areas [Note (c)]; (iv) Gibraltarian refugees.		Arrangements by Hospital Officer Arrangements by local official

* Issued to local authorities only.   † Issued to voluntary hospitals only.

APPENDIX IV—contd.

CLASSES OF E.M.S. PATIENTS

B. Patients entitled to Treatment as E.M.S. Patients, but subject to contribution according to their ability to pay. (This may be discharged by production of Contributory Scheme, etc., Vouchers as indicated in Circulars 1938*, 1938A†, 2346A†, 2364*, 2516, 2572, 2779)

Group	Description of class	Relevant Circulars, etc.	Documents or evidence establishing title
B.1	*Fracture cases and certain other injuries among* (i) whole-time Civil Defence workers; (ii) Manual workers in certain industries and all factories.	Circs. 2346*, 2346A†, 2876 Circ. 2795	Enquiry in case of doubt, or card from employer or organisation
B.2	*Sick Civilians transferred* from other hospitals, etc. (i) with Form E.M.S. 116 [Note (j)] (ii) not with Form E.M.S. 116, but at the direction of Hospital or Sector Hospital Officer with nominal roll [Note (j)] (iii) sick civilians removed from shelters, rest and feeding centres and private houses, after first three months from date of evacuation (cf. A.3 (iii))	Circs. 1938*, 1938A†, 2346*, 2346A†	Form E.M.S. 116 Nominal roll. Instructions from Hospital Officer
B.3	*Transferred War Workers* sick or injured, other than by enemy action, including (i) men and women transferred away from home as war workers at the instance of a Government Department, including Ministry of Labour trainees, workers from Eire and Northern Ireland, agricultural workers in hostels and billets, Women's Land Army members (including Forestry Corps) Canadian teachers and social workers on loan to this Country (ii) boys and girls in harvest camps; workers at Ministry of Supply Production camps and Volunteer Agricultural camps. (iii) whole-time Civil Defence workers transferred away from home (iv) officers and men of the Merchant Navy away from home port and of foreign merchant navies (when not covered by A.2 (vi))	Circs. 2228, 2416, 2346*, 2346A†, 2690 Circ. 2572, 46/44 Circs. 2228, 2416 Circs. 2346*, 2346A†, 2467	Card from employer or organisation or enquiry Note from Camp Commandant Enquiry from local head of Service in case of doubt Certificates of Service or competency
B.4	*Evacuees* (other than unaccompanied children evacuated under the Government Scheme, see A. 3(ii)) whether privately or officially evacuated. (*See*, however, paragraph 14 of Circ. 2283.)	Circs. 2346*, 2346A†	Billeting form plus enquiry
B.5	*Refugees* from Abroad, including Channel Islanders but not Gibraltarians (as to whom see A.3 (iv)) and only until settled in this Country.	Circ. 2051	Enquiry

* Issued to local authorities only. † Issued to voluntary hospitals only.

NOTES

(a) Officers of both sexes, including Nursing Sisters of the Naval, Army and Air Force Nursing Services, but not officers of the Home Guard, are to be treated in Officers' wards or private wards. The position as to other E.M.S. patients wishing to be treated in private wards is set out in Circular 2438†, (2438A)*.
(b) Contribution is collected in respect of these children by other means.
(c) Free for first three months only; after that, assessable.
(d) Police Sick are not an E.M.S. responsibility. Women Police are treated as Regular Police.
(e) Members of N.A.A.F.I. staff are civilians unless they have been enrolled for service overseas. They are then treated as Service cases. Women employees of N.A.A.F.I. who have been directed to that employment by the Ministry of Labour and National Service are to be treated as transferred War workers.
(f) Royal Marine Police Special Reserve employed in Naval Dockyards are regarded as Service personnel.
(g) Men and Women in Class W and Class W(T) Army Reserve and A.T.S. members relegated to the "Unemployed list" of that Service are not entitled to be treated as members of the Services; nor are men who have received a calling up notice; but have not joined their units, unless they are referred by the Service authority for special examination.
(h) Civilian students at A.A. Radio School are not an E.M.S. responsibility.
(i) Hospital staff (doctors and nurses) who fall sick and are warded are to be treated in accordance with the custom of their parent hospital if transferred staff, or of the hospital service if directly appointed. This still applies if they are transferred to another hospital for treatment. Women undergoing 14 days' preliminary training as members of the C.N.R. are counted as nurses for this purpose.
(j) Cases transferred are to be dealt with as regards assessment as they would have been in the Hospital of origin. All other assessable cases are to be dealt with as if they were patients for whom the Hospital of treatment was responsible.
(k) Includes First Aid Nursing Yeomanry members only when in the A.T.S.
(l) Ferry Pilots (Air Transport Auxiliaries) are civilians.
(m) Personnel of War Department Fleet are civilians only exceptionally entitled to free hospital treatment, and in such cases will produce Form A.F.O. 1668.

APPENDIX V

EXTRACT FROM MEMORANDUM "MEDICAL ARRANGEMENTS IN REGION IV AND NOTES ON THE ACTION TO BE TAKEN IN INVASION OR SEVERE ENEMY ACTION FROM THE AIR".
(APRIL 1942)

ACTION TO BE TAKEN ON INVASION

ON PRELIMINARY WARNING

(1) *Primary Clearance of Hospitals.* On the receipt of instructions from the Ministry of Health, Whitehall, the medical officers of health concerned will be instructed by the Hospital Officer to clear hospitals in the 20 mile 'coastal belt' and certain base hospitals in close proximity to the coastal belt called the '*green belt*'. If possible the clearance will be made in two stages—

(a) A reduction of bed occupancy to ease the problem.
(b) A complete clearance.

The preliminary reduction of bed occupancy will probably be to 50 per cent. in the 'coastal belt' and 60 per cent. in the 'green belt', and the second a clearance of all patients fit to be moved in the 'coastal belt', and reductions of bed occupancy in the 'green belt' to 40 per cent. The first stage will be effected by sending patients home who require no further hospital treatment, by restricting admissions and by transferring by ambulance transport, patients to other hospitals outside the areas concerned. The second stage will entail the moving of all patients fit to be moved by ambulance transport to entraining points for ambulance trains in accordance with the Ministry's existing plans. The medical and nursing staffs of these hospitals will remain at their posts.

Hospitals should prepare nominal rolls of those transferred and these nominal rolls should be sent with the patients. Patients should also take food for twenty-four hours. If patients have been transferred by bus ambulances, the discharging hospital should send a nurse with each ambulance and such nursing requisites as may be necessary for the journey. Every effort will be made to return these articles as soon as possible, but it would be well if the hospitals would affix their name to each article. No chronic sick, mental or incurable T.B. cases should be transferred unless specific instructions to do so are issued.

Care should be taken that no patient is sent away either by ambulance or train who obviously cannot stand the journey. A certain number of patients will be too ill to move, but it is unlikely that the number will exceed 10 per cent. of the occupied beds.

(2) *Lines of Evacuation.* Certain planned lines of evacuation to be brought into operation during enemy action were drawn up from time to time on the assumption that invasion would be from the sea. It is now thought that invasion may be by airborne troops and that these may be dropped far inland

and that this will be combined with invasion from the sea. For this reason, set plans for evacuation have been cancelled. Medical officers of health will now have to determine the lines of evacuation in their areas in accordance with the military position and keep in close touch with their neighbouring medical officers of health so that transfers from one area to another may be arranged. All such plans must be flexible and capable of adjustment to the military situation.

All plans in the past were drawn up on the assumption that it would be possible to evacuate casualties from front line hospitals to base hospitals in the rear, but recent military exercises have indicated that it may be difficult to evacuate casualties in this way in any numbers. The military situation may change so rapidly that it may not be feasible to use convoys of ambulances while fighting is in progress. It may be possible, however, in certain areas for ambulances to be moved, but in other areas this procedure may only be justifiable in exceptional circumstances. When it is possible and desirable to move patients by ambulance they should never be moved in convoys, but ambulances should be despatched in ones and twos. Small four-stretcher ambulances may, however, be moved in numbers not exceeding five. Drivers should be given written instructions as to hospitals to which they are to proceed and as to their further movements.

From this it necessarily follows that some hospitals may become overcrowded and they must be prepared for this; patients must be held until the situation clarifies. The number of casualties may be very great and the hospital authorities in consultation with the medical officers of health should, in addition to the reserve hospitals, now review schools, church halls and large houses in their vicinity into which the overflow of patients could be put. It is not intended at this stage to requisition these buildings, but possible places should be listed so that there will be no delay when the need arises.

It may even be impracticable to transfer patients from first-aid posts to hospitals and first-aid posts must be prepared to hold casualties. This applies particularly to first-aid posts in smaller towns where there are no hospitals and in these cases medical officers of health should review the possibility of using schools, church halls, etc., for the retention of casualties. In these areas, and in country areas where there are only first-aid points, medical officers of health should stimulate Parish Invasion Committees to take similar action to draw up lists of nursing requisites, sheets, blankets, beds, etc., which could be supplied by the civil population. Detailed instructions regarding this procedure have already been issued with regard to "Defended Places", etc.

(3) *Evacuation of Particular Hospitals.* If the complete evacuation of any particular hospital is required (patients, staff and equipment) for military reasons, pre-arranged plans for doing so will be put into operation by the Hospital Authority on receipt of specific instructions.

(4) *Opening of Reserve Hospitals.* Reserve hospitals may be taken possession of at this stage on the receipt of instructions from the Ministry of Health. If this is decided on 'parent' hospitals will be warned to be ready to put into operation plans for the staffing and administering of these hospitals and the Ministry will arrange for the despatch of the necessary equipment which is not already on the premises.

(5) *Opening of Reserve 'B' Beds in Hospitals.* Hospitals may be instructed to set up their Reserve 'B' beds; the necessary equipment will then be supplied by the Ministry from Regional Stores and steps will be taken by the Hospital Officer to augment the medical and nursing staff to the extent required.

(6) *General Clearance of Class I or II Beds or Both.* The Hospital Officer will instruct medical officers of health to 'clear' all hospitals when he is instructed to do so and hospitals will be informed by telegram. This clearance will be effected by sending patients home who require little or no further treatment and, if instructed to do so, by transferring appropriate cases to Red Cross convalescent hospitals. Non-E.M.S. cases in such hospitals who have been temporarily accommodated there should be evacuated to their homes.

(7) *Re-opening of First-aid Posts.* The question of re-opening first-aid posts which are on a " care and maintenance" basis will be considered and instructions issued to Scheme-making authorities.

(8) *Gas Cleansing Arrangements at Hospitals.* Gas cleansing arrangements at hospitals will be reviewed by the hospital authorities on the receipt of instructions from the Hospital Officer. It will be appreciated that the patient's welfare is the chief consideration and that the injury may be more important than the contamination. If the casualty is seriously injured and suffering from shock, all that is necessary is to remove the outer clothing and wipe off obvious patches of contamination. The patient should immediately thereafter be taken to the resuscitation ward. Provided the outer clothing has been removed there is little danger of carrying contamination into the wards.

(9) *Defended Places.* Local authorities may be required to check the preparations at first-aid posts, etc., in such places and for putting improvised hospital accommodation into readiness.

(10) *Hospital Supplies.* Hospitals should review their stocks of non-perishable foods, drugs and dressings and arrange to have a reserve of one month's supply.

(11) *Allocation of Hospital Staffs.* It is essential that medical officers of health should arrange for the allocation of medical and surgical staffs between hospitals to the best possible advantage. This can be done by consultation with the staffs of hospitals and should be arranged in advance of invasion. It has already been done in some cases, but where it has not been done steps should be taken at once to complete the arrangements and the Hospital Officer should be informed. Arrangements have been made by the Hospital Officer in an emergency to transfer house officers, staff and nurses from hospitals where there is little activity, to hospitals which are hard-pressed. This transferred staff will remain until the position eases when it will be returned to its own hospital. This arrangement is not confined to this Region but is national and help of this kind may be obtained from any part of the country.

(12) *Relief of Surgical Staff, etc.* In invasion, even more than in 'blitz' conditions, it is essential that the medical officer in charge of a hospital should be alive to the question of fatigue amongst staff and he should have definite plans for relieving them and should be aware of the arrangements for calling up mobile surgical and resuscitation teams and supplies of plasma and whole blood. Every member of the hospital staff down to orderlies and porters should be told in advance what part they are to play in the general plan. The

Hospital Officer will endeavour to meet every demand for surgical, resuscitation or nursing teams even if it means asking the Army to send them under escort.

(13) *Methods of Communication.* If communications, e.g., telephones, break down, there may be difficulty in forwarding messages. Arrangements have been made to supply each hospital with a runner and, in the case of hospitals at some distance from the control centre, with despatch riders, and messages should be sent to the nearest control centre with the request that the message be forwarded.

(14) *Towns cut off by the Enemy.* Towns may be cut off by the enemy and even if it is possible to evacuate patients from hospitals before the town is surrounded, adequate medical and nursing staff must be prepared to remain on duty to look after patients not evacuated and other casualties who may be brought in later.

(15) *Liaison with the Services.* The closest liaison has been established between the Ministry of Health and the Services and so far as is possible mutual assistance has been arranged. For example, the Navy has made arrangements to send a surgical team to the Lowestoft Hospital. Arrangements have been made for Service ambulances to pick up civilian casualties of either sex and either to take them to an E.M.S. hospital, a first-aid post or to a military main dressing station according to the military situation. Similarly, it has been agreed that civil defence ambulances will collect Service casualties and the Services will apply for the use of civil defence ambulances when necessary to the medical officers of health or civil defence controllers. If the demands on the civil defence ambulances are numerous, both from the Army and from the Civil Defence Services, each application must be taken in order of priority and no distinction must be made between the two classes of casualty.

(16) *Liaison with Sector Group Officers.* From 'Preliminary Warning' onwards, hospitals in this Region administered by the Sector Group Officers will render 'bedstates' to the Hospital Officer as well as to the Sector Group Officer, in order that he may make full use of these hospitals, but if circumstances permit, the Group Officer will be notified of the numbers of patients it is proposed to transfer to their hospitals.

On 'Stand-To'.

(17) *Leave.* All leave will be stopped and the pre-arranged plans for augmenting the staffs of hospitals and providing reliefs will be put into force.

(18) *Fifth Columnists.* Medical officers of health and hospital authorities must be on their guard against fifth columnists. Efforts must be taken to prove the authenticity of important messages received. This can be done by ringing back to the office from where the message purports to have emanated. Visitors to hospitals who are unknown should be asked to produce their identity cards.

(19) *Advanced Medical Control Centres.* Advanced medical control centres will be established at the following places:

    (a) The Public Health Department, St. Giles' Street, Norwich.
        Telephone Number—Norwich 3800.

    (b) The Public Health Department, Westgate Street, Bury St. Edmunds.
        Telephone Number—Bury St. Edmunds 508.

(c) The County Hall, Chelmsford.
Telephone Number—Chelmsford 3931.

These centres will be staffed by the medical officer of health or one of his deputies, a Military Medical Liaison Officer deputed by the D.D.M.S. Eastern Command and an Assistant Hospital Officer. The Assistant Hospital Officer will act primarily in an advisory capacity to the medical officer of health and will normally only take action at the request of the medical officer of health or if the latter becomes a casualty. He will, as far as circumstances permit, keep in touch with Cambridge, the other advanced control centres and in the case of the centre at Chelmsford, with Sector 3 headquarters. The Group Officer, Sector 3 will act in operations on behalf of Sectors 2, 3 and 4. The Assistant Hospital Officer will assist the medical officer of health by making arrangements for the transfer of patients from one area to another and will make decisions on the spot without reference to Cambridge. The Military Liaison Officer's chief function is to keep the medical officer of health informed as to the general military situation and as to the number of casualties expected or occurring in any locality.

On 'Action Stations'.

(20) *Bedstates.* Hospitals should during hostilities endeavour to send three-hourly bedstates to the medical officer of health in whose area they are situated. The medical officer in charge of the hospital should inform the medical officer of health when 75 per cent. of the beds are occupied so that if possible ambulances may be diverted elsewhere.

(21) *Mobilisation of Doctors in an Emergency.* Arrangements have been made whereby nearly every doctor in the Region has been assigned some special duty in the event of an emergency and the details are in the possession of the medical officers of health concerned. These doctors will be mobilised on 'Action Stations' and directed to take up the duties which have been allotted to them.

APPENDIX VI

CLASSES OF E.M.S. PATIENTS IN HOSPITAL

In-Patients

Group	No. as at June 30, 1943	No. as at June 28, 1944	No. as at June 27, 1945	No. as at December 26, 1945
A·1	1,232	4,088	2,027	716
A·2	20,600	30,393	34,411	19,865
A·3	978	1,136	348	146
B·1	918	1,119	1,082	1,140
B·2	15,812	8,587	10,232	6,819
B·3	726	596	552	421
B·4	1,233	883	949	673
B·5	248	229	126	26
Totals	41,747	47,031	49,727	29,806

Out-Patients

Group	No. as at June 30, 1943	No. as at June 28, 1944	No. as at June 27, 1945	No. as at December 26, 1945
A·1	586	1,552	426	172
A·2	3,275	3,690	3,964	2,079
A·3	158	106	47	3
B·1	616	1,151	993	310
B·2	270	358	222	201
B·3	397	237	296	70
B·4	85	134	91	15
B·5	16	17	11	3
Totals	5,403	7,245	6,050	2,853

NOTE: For Classification of Groups, see Appendix IV.

APPENDIX VII

ESTIMATED NUMBER OF PATIENTS ADMITTED TO E.M.S. HOSPITALS FOR DISABILITIES NOT DUE TO ENEMY ACTION 1943–45

Categories	1943 Based on 28 days bed occupancy	1944 Based on 28 days bed occupancy	1945 Based on 28 days bed occupancy
A3. (1) Unaccompanied child evacuees (2) Mothers and children for 48 hours' rest and shelter (3) Sick civilians from shelters (4) Gibraltar refugees	11,162	13,382	8,707
B1. Fracture cases among— (1) Whole-time civil defence workers (2) Manual workers in certain industries and all factories	15,407	17,910	14,834
B2. Sick civilians transferred from other hospitals	191,205	151,808	141,395
B3. Transferred war workers, injured other than by enemy action (1) Men and women transferred away from home (2) Boys and girls in labour camps (3) Whole-time C.D. workers away from home (4) Officers and men of Merchant Navy away from home port and of foreign Merchant Navies	9,532	8,243	7,304
B4. Evacuees other than unaccompanied children	14,769	16,562	16,216
B5. Refugees from abroad, including Channel Islands but not Gibraltar	2,846	2,401	1,547

APPENDIX VIII

ESTIMATED NUMBER OF PATIENTS ADMITTED TO E.M.S. HOSPITALS FOR DISABILITIES DUE TO ENEMY ACTION, 1939–45

Year	Civilians	Civil Defence Personnel (including Police)	Merchant Navy Personnel (including any passengers)	Totals
1939	60	45	465	570
1940	28,925	1,890	1,195	32,010
1941	20,495	1,660	810	22,965
1942	3,640	635	255	4,530
1943	3,265	430	135	3,830
1944	18,410	540	115	19,065
1945	3,305	20	45	3,370
Totals	78,100	5,220	3,020	86,340

PART II

The Ancillary Services

CHAPTER 7
THE CIVIL DEFENCE CASUALTY SERVICES

by

LT. COLONEL E. S. GOSS

M.C., I.M.S. (ret.)

Assistant to the Consultant Adviser, Casualty Services

SECTION I: EARLY ORGANISATION AND POLICY, 1925-39

FIRST REPORT ON CASUALTY SERVICES REQUIREMENTS FOR LONDON

IN the years preceding the war much work had been done to provide an efficient casualty service for Great Britain should an emergency arise, and the year 1925 may be taken as that in which the foundations of such a service were laid. In July of that year the Air Staff furnished to the Committee of Imperial Defence an estimate of the casualties which they considered likely to occur in the London area as a result of enemy air bombing, basing their calculation on the assumption that 17 persons would be killed and 33 wounded per ton of bombs dropped. On this estimate the first report on the Casualty Services which would be required for the London area was prepared.

This report, which was drawn up by Colonel P. G. Stock of the Ministry of Health, and submitted on February 23, 1926, may be considered as the initial stage in the organisation of the casualty services. The establishment of stretcher parties, casualty dressing stations, an ambulance service and the provision of hospital accommodation and equipment were fully considered in this report, and among its many recommendations was one that a special A.R.P. sub-committee should be formed, on which the Ministry of Health, the War Office and the Police should be represented. This sub-committee was formed and the question of responsibility for the collection and treatment of casualties was discussed. The Ministry of Health considered that the Army should accept this responsibility, as military casualties were likely at first to be light, while civilian casualties would be heavy. The War Office, however, did not accept this view and emphasised that the military situation would probably not permit of the Army's dealing with civilian casualties as well as its own.

THE FRANCIS SUB-COMMITTEE

The Ministry of Health finally gave way on this point and an interdepartmental sub-committee was set up, under a chairman appointed by the Ministry of Health, to work out a scheme for the medical services in London. This sub-committee, which was known as the Francis Subcommittee (see Introduction) from the name of its Chairman, Mr. H. W. S. Francis, C.B., O.B.E., a Principal Assistant Secretary of the Ministry of Health, included representatives of the Ministry of Health, the War Office, the Home Office, and the Ministry of Transport. Its terms of reference were, to draw up a scheme to apply to the Metropolitan Police district and the City of London for:

(*a*) The medical treatment of casualties, including co-ordination of the existing ambulance services, and their expansion if necessary;
(*b*) Hospital accommodation;
(*c*) The evacuation of wounded in the area of bombardment;
(*d*) To report with estimates of the personnel and material required.

The first report of the Francis Sub-committee was produced in July 1927, and between that date and the year 1934 a further number of reports was made to the Organisations Sub-committee of the Committee of Imperial Defence. In these reports further schemes for the treatment of casualties were submitted, and among the duties of the casualty services, the cleansing of persons contaminated by poison gases, as distinct from the decontamination of material, was included. The sub-committee recommended the establishment of first-aid posts, and that on each there should be based first-aid parties of four men per shift, provided with special first-aid equipment, to go out to incidents. At incidents these first-aid parties would meet the ambulances. Slightly injured casualties, after essential first aid, were to go on foot, or would be sent in sitting-case cars to the nearest first-aid and cleansing centres, while seriously injured persons would receive necessary first-aid treatment on the spot and then be sent by ambulance to the casualty clearing hospitals. It was also recommended that there should be combined first-aid and cleansing centres, and a layout for such premises was submitted. This was the forerunner of the more elaborate plans which were adopted later. The question of staffing first-aid parties was also considered, and the use of members of the St. John Ambulance Brigade and the British Red Cross Society recommended. In the draft handbook on Passive Air Defence dated May 1934, first-aid parties were described as being stationed at selected posts throughout the Metropolitan District. Wherever possible, persons contaminated by poison gas, but not otherwise injured, would also be dealt with at first-aid stations. In London, it was proposed to establish 212 first-aid stations within a radius of distances varying from 4–15 miles of Charing Cross, and that the staff for them should be found from the St. John Ambulance Brigade and the British Red Cross Society.

ORGANISATION OF AIR RAID PRECAUTIONS

From the above short summary it will be seen that by 1934 the Francis Sub-committee had worked out a comprehensive scheme for the first-aid treatment of casualties and their removal to hospital, as well as provision for combined first-aid posts and cleansing centres, in the London area. Up to that date enquiries had to be made under a strict rule of secrecy; and therefore information had been only obtained with considerable difficulty. In April 1935, the veil of secrecy was lifted, and the organisation of Air Raid Precautions in the United Kingdom was begun, the responsibility for its development being placed in the first instance upon the Home Office. So far as the main organisation was concerned, it was decided at the outset that Air Raid Precautions (A.R.P.) should be a local service and that the responsibility for its development should rest upon the local authorities, acting under the general direction of the Home Office.

LOCAL AUTHORITIES AND THE CASUALTY SERVICES

In July 1935, local authorities throughout Great Britain were informed of the above scheme. The circular [1] which was issued required local authorities to make provision for the mobilisation of the medical and first-aid resources of each area, so as to provide first-aid posts and hospitals for more extended treatment, together with an adequate ambulance service. The voluntary aid societies were to help with the enrolment and training of personnel, but were to assume no administrative responsibility for recruits. Guidance to local authorities was further strengthened by the publication of A.R.P. Memorandum No. 1 (first edition) in 1935, in which as an example, the casualty service organisation needed for a county borough was described. (See Part I, Appendix I). The establishment of first-aid parties (on a scale of 12–15 parties, with 25 per cent. reserve in towns, for a population of 100,000), first-aid and decontamination centres (later called first-aid posts), casualty clearing and base hospitals and ambulance services were laid down in this publication. A second edition of this memorandum was published in the following year, and in this edition first-aid and decontamination centres were designated as first-aid posts, and a complete layout for a combined first-aid post and cleansing section was included. (See Fig. 5.)

AIR RAID PRECAUTIONS ACT, 1937

For the next two years work was mainly of a preparatory nature; including the breaking down of prejudice or apathy on the part of certain sections of the general public, and enlisting the co-operation of local authorities. At this time it was realised that the possibility of gas attacks on a population not provided with any means of protection constituted a serious menace, and emphasis was laid upon anti-gas training. A.R.P. handbooks Nos. 1, 2 and 3 were published and the war-time *Atlas of Gas Poisoning* republished in 1936.

Ten, later increased to sixteen, specially selected medical men were trained and appointed as medical instructors in anti-gas measures, to train medical, dental and veterinary practitioners and students. In the same year a civilian anti-gas school was opened at Falfield in Gloucestershire, and in 1937, a second school at Easingwold in Yorkshire. Many

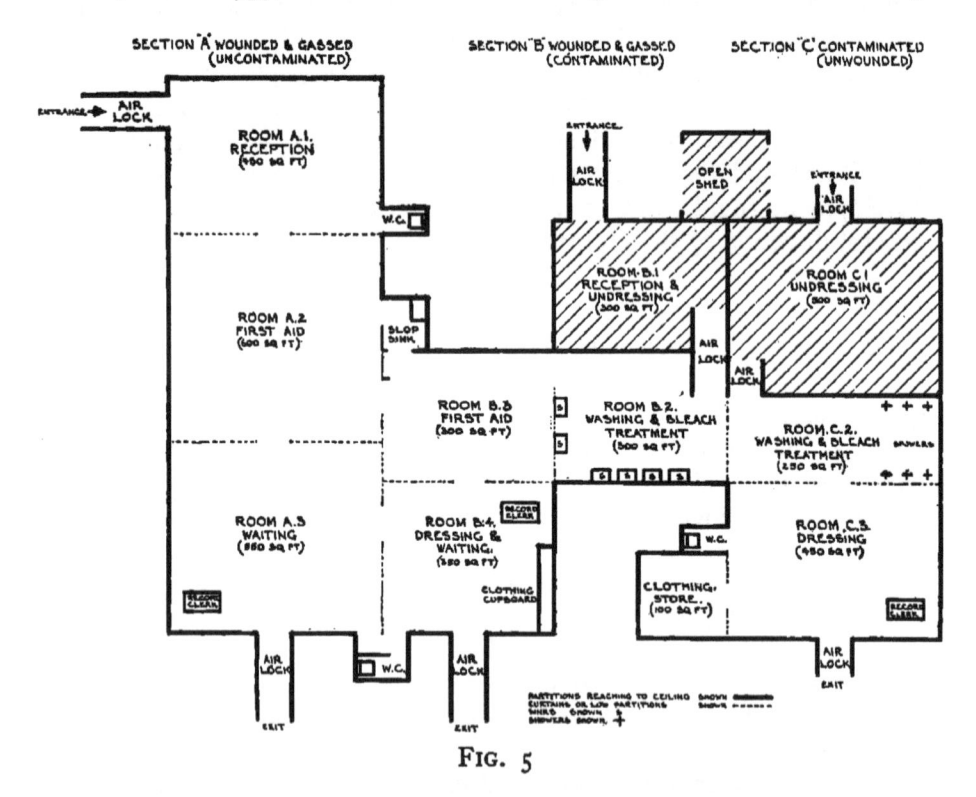

FIG. 5

local authorities prepared schemes; a few, however, were non-co-operative, and no compulsion could be laid upon them until the passing of the Air Raid Precautions Act of December, 1937. That Act, which became law on January 1, 1938, laid upon county councils and county boroughs in England and Wales, and upon county councils and large burghs in Scotland (known as 'Scheme-making Authorities'), a responsibility to prepare general air raid precautions schemes for their areas as prescribed by the Act. This responsibility included the establishment of first-aid posts, first-aid points, first-aid parties with essential transport, and an ambulance service. General control of these services would rest with the A.R.P. Department of the Home Office.[2] First-aid posts at that time were envisaged as a purely local organisation not necessarily related to the hospital system of the area.

ENROLMENT OF PERSONNEL FOR CASUALTY SERVICES

After the passing of the 1937 A.R.P. Act, the scheme-making authorities had a statutory obligation to organise their own casualty services and, in consequence, some confusion arose between them and the uniformed societies which had previously provided the trained personnel. After several meetings, an agreement was finally reached between the two parties and an important circular was issued by the Home Office A.R.P. Department to local authorities in August 1938, announcing the arrangements for the recruitment, instruction and training of personnel to form a scheme-making authority's casualty service. This circular, which was the first document to set out the stages in the formation of such a service, also made it clear once and for all that the scheme-making authority must be responsible for the organisation of the casualty services.[3] This did not mean that the uniformed societies would be cut off from this sphere of their activities. They were still to help and to receive a grant for their services (paragraph 7 of the above circular).

In spite of this circular, which did much to clarify the situation, the recruitment for the casualty services was far from satisfactory, and there was a serious deficiency in the numbers of persons who had enrolled for these services; this was particularly noticeable in first-aid parties. Several reasons have been advanced for this condition, the most cogent being:

(*a*) The late start in recruiting and lack of precision regarding responsibility before August 1938.

(*b*) Many of these, recruited from the St. John Ambulance Brigade in England and Wales, and from the St. Andrew's Ambulance Association in Scotland had melted away, some to the Fighting Services and others to industry where they could obtain good wages.

(*c*) The casualty services were not popular as there was little glamour attached to them and they were not provided with uniforms. Moreover, the service was without officers, with the result that there was no one between the man on the ground and the medical officer of health who was in control of the service. The Government was not satisfied that there was any need for officer and N.C.O. ranks and rates of pay until this had been demonstrated later in operations.

MINISTRY OF HEALTH AND THE CASUALTY SERVICES

During 1938 a change occurred in the general outlook, and it became clear that the first-aid post and ambulance services should be closely related to the hospital service, and it would therefore be more convenient that these services should be administered by the Ministry of Health rather than by the Home Office.

The early conception by the Home Office of a first-aid post was a place, to be built according to a model plan, to which lightly injured casualties should be brought by first-aid party personnel who, after giving minimal first aid, would decide at the incident whether casualties were to be sent to a post or to a hospital. It was not considered necessary to have doctors at first-aid posts, as few general practitioners had any experience in war wounds or war surgery and would not be substantially more valuable than experienced and highly trained first-aid personnel, whereas they would be of definite use in hospitals working with more experienced surgeons. A prominent place in the plan was given to the cleansing of people contaminated by persistent gases, in conformity with the general policy at that time of concentrating air raid precautions largely on measures for meeting anticipated gas attacks. First-aid posts were thus designed to shield the hospitals from a rush of casualties, many of whom would be lightly injured, or not injured at all, and would not require in-patient treatment. As regards first-aid parties, these were to consist of men only and would be stationed at first-aid posts and undergo the same first-aid training as women auxiliary nurses in the posts. When called out to incidents the first-aid parties would deal with the casualties on the spot, bringing back or sending lightly injured to the post and transferring seriously injured to hospitals in ambulances. The first-aid post, party and ambulance service were to be under the local authority and organised, trained and controlled by the medical officer of health and A.R.P. officer, who were servants of the authority; during operations they would be under the control of the local control centre; general direction only was to be exercised by the Home Office. First-aid party personnel were trained in all other aspects of A.R.P. in addition to first aid (such as incendiary bomb control and high explosive bombs, anti-gas measures, etc.), and, like the personnel of first-aid posts, were chiefly recruited by the local authority from one of the uniformed first-aid bodies (e.g. St. John Ambulance Brigade, British Red Cross Society, etc.).

The view of the Ministry of Health was that first-aid posts or 'dressing stations' as they preferred to call them, should possess greater facilities for the treatment of casualties and have doctors in attendance and perhaps a small number of beds for very urgent cases. It was considered that reliance could not be placed on first-aid workers alone to distinguish between cases, as the diagnosis of war injuries was not easy. Dressing stations, as a first choice, should be buildings already in use for medical purposes, such as clinics and the smaller special hospitals which would be suitably adapted, and mobile surgical teams might be formed to work in them. The doctor in charge of a post could be responsible for the individual and team training of the personnel of the post and first-aid parties located at his post, most of whom were members of one or other of the uniformed first-aid bodies. First-aid points, as small treatment centres in villages, were also contemplated.

The main points in the discussions which followed were whether the control of the casualty service as a whole should be transferred from the

Home Office to the Ministry of Health, or whether only the first-aid post, first-aid point and ambulance services should be so transferred, leaving the control of the first-aid party service with the Home Office.

The Ministry of Health took the view that, logically, all units dealing with casualties should be considered as under their control, as a medical department, and referred to the possible effect on the public of placing casualties under the control of the Home Office, which had not a comprehensive medical department. They urged that they were looking at the whole question from the point of view of casualties and that, unless the treatment of casualties was under the control of one department, they would suffer by coming under two departments at different stages in their treatment. They agreed that first-aid posts should act as filters for hospitals to prevent them from being swamped by the simultaneous reception of both lightly and seriously injured casualties; and pointed out that another reason for associating the first-aid post service more closely with the hospital service was the importance of ensuring that a number of first-aid posts should be capable of functioning at very short notice. This would be easily effected only in buildings which were in regular use for medical purposes.

The Home Office did not agree that all units of the casualty service should be transferred to the Ministry of Health, but were willing to concede that this might be done with first-aid posts, first-aid points and ambulances only, as these were closely associated with hospitals, provided that control of the first-aid parties remained with the Home Office, even though this involved a system of dual control. They pointed out that the work of first-aid parties was intimately bound up with other 'outdoor' A.R.P. services, such as rescue parties, wardens, fire services, etc., and parties must be stationed and controlled so as to be immediately available under the local report centre organisation. Their duties were specific and their training should be in the hands of the department which had studied the specific medical and first-aid implications of aerial attack and the tactical control of A.R.P. Services for several years, when the Ministry of Health had not been concerned with such matters.

After due consideration, a change was decided upon, and on December 23, 1938, an announcement was issued by the Lord Privy Seal that from December 1938, the Ministry of Health was assuming responsibility in England and Wales for approving, under the Air Raid Precautions Act of 1937, the provisions in local authorities schemes for first-aid posts, first-aid points and the ambulance service. The A.R.P. Department of the Home Office continued to be responsible for questions of recruiting personnel and of their preliminary training in first aid, and the control of first-aid parties remained with that department.[4] Administration of the transferred casualty services was vested in a newly created Division of the Ministry of Health and in the Medical Section under Dr. J. H. Hebb. As might have been expected, the Ministries' decision evoked a good deal of criticism, particularly from medical officers of health, and, also, from some local authority controllers and their committees.

All were agreed that unified control was essential in order to secure efficiency in administration and obviate obstruction and delays. Cases were mentioned where first-aid party and first-aid post personnel were occupying the same buildings and, when measures for alteration or protection of the building had to be carried out, groups of county surveyors and valuers would report on those parts of the buildings occupied by the first-aid posts, and other groups would follow on their tracks and report on the parts of the buildings occupied by the first-aid parties.

Most medical officers of health and many local authorities were in favour of the Ministry of Health's assuming control of all the casualty services, but some local authority controllers were strongly for a continuance of Home Office control as they found it very satisfactory in their A.R.P. organisation.

Representations made to the Government on the need for unified control of all first-aid services received the reply that the change over had only been made after the most careful consideration, and that there was no prospect of complete unification of control under a single department.

It cannot be denied that delays as foreshadowed were frequent, but they could not always be attributed to the system of dual control; in many cases they were due to the tardy action of a local authority or of one Ministry only, and this might equally have occurred under unified control. The position was greatly improved when first-aid parties were separated from first-aid posts and placed in separate depots. Later, this improvement was extended when Assistant Hospital Officers were appointed in April 1940, as these formed a close link between local authorities and the Ministries.

ADDITION OF MOBILE UNITS TO CASUALTY SERVICES

The Ministry of Health continued to regard the various memoranda and circulars which had been issued from time to time by the Home Office as the basis upon which the first-aid service should be organised, and did not call for fresh schemes where these had already been submitted by local authorities. These authorities were, however, told that consideration was being given by the Ministry to supplementing the fixed posts in less densely developed areas by mobile units which could be used, in effect, to set up first-aid posts as and where required. Experiments were being made and a further communication would be addressed to local authorities as soon as possible. Mobile units were added to the casualty services organisation in March, 1939[5] and a circular was issued to local authorities saying that a doctor should be allocated to every fixed first-aid post and mobile unit and, further, that first-aid posts should, wherever possible, be located at hospitals.[6]

ISSUE OF ALL-METAL STRETCHERS FOR CASUALTY SERVICES

In January 1939, all-metal stretchers were issued to all local authorities as the standard pattern of stretcher for the A.R.P. casualty services. Local authorities had been notified in a previous circular, to expect the issue of this type of stretcher. The initial issue to all scheme-making authorities was on a scale of 25 stretchers per 100,000 population.

PREPAREDNESS OF CASUALTY SERVICES PRIOR TO THE OUTBREAK OF WAR

At the time of the Munich crisis in September 1938, the Air Raid Precautions Scheme was still in an elementary stage throughout the country. Had war been declared then, it would have been necessary to depend almost entirely upon the voluntary aid societies to deal with casualties, as well-organised casualty services were practically non-existent, except in some areas, and then mainly on paper. Some buildings had been earmarked as depots and first-aid posts by local authorities, but few had been adapted. The out-patient departments of hospitals were the only places in which lightly injured casualties could have been adequately attended to; no organised ambulance service existed. The only preparations which were in any way advanced were anti-gas measures. Following the crisis, the country appeared to awake to the seriousness of the situation and active steps were taken to put the air raid precautions into operation. Enrolment and training for the casualty services were speeded up. Work on adapting buildings as ambulance and first-aid party depots and for first-aid posts was commenced in earnest, and separate ambulance services were organised. From January 1939, great strides were made. During the spring and summer, courses were held at a recently opened A.R.P. Staff School in London for medical and other officers concerned with first-aid parties. These courses prepared officers for administrative, executive and staff duties, in addition to training instructors in the specialised first-aid applicable under war conditions.[7]

PROVISION OF UNIFORMS FOR A.R.P. SERVICES

As the result of the widespread desire among members of the air raid precautions services for some form of uniform, the Government decided to place local authorities in a position to provide free uniform for their services on a grant-aided basis. The uniforms proposed were, for men volunteers, a uniform overall (combination suit) in dark blue heavy drill cloth, with a red A.R.P. badge on the left breast; for women drivers and attendants of ambulances and drivers of sitting-case cars, a light coat of the same material with a similar badge and a soft peaked cap; for women members of first-aid posts, a nursing overall as provided for nursing auxiliaries, but bearing the letters A.R.P.

PUBLICATION OF A.R.P. HANDBOOK NO. 10 AND FIRST-AID TRAINING

In September 1939, A.R.P. Handbook No. 10 (The training and work of first-aid parties) was published by the A.R.P. Department of the Home Office. This book described the local training and tactical organisation for first-aid parties (in London Region, 'stretcher parties') and stressed the necessity for the combined training of first-aid party personnel with other A.R.P. services, such as rescue parties. The aim of the book was to teach the application to war-time needs of the principles of pure first aid until its publication. The theoretical instruction in first aid had been that of the St. John Ambulance and British Red Cross type which was more suited to pre-war emergencies.

CASUALTY SERVICES AT THE OUTBREAK OF THE WAR

When war was declared, the casualty service organisation was fairly complete and capable of functioning efficiently, although not fully manned, especially the first-aid parties.

Fixed First-aid Posts. As mentioned earlier, the A.R.P. Department of the Home Office had given a lead to local authorities in preparing schemes for units of their casualty services, and directions, together with model plans for combined first-aid post and cleansing centres, had been issued in a memorandum.[8]

In several places first-aid posts had been built according to these plans and were very satisfactory; they were mostly constructed of brick and concrete and had good overhead and lateral protection, but in others, instead of following these plans, a policy of improvisation was adopted. Any kind of structure which was vacant or could be rendered vacant was selected and earmarked, without sufficient regard to the practicability of adapting it to its new purpose. Such buildings as public swimming baths with high glass roofs, schools with high roofs and windows and glass partitions between the rooms, sports pavilions built of wood, disused and sometimes derelict, and other types of buildings of poor structure were taken over and adapted for use as first-aid posts. In a few instances, however, satisfactory buildings such as child welfare clinics, well constructed and solid, were used.

This policy of improvisation might have been justified by the apparent stress and urgency of the situation, and had the places chosen been looked upon as some sort of shelter where first aid could be carried out until something better was provided, no criticism could have been made.

Had more consideration been given to the essential minimum requirements for first-aid posts, those found unsuitable could have been retained only until they could be replaced by new buildings, or by existing buildings suitable for adaptation, at a time when labour and material were more readily available and comparatively cheap. By this means greater efficiency would have been achieved and much money saved.

As it was, there began a piecemeal, patchwork system of adaptation. Where possible, roofs were strutted to provide overhead cover, sandbags were tried to provide lateral cover, but from faulty laying and lack of protection from damp, in many places these rapidly disintegrated. They were to be replaced later by brick revetments, and in many cases this was ultimately done, although not without difficulty. Many local authorities had realised the importance of building brick revetments in the first instance and had erected them.

Other improvements were adopted until in most places it was decided that no more could be done, especially since labour and material were more difficult to obtain and their cost had increased. In consequence, many of these adapted buildings had little or no protection against blast and splinters of bombs or A.A. shells, although most of them were more or less proof against gas.

By contrast, the interior layout of the buildings was, on the whole, extremely good and due regard had been paid to the easy progress of casualties so as to avoid congestion and delay. It was inevitable that some posts should be better than others, and that there would be some which did not come up to the required standard. It can be said, however, that much thought had been given to the interior organisation of first-aid posts and that, in most cases, available space and material had been utilised to the best advantage.

It would have been satisfactory to base first-aid posts in or near casualty receiving hospitals, as was done in many cases,[9] one of the advantages being that everyone knew where hospitals were and casualties could reach them quickly, whereas there could be delay in finding isolated first-aid posts, especially in the dark, in spite of the system of sign posting generally in use. It was obvious however, that hospitals alone would not be sufficient, so first-aid posts were provided on the scale of six posts per 100,000 population,[10] and in urban districts not more than one mile apart.

Each post was divided into two sections, one for first aid and one for gas cleansing, separate accommodation being provided for each sex.

Equipment. A circular issued in October 1938, by the Home Office, set out schedules of the stores and equipment suggested for first-aid posts. These schedules were revised when the Ministry of Health assumed control.

The equipment provided was ample and of good quality. In some circles, especially medical, fears were expressed that it was too lavish for pure first aid and might tend to encourage operative measures which were undesirable at first-aid posts, and to delay the despatch of serious cases to hospital.

First-aid posts were graded as follows: A large post for a population of 30,000 to 60,000; a medium post for a population of 20,000 to 30,000; a small post for a population of 3,000 to 20,000.

Personnel. It was intended that the staffs of first-aid posts should consist mainly of part-time volunteers, and in March 1939, it was laid down that large posts in the most congested areas should have a personnel of 60 (10 men and 50 women), and for the remaining types of posts a staff of 40 (7 men and 33 women), all working on three 8-hour shifts. In addition, a doctor and trained nurse were attached to each post. Later, it was found necessary to increase the number of whole-time personnel in first-aid posts. By September 3, 1939, 150,000 persons had been enrolled for first-aid posts and mobile units, 10,000 men and 35,000 women being whole-time, the rest part-time. Out of a total of 2,180 first-aid posts which had been approved for England and Wales 1,912 were ready, and the remainder on the way to completion by September 3, 1939.

First-aid Points. In rural and semi-rural districts first-aid points had been established. Each of these consisted of a box of first-aid equipment costing 25s., which was kept in some convenient and accessible place, usually in a doctor's surgery, a vicarage, or in a selected private country house. This formed a centre where part-time volunteers met and trained in first aid, so that they could deal with lightly injured persons when the need arose. No doctor, trained nurse or paid personnel were attached to a point, and the maintenance cost, except for replacement of dressings used for casualties, was nil. Training in first aid was usually conducted by a member of one of the voluntary aid societies or by a local doctor. On the outbreak of war there were about 6,500 first-aid points throughout England and Wales.

Mobile Units (later Mobile First-aid Units). A total of 783 of these units had been approved and were mostly ready. Each consisted of a motor vehicle, such as a Bedford truck, a furniture van or even a single-decker passenger bus, in which the equipment of a fixed first-aid post and the medical staff of the unit were carried; the auxiliary personnel travelled separately. These vehicles were most suitably stationed at hospitals and would go out from them when summoned to an incident. When it was not possible to locate them at hospitals, they were placed at convenient centres, regard being paid to the fact that linking up with a doctor was essential. First aid was not to be carried out inside these vehicles.

The main functions of a mobile unit were:

(i) To go to an incident and set up a first-aid post in some convenient previously earmarked building (e.g. a school or public house), or even in the open air near to where the incident had occurred, provided that there was not already a fixed first-aid post in the vicinity to deal with casualties.

(ii) To reinforce an overworked fixed first-aid post or to take over from one damaged or destroyed.

(iii) To provide supervision, classification of injuries and skilled treatment by a doctor and nurses at the scene of an incident.

(iv) To set up and act as a temporary casualty receiving hospital, where such a hospital had been damaged or destroyed. Most valuable work could be done in this way, especially if this temporary hospital was used by a mobile surgical team.

Personnel. The personnel of a mobile unit consisted of eighteen women nursing auxiliaries (for three shifts of eight hours each), in addition to a doctor and trained nurse and two men drivers.

Ambulance Service. Before 1935 ambulance services were maintained by local authorities for ordinary duties, e.g. the transport of accident cases, cases of illness and infectious disease, etc., to hospital. This service was augmented by ambulances belonging to the Order of St. John, the British Red Cross Society and other voluntary aid bodies and there was no uniformity in design. An even greater handicap was that the stretchers with which the different types of ambulances were equipped were not interchangeable. In London the position was further complicated by the maintenance of one ambulance service by the London County Council for the Administrative County of London, and many others by local authorities for their own districts outside this area.

It had already been recommended by the Francis Sub-Committee that co-ordination should be secured by placing all ambulances under unified control; but it was not until 1935 that local authorities were asked by the Government to review their existing ambulance services and to make arrangements to organise services for the transport of air raid casualties, in addition to ordinary peace-time duties. For this purpose the existing services were to be expanded, if necessary, by obtaining and adapting extra vehicles to carry stretcher cases when required by an emergency. It was strongly recommended that when new ambulances were ordered, whether by local authorities or by private bodies, they should be fitted to take any kind of stretcher in general civilian use. Later, in 1936, the standard army pattern of stretcher was included.

Under the Air Raid Precautions Act of 1937, the emergency ambulance service, i.e. the street service for picking up air-raid casualties, became the responsibility of local authorities. The original plans made before the war were usually based on the idea that suitable commercial vehicles, e.g. tradesmen's vans, should be earmarked and have stretcher-carrying fitments made for them, so that in the event of an emergency they could be taken over and used as part-time ambulances after installing the fitments.

Cars were also earmarked for conveying sitting casualties. These plans were designed to avoid heavy capital expenditure on a large number of special vehicles in time of peace, and ensured that the requisite service would be immediately forthcoming on the outbreak of war.

About 6,000 trade vehicles were to be provided on these terms in England and Wales, although this arrangement proved more difficult to put into practice than had been expected. The earmarking of vehicles was being undertaken independently by Government departments and the Services as well as by local authorities, and it was by no means uncommon for the same vehicles to be earmarked by more than one authority.

Few commercial vehicles were really suitable for use as ambulances, some were too small to accommodate stretchers, others too large to be accommodated in garages and the engines too heavy for women to start by hand, no self-starter generally being provided. Vehicles were constantly changing ownership, and it was impossible to keep the list of earmarked vehicles up to date, as owners seldom notified the local authorities of any change of ownership.

When hostilities began these vehicles were called in, many fewer appeared than was expected and most of the best of them were claimed by the Services and by Government Departments who had a higher priority than the A.R.P. services. Those obtained as ambulances were often in poor mechanical condition, unsuitable for the purpose and too heavy for women to drive. The rates of hire for these vehicles were fixed by the Ministry of War Transport and were high; in addition, the cost of maintaining large numbers of these vehicles in running order was enormous. It was estimated that the annual expenditure would be in the neighbourhood of £900,000, possibly more.

In October 1939, therefore, the Minister of Health directed local authorities to buy suitable secondhand cars and convert them into ambulances in place of the hired trade vans.[11] This arrangement, considered as a war-time measure, was satisfactory except that local authorities were not at first allowed to spend more than £30 for the vehicle and another £20–£30 on its conversion to an ambulance, in all not more than £60 for the completed vehicle. About the same time the Minister of Home Security authorised local authorities to purchase secondhand cars for conveying first-aid and light rescue party personnel and here also the cost per car was not to exceed £30.[12] The total establishment of ambulances had been laid down by the Home Office in January 1939, as approximately 19,000, and by the end of December 1939, about half of the 6,000 trade vehicles had been replaced by converted-car ambulances, effecting a substantial saving in expenditure. While the actual conversion of cars into ambulances presented little difficulty in the early days, buying satisfactory vehicles was a difficult problem. Those local authorities which got in early had the advantage, and there is no doubt that some vehicles which were in really sound mechanical condition were bought at bargain prices; in addition, some excellent cars were donated by private persons. It quickly became known, however, that local authorities were buying vehicles on a large scale and this had the immediate effect of putting the prices up. As local authorities were still tied to the £30 per purchase, they could only obtain the older vehicles, which were frequently mechanically unsound, with the result that maintenance costs were high and, as it turned out, vehicles had to be replaced in large numbers after a year or two. A high percentage of such cars needed an extensive overhaul after a short spell of use; each local authority had to maintain a staff of mechanics to keep them in running order, and their actual cost after counting repairs and reconditioning was often more than it would have cost to buy new cars. The position with regard to cars for sitting cases was if anything rather worse. The maximum price allowed by Government being £30 the best cars were naturally converted into ambulances and those in a poorer mechanical condition were used for sitting cases. Again, this led to high maintenance costs, and a large replacement programme after a year or two could be expected.

From this unpromising material an efficient service was eventually built up and, as its later history shows, stood up well to the calls made upon it. Most of the drivers and attendants were young women and it was largely due to the care and attention which they bestowed upon their vehicles, to their high morale and disregard of danger whilst driving them under all conditions, that the ambulance service achieved such a notable success. No amount of praise can be too high for the personnel of the ambulance service.

Two types of ambulances were required for the Casualty Service organisation:

> Large ambulances: used mainly for inter-hospital work and described elsewhere. (Chap. 8).
>
> Small ambulances; carrying two to four stretchers, used principally for picking up casualties in the street and clearing first-aid posts. Local authorities were responsible for providing these and for having stretcher carrying fitments made for them. For this a percentage grant was paid by Government under the Air Raid Precautions Act.[13]

Experience showed the undesirability of using ambulances of varying capacities, as it added to the difficulty of controllers in deciding how many ambulances should be sent to incidents.

On September 3, 1939, 1,600 whole-time and about 150 part-time local authority ambulances were ready in the London Region, and 5,300 whole-time and 5,200 part-time in the provinces in England and Wales. By the end of December, 1939, whole-time and part-time local authority ambulances in London numbered 1,902 and 215 respectively and in the provinces 5,181 and 5,945. At this time sitting-case cars in London numbered 1,310 whole-time and 1,122 part-time, the strength in the provinces being 1,022 and 11,402 respectively.

Personnel. The total personnel of the ambulance services in England and Wales, comprising drivers and attendants for ambulances and drivers for sitting-case cars, was originally laid down in January 1939, as 129,600, the whole to be composed of women only.[14] This figure had lost any real significance on account of the change in vehicular establishment, and the split between whole-time ambulances and part-time auxiliaries; also because the service had been opened to men as well as to women. It was found impracticable to assess a requisite personnel establishment where there was no uniform standard in the periods of duty of part-time unpaid volunteers. Figures at December 31, 1939, show that the total personnel, whole-time and part-time, men and women, in England and Wales, was about 80,900 (of which London Region provided 17,344). The total number of whole-time men and women was 26,900 as against 54,000 part-time.

Recruitments of drivers and attendants had on the whole been unsatisfactory, due in many cases to apathy and lack of uniforms and badges; moreover, there was a great demand for labour carrying good wages. In many large cities recruitment had been particularly disappointing.

First-aid Party Service (in London Region, 'stretcher party'). When war broke out, the first-aid party service was still under the control of the Home Office (A.R.P. Dept.). Scheme-making authorities were responsible for the enrolment of suitable volunteers, each of whom was obliged to hold a certificate in first aid from one of the recognised voluntary aid bodies (e.g. St. John Ambulance Association, British Red Cross Society, the St. Andrew's Ambulance Association, etc.). These volunteers after enrolment and a short basic training in general A.R.P. subjects, were trained in first aid and anti-gas measures, and practical and collective training together with combined training with other A.R.P. services were carried out. Classes were arranged for volunteers not in possession of certificates before they could be allocated to first-aid parties.

First-aid and stretcher parties each consisted of four men, with a car and a driver. Parties on duty were stationed in first-aid party depots, protected as far as possible from blast, splinters and gas. These depots were tactically distributed over an area so that any part of it could be reached with the shortest delay, and were in telephonic communication with the local control centre. The number of parties allotted to each depot depended on local conditions, but in urban areas they were never less than two. From these depots parties would go out in their own transport to incidents, when summoned by the local control centre, or, exceptionally, as the result of direct calls by wardens, police, etc. (in such cases the control centre was always to be notified).

Each party had a leader, selected usually by the personnel themselves, who would direct the activities of the party. Each member of the party carried a first-aid pouch containing first-aid equipment, and in addition a water-bottle and an electric handlamp. Each party carried a haversack which contained a greater quantity of equipment and included sectional splints, wooden thigh splints with straps, spare respirators (usually five), eight blankets and four metal stretchers, the last named later carried on the roof of the car in a special fitment.

Personnel. Reference has already been made to the shortage of personnel in the first-aid party service, and little improvement had taken place when war broke out. In many of the more important and vulnerable areas the problem of obtaining this personnel, especially wholetime, presented the greatest difficulty. Many of these places were industrial areas in which large numbers of men were in reserved occupations, and there was a tendency for them to hold back from any A.R.P. obligation on account of their long hours of work and of the expectation of good wages in industry. In less industrialised areas the problem of obtaining whole-time personnel was somewhat easier, but it was seldom an easy one. In 1938 first-aid parties had been established on a scale of 12–15 parties (with 25 per cent. reserve in towns) per 100,000 population. After further consideration, however, the conclusion was reached that these provisions were likely to be quite insufficient, especially in thickly populated areas and, later, in 1939, the whole basis of calculation was changed in order to distinguish between requirements for areas of different vulnerability. A new scale was worked out and parties were allocated on a scale of 66 per 100,000 population in most vulnerable areas, 33 in highly vulnerable areas, 26 in less vulnerable areas and 20 in least vulnerable areas.

A war establishment figure of 117,500 personnel had been provisionally fixed for the whole country early in 1939, but in August 1939 there was actually a shortage of about 44 per cent., leaving a total strength of roughly 66,000 available personnel, so that it can be seen that the position was serious. This had already been pointed out in a memorandum to the Lord Privy Seal on July 25.

The Rescue Party Service. Although not at that time classed as a branch of the Casualty Service organisation, mention must be made of this Service, as it was designed to work in close co-operation with the first-aid party service at incidents, and reference will be made to it later. Rescue parties, each consisting of six or eight men with their own transport, were enrolled partly from local authorities' staff and partly from employees of building contractors, and were under the control of the local authority engineer or surveyor. They were originally established on a scale of 6 parties per 100,000 population in urban areas. As was done for first-aid parties, a new scale was worked out and heavy and light rescue parties were constituted and allocated on a scale of 6 heavy parties of 9 men each and 24 light parties of 7 men each per 100,000 population in most vulnerable areas, 3 heavy and 12 light parties in highly vulnerable areas, and 1 heavy and 9 light parties in less vulnerable areas, and 1 heavy and 6 light parties in least vulnerable areas. Their main duties were to extricate casualties from damaged buildings, demolition work and remove debris. Each party was under a leader skilled in his work. They were based on depots similar to those of first-aid parties.

First Aid in Industry. In 1936 the Home Office had published a useful and instructive pamphlet to guide occupiers of factories and workshops in establishing at their works a satisfactory first-aid and ambulance service.[15] In 1937 the Home Office (A.R.P. Dept.) published a handbook dealing with the air raid precautions which should be taken in factories and business premises.[16] This handbook stressed the responsibility of employers of labour for the protection of their employees whilst at work, and the safeguarding of their property. Space was devoted to the provision of first-aid posts, gas-cleansing centres, first-aid parties, ambulance transport and the training of personnel in first aid, and it was suggested that at least one out of every twenty work people should be trained in first aid and anti-gas precautions. The Civil Defence Act of 1939 required all commercial and industrial undertakings which employed more than thirty persons to ensure that all their employees knew what to do in the event of air raids and that necessary personnel should be trained in first aid, anti-gas measures and fire-fighting, and that equipment should be provided for these purposes. A suggested scale of personal protective equipment for use by personnel so employed was suggested. Many factories and commercial undertakings throughout the country already possessed elaborate and very efficient provision for first aid, and only in some cases were changes necessary. As regards gas cleansing, more extensive measures had to be taken. Training in first aid was carried out among the employees, classes being conducted by the factory doctor, if there was one, by the trained nurse present in most factories of any size, or by trained instructors of one of the voluntary aid bodies. At the beginning of the war many of the larger factories and commercial concerns had very seriously taken up the provision of first aid, as well as other A.R.P. measures, and on the whole arrangements were fairly satisfactory. Little official guidance and supervision had however been given in the construction and administration of first aid and gas-cleansing measures at this stage, and co-operation was sadly lacking between the A.R.P. Casualty Services in factories and commercial undertakings and those of local authorities.

THE MORTUARY SERVICE

The duty of providing special arrangements to deal with the bodies of civilians killed by enemy action was laid upon local authorities by the

Ministry of Health and by Defence Regulations.[17] The circular laid down that bodies would be placed in a secluded place by rescue or first-aid personnel and later collected and removed in a special mortuary van to a mortuary. The personnel of the Mortuary Service, mainly part-time, might already be in the service of a local authority, or be specially recruited for the purpose. The transport, which should consist of suitable covered vehicles, was to be either hired or requisitioned. Arrangements were to be made to separate gas-contaminated bodies from others and for their cleansing. Accommodation for relatives who came to identify bodies, and for the temporary storage of personal effects recovered from the bodies, was to be provided. Mortuaries were to be under the charge of competent whole-time superintendents, and in vulnerable areas with a population of over 30,000 would be fully equipped and located in buildings which could be adapted on a scale of provision for 400 bodies per 100,000 population. In less vulnerable areas provision would be less, and in rural districts and small urban areas earmarking of premises to be used as mortuaries was considered sufficient. At the beginning of the war the Mortuary Service was one of the more difficult problems with which the Ministry of Health had to deal. This was mainly due to the unattractiveness of the Service for volunteers, and the expansion of the Service for war-time requirements was much greater than could be covered by pre-war personnel. A considerable provision of additional mortuaries was necessary and suitable buildings were hard to find. The duties required of the mortuary staff were also very exacting; gruesome and distressing services had to be carried out, and the reception of relatives and the recording of particulars of dead bodies had to be most carefully conducted. There was at the beginning and throughout the war a shortage of suitable vehicles for transport of bodies to the mortuaries, and it was expected that ambulances would on occasions perforce have to be used. In the circumstances of modern bombing it was realised that the identification of corpses could not always be secured. In the more vulnerable areas a number of spaces for graves were made ready in advance.

TRANSFER OF DIRECTION OF TECHNICAL TRAINING

In December 1939, the training branch of the A.R.P. Department was re-constituted, and although the general responsibility for the individual training of first-aid and stretcher parties remained with the A.R.P. Department, the responsibility for the technical oversight and direction of training and exercises passed in England and Wales to the Director-General of the Emergency Medical Services (Dr. J. H. Hebb), who was responsible in this latter to the Minister of Home Security. Dr. N. W. Hammer (later Lt. Colonel) was transferred from the A.R.P. Department of the Home Office, to the Ministry of Health to work under Dr. Hebb, in close collaboration with the A.R.P. Training Branch.

Medical Officers of Health of local authorities were responsible to the Director-General of the Emergency Medical Services, through Regional Hospital Officers, for carrying out the above work.

FORMATION OF THE MINISTRY OF HOME SECURITY

On the outbreak of war, the then Lord Privy Seal (Sir John Anderson) became Home Secretary and also Minister of Home Security, and a separate Ministry was formed under the title of 'The Ministry of Home Security' to co-ordinate civil defence throughout the country. This replaced the A.R.P. Department of the Home Office.

SECTION II: FIRST YEAR OF ACTIVE WARFARE, 1940-41

CONSOLIDATION AND TRAINING OF THE CASUALTY SERVICES

MODIFICATIONS IN FIRST-AID TRAINING

No enemy air raids occurred during the early part of 1940, during which the expansion and consolidation of the Casualty Service and the training of its personnel in first aid were continued. Ideas for teaching this subject had undergone a great change. It was being realised that first aid as formerly practised in dealing with accident cases, generally unattended with any danger to rescuers, would not fully meet the case of casualties caused by enemy action. Large numbers of persons would probably be involved and those rendering first aid might be exposed to extreme danger and would have to work under very difficult circumstances. Not only the Casualty Service but the entire population of the United Kingdom owes an immense debt to the voluntary aid societies for their system of training, without which we should have been hard put to it when war broke out, but it was found that considerable modifications would be necessary under the abnormal conditions which bombing raids would produce. In air raids, which would frequently occur at night, first aid must often be given in darkness, in dirt, and in the confusion caused by the noise of explosions and the destruction of buildings. The supreme need in dealing with casualties under such conditions is the saving of time. Ultimate recovery, after a stay in hospital and a smooth convalescence, depends upon getting a seriously injured casualty to hospital as soon as possible, so that resuscitation and effective surgical treatment can be carried out within a short time of wounding. It is here that training is valuable. The main considerations in dealing with casualties at incidents are: to save life by correct and prompt treatment; to treat shock; to handle injured persons judiciously and carefully so as to prevent their injuries from becoming worse and to remove them swiftly to shelter and skilled care. The exercise of these principles of first-aid treatment requires the omission of much elaborate splinting and meticulous bandaging, which are both time-consuming and dependent on reasonably safe circumstances.

The modified system of first aid, admirably laid down in A.R.P. Handbook No. 10 (1st Edition), 1939, and which was being taught to personnel of the first-aid party service, was based on those principles. Personnel of the first-aid posts, points and ambulance services continued to be trained in the British Red Cross Society, St. John, and St. Andrew's Ambulance methods.

The memorandum issued by the Ministry of Health in 1939 for the guidance of medical officers and other personnel at first-aid posts had perhaps proved rather misleading, as after laying down correctly the functions of first-aid posts and stressing the importance of minimal first aid being carried out in them, it described forms of treatment for certain conditions which later experience showed to be too elaborate and ambitious for the facilities available. Treatment of such cases should have been carried out only in hospitals.

Instructions for giving tetanus anti-toxin (A.T.S.) to all casualties with open wounds were given in this memorandum, a measure of extreme importance. These instructions were subsequently emphasised and amplified in E.M.S. Instruction 351 of March 1942.

TOURNIQUETS

A controversy with regard to tourniquets, particularly the Samway type, in which Sir Thomas Lewis, C.B.E., M.D., F.R.C.P. had taken a prominent part, was referred by the Ministry of Home Security to the Ministry of Health in January 1940. In spite, however, of general agreement on the dangers of the over-use of this tourniquet, it was not considered necessary to scrap the large number (290,000) which had been issued for the A.R.P. Services, but it was considered desirable that every opportunity should be taken for first-aid parties to be given special instruction on the use and misuse of tourniquets in general.

APPOINTMENT OF ASSISTANT HOSPITAL OFFICERS

In April 1940, in order to assist Regional Hospital Officers in the discharge of their responsibilities to the A.R.P. Casualty Services, a medical officer was appointed to each Region to act as a staff officer to the Hospital Officer, after a course of instruction in A.R.P. subjects held at Westminster Hospital.

The main duties of these Assistant Hospital Officers were to supervise the training of the local casualty services and to bring them to the highest possible state of operational efficiency. They would also assist in the technical training of first-aid parties and, if required, in the first-aid training of the rescue services. During combined exercises or actual operations, Assistant Hospital Officers would act as staff officers of the

Regional Commissioners for the control of the Casualty Services. In May 1940, a comprehensive and most instructive E.M.S.I. was issued by the Ministry to all Hospital and Assistant Hospital Officers and to Group Officers, about this new appointment and the various duties attached to it.[18] The appointment of these Assistant Hospital Officers was an extremely wise move to ensure an improvement not only in the first-aid training of the Casualty Services but also in all matters connected with their administration and welfare. These officers also formed a valuable personal link between medical officers of health of local authorities and Regional headquarters.

Unfortunately, the misnomer of 'Assistant Hospital Officer' tended to prevent full effect being given to their functions as defined. They were in fact regarded for a time as little more than one of the 'assistants' of Hospital Officers, whereas their duties did not lie in hospitals but in the field.

FIRST AIR RAIDS ON ENGLAND

The first bombs fell on England in May 1940, doing little damage, but after the collapse of France in June, frequent attacks were made on various places and an increasing number of casualties resulted. During this period the casualty services, in common with other A.R.P. services, were finding their feet and putting into practice what they had learnt in their training. Very good reports of their work were received from many parts of the country. After the opening of the Battle of Britain, heavy bombing attacks were made on convoys, aerodromes and aircraft factories, as well as on several large towns. Many severe attacks were directed against London during the last four months of the year.

APPOINTMENT OF CONSULTANT ADVISER FOR CASUALTY SERVICES

On June 11, Mr. E. Rock Carling, F.R.C.S. (later Sir Ernest Rock Carling) was appointed Consultant Adviser to the Ministers of Health and of Home Security for the Casualty Services.

INTENSIFICATION OF FIRST-AID TRAINING

All over the country the training of A.R.P. personnel in the various branches of the Casualty Service was intensified and frequent combined exercises were held by day and by night, especially in places where bombing attacks had been made and were likely to recur. In April 1940, it was laid down that rescue parties (which now should each consist of ten men, including a leader and driver) would be supplied with first-aid equipment and that not less than half their number would be trained in first aid.

About this time the faking of injuries on 'casualties' and the using of damaged or demolished buildings at exercises were seriously taken up as expedients for training first-aid parties. Realism was thus introduced and interest in instruction stimulated.

'WILLESDEN TRIGGLIFT' (WEBBING BANDS)

In July 1940, a most important article of equipment, consisting of a set of four webbing bands with metal handles, was sanctioned for issue to rescue parties on the scale of two sets per party, after demonstrations of these webbing bands had been given to representatives of the Ministry of Health and of the voluntary aid bodies. This equipment, which was devised by Mr. A. G. T. Trigg, of Chiswick (since deceased), was to be used for carrying casualties in narrow or awkward situations where rigid stretchers were found impracticable.

METHOD OF BLANKETING STRETCHERS

In November a method of blanketing A.R.P. or other types of stretcher which had been evolved by stretcher party leaders and personnel at Wanstead and Woodford, and required two blankets only, was described in the *British Medical Journal* by Dr. E. B. Grogono, Medical Officer for Civil Defence at Wanstead and Woodford.[19] A further reference will be made to this later.

MALE PERSONNEL OF FIRST-AID POST AND AMBULANCE SERVICES

A tendency having appeared for male members of the first-aid post and ambulance services to resign and seek more lucrative work in other Government departments, a circular was issued by the Ministry of Health to local authorities drawing attention to Civil Defence (Employment) (No. 2) Order of September 12, 1940, which had been made by the Minister under Regulation 29B of the Defence (General) Regulations, 1939. The general effect of this was to require all male whole-time personnel of the first-aid post and ambulance services to continue in that employment until their services were dispensed with in accordance with the Order.[20]

FIRST-AID PARTY EQUIPMENT PANEL

Mention must be made of this very important panel which was formed in November 1940, on similar lines to the Rescue Equipment Panel already in existence.

The panel, whose chairman was Mr. E. Rock Carling, consisted of representatives of the Ministry of Health (including Regional representatives), the Ministry of Home Security (Supply Policy Division), the Ministry of Works and Buildings and the Department of Health for Scotland and Welsh Board of Health. At frequent meetings in London, questions of change of, additions to, and improvements in, the equipment of all branches of the casualty services were discussed and recommendations made. This panel was responsible for many improvements in the equipment of these services from time to time.

CONTINUANCE OF HEAVY RAIDS—JANUARY–MAY, 1941

The year 1941 opened with a continuance of heavy raids on London and on arms production towns and cities, as described elsewhere in this History. From the middle of May until the end of the year, London enjoyed comparative freedom from heavy raids, although several were made on other parts of the country.

ANTI-GAS PRECAUTIONS

After anxiety had been expressed by the Government as to the adequacy of existing anti-gas measures to meet a possible emergency, there was a general tightening up of these measures in all likely target areas throughout the country. Many cleansing sections of first-aid posts and public cleansing centres, which had hitherto been incomplete or not properly equipped, were put in order, and, where necessary, built as *ad hoc* buildings, and other measures for the cleansing of contaminated persons and the decontamination of their clothing were instituted.

UNIFORMS FOR FIRST-AID PARTIES AND RESCUE PARTIES

In February notice was given by the Minister of Home Security to local authorities that arrangements had been made for the provision of heavy uniforms of battle-dress design for members of first-aid parties and rescue parties.

METHOD OF SECURING A PATIENT TO A STRETCHER

In March, a method of securing a patient to an A.R.P. stretcher by means of seven triangular bandages, devised by Mr. H. F. Hodges, Staff Officer for stretcher parties, and Dr. E. B. Grogono, Medical Officer for Civil Defence, Wanstead and Woodford, was described in the *Lancet*.

The 'Neil-Robertson stretcher' which had proved valuable in the Navy for removing wounded men from turrets and stokeholes, or from ship to ship, was also described.[21] Although these stretchers had not been approved for issue as A.R.P. equipment, several local authorities, notably in the London Region, had obtained them and they were found of great value in rescue work.

INTERCHANGEABILITY OF FIRST-AID, RESCUE AND DECONTAMINATION PARTIES

In February, the training policy of these services underwent a change. As a result of experience it was found that the Rescue Party Service, next to the Fire Service, had had the heaviest burden at incidents, and it was realised how useful it would have been if members of first-aid parties had been trained in rescue work, and rescue parties in first aid, so that they would be familiar with and able to undertake each other's duties. The first-aid parties had not been so heavily pressed after raids as the rescue parties, whose work of extricating persons trapped in debris, cellars, basements, etc., and the recovery of bodies, sometimes extended over several days and nights after incidents. Where rescue operations were handicapped by a shortage of rescue personnel, first-aid parties trained in rescue work would have materially helped to accelerate the release of the casualties. Furthermore, a great saving of man-power would be effected by adopting a system of interchangeability. The Ministry of Home Security issued an important circular to local authorities, which set out the training programme which should be arranged for inter-service training of the first-aid, rescue and decontamination parties.[22]

INTER-SERVICE TRAINING OF FIRST-AID, RESCUE AND DECONTAMINATION SERVICES

In order to give effect to the circular referred to above, a conference was called by the Ministry of Home Security at Peel House, Vincent Square, from April 22–26, 1941. This conference, which was familiarly called 'The Peel House Conference', was attended by rescue and first-aid party instructors from all Regions, and also by some training officers. The programme consisted of two syllabuses of specimen lectures and demonstrations drawn up by the training branch of the Ministry of Home Security, in collaboration with the casualty service branch of the Ministry of Health, and were given by selected teachers in first aid and rescue work. The teaching was followed by free discussions as to the suitability for inclusion, in whole or in part, of the subjects dealt with in the training programme for the joint service. The syllabuses which were drawn up were based entirely on the experience gained during enemy raiding, and differed in many respects from training programmes up to that time. Among the demonstrations given at the conference were the Trigglift (webbing bands), the Wanstead and Woodford method of blanketing a stretcher, and the method of securing a patient to a stretcher with triangular bandages. The two latter were subsequently adopted as standard methods for A.R.P. Services; the Trigglift had already been approved. The two approved syllabuses which were for courses to be inaugurated for rescue party leaders and for first-aid party leaders at the rescue party schools, set up in the previous year, were published in August 1941.[23]

THE INCIDENT DOCTOR

The desirability of having a doctor present at every incident had been recognised early in the war, and scheme-making authorities had been directed to discuss with Hospital Officers how arrangements for this should be made. A reference had also been made to the question of having additional medical men for duty with first-aid posts and mobile units. During an intensive raid on Cardiff early in January 1941, several doctors, unconnected with any of the casualty services, were called out by the wardens and did very useful work in the streets and among trapped casualties at the height of the 'blitz'. In this work they were ably assisted by many medical students who volunteered to help them. The Incident Doctor was officially recognised in May 1941, and it was laid down that he could claim a fee, on a sessional basis, for services rendered. Rotas of doctors who were not members of the casualty service organisation, but were willing to attend at incidents, were maintained by medical officers of health, generally at control centres but sometimes at wardens' posts. From there these incident doctors were called out when required.

MOBILE GAS-CLEANSING UNITS

The Ministry of Health decided to supplement facilities for the cleansing of gas contaminated persons in vulnerable areas, by lending mobile gas-cleansing units to local authorities. Notice was sent to these authorities that production of these units had begun. Later, the Ministry of Health notified Regional authorities that the original order of 500 mobile gas-cleansing units had been increased by a further 500 and that 40 complete units would be available for each Region.

UPGRADING OF FIRST-AID POINTS

In the light of air-raid experience and the changed conditions that followed the dispersal of industry and of the civilian population since the outbreak of war, the Ministry of Health decided in June to upgrade certain first-aid points in semi-rural areas near target cities, and in rural areas with small country towns and large villages near aircraft factories, munition works, aerodromes, etc., which might be subject to intense bombing. Such upgraded first-aid points would have a special increased equipment and would be larger than a point but not so large as a first-aid post. A trained nurse and a staff of ten volunteers would man these upgraded points, and a doctor would be on call.

FORMATION OF HEADQUARTERS STAFF FOR CASUALTY SERVICES

In order to strengthen the relations between the Ministries of Health and of Home Security at Headquarters and in Regions, a small Headquarters Casualty Service Staff was appointed by the D.G.E.M.S. in July 1941, under an officer with the title of Deputy Director-General Emergency Medical Services (for Casualty Services). The main functions of this staff were to maintain the closest contact with the Inspector General's Department of the Ministry of Home Security on all matters connected with the A.R.P. Casualty and General Services;

to pay frequent visits to Regions and report on all problems connected with the services therein; to hold conferences at regular intervals at headquarters which would be attended by Regional Assistant Hospital Officers and administrative officers of the Ministry of Health.

LIGHT MOBILE FIRST-AID UNITS AND REDUCTION OF NUMBERS OF FIXED FIRST-AID POSTS

As the result of a review by the Ministry of Health of fixed first-aid posts, it was evident that the numbers of slightly injured persons had not proved so large that separate first-aid posts were needed to prevent hospitals from being swamped with casualties. It was therefore suggested in July 1941, that the number of fixed first-aid posts could safely, especially in residential areas, be put on a care and maintenance basis, or reduced to the status of upgraded first-aid points. This would necessitate a fuller use of mobile units, and it was suggested that some of these could probably be reduced to light units, consisting of a doctor, a trained nurse with a couple of auxiliaries, with simple portable equipment, who would go to incidents in a light vehicle, possibly the doctor's own car.

In December 1941, the Light Mobile First-aid Unit was approved and a schedule of equipment issued for it.

ADAPTATION OF STRETCHER FITMENTS FOR AMBULANCES

In order to convert the standard A.R.P. ambulances to dual-purpose vehicles to convey either sitting or stretcher cases, or both, a modification of the stretcher fitment was designed in August 1941, so that by placing the upper stretchers upon the lower ones the upper stretcher racks which had been hinged could be lifted upwards and secured to the sides of vehicles. When the upper stretcher racks had been so secured, patients travelling in the ambulances would use the stretchers as seats. This important measure tended towards economy in the use of separate cars for sitting cases; it also avoided the risk of using upholstered cars for the conveyance of casualties contaminated by blister gas. Not more than six sitting cases were to be carried in the vehicle at one time.

CHANGE OF TITLE OF A.R.P. SERVICES AND INTRODUCTION OF SERVICE BADGES AND MARKINGS

In order to emphasise the growth and increased importance of what were known originally as the A.R.P. General Services, and their essential unity with other branches of civil defence, it was decided in September 1941, to adopt the title 'Civil Defence' in place of 'A.R.P.' for these services. In connexion also with the issue of improved uniforms for members of the civil defence general services earlier in the year, it was decided to introduce at the same time new service badges and markings, and a national system of badges of rank. Thus the title 'Civil

Defence' was prefixed to each branch of the Casualty Service (e.g. Civil Defence Ambulance Service) as for other branches of the general services. Uniforms were also sanctioned for medical officers at first-aid posts.

CO-ORDINATION OF CIVIL DEFENCE CASUALTY SERVICE WITH THE HOME GUARD MEDICAL ORGANISATION

After conferences between representatives of the Ministry of Health and of the War Office, it was decided that the Civil Defence Casualty Services should be responsible for the treatment of casualties from the Home Guard, and that arrangements must be made between medical officers of the Home Guard and medical officers of health of local authorities to ensure the full co-ordination of the Civil Defence Casualty Services with the Home Guard medical organisation. The principles which had been observed in the preparation of schemes for this object were published in a Ministry of Health circular to scheme-making authorities in September 1941.

CO-ORDINATION OF AIR RAID PRECAUTIONS OF INDUSTRIAL UNDERTAKINGS WITH THOSE OF A.R.P. SCHEMES

In August 1941, instructions were issued to scheme-making authorities that it was the duty of A.R.P. controllers to see that co-ordination was secured between the A.R.P. services and the arrangements made by industrial undertakings for dealing with their casualties. It was stressed in a circular issued in August by the Ministry of Health that officers of the scheme-making authorities, and in particular medical officers of health, should become fully acquainted with the arrangements of industrial undertakings for dealing with casualties, including gas casualties, among their employees.

AUTHORISED UNIT ESTABLISHMENTS FOR FIRST-AID POST AND AMBULANCE SERVICES

With close regard to the paramount need of conserving man-power and woman-power, thus releasing more men and women to the Forces and to industry, the Ministry of Health in October 1941, fixed the maximum number of members of the civil defence first-aid post and ambulance services (whole-time or part-time), which local authorities should have on duty at any one time, when full manning was needed. This was known as the 'unit establishment', and Regional Commissioners were requested to authorise unit establishments in the following services up to the maximum laid down:

(*a*) Fixed first-aid posts (including gas cleansing sections);
(*b*) Mobile first-aid posts (later, mobile first-aid units);
(*c*) Mobile light units (later, light mobile first-aid units);
(*d*) Ambulances and sitting-case cars.

THE CIVIL DEFENCE RESERVE

In view of the increasing difficulty in maintaining the numbers of part-time and, to a lesser but appreciable extent, of whole-time personnel in the civil defence general services, Regions were asked in October 1941, by the Ministry of Home Security to consider forming in their areas regional mobile reserves of the principal mobile services, namely first-aid rescue, decontamination, and ambulance (together with a small number of dispatch rider messengers). Such was the beginning of a very valuable mobile force which came into being later.

SEPARATION OF LOCAL AMBULANCE SERVICES FROM FIRE SERVICE CONTROL

In November 1941, in order to free the National Fire Service from the ambulance duties which had hitherto been under their control, it was decided as a war-time measure to transfer this responsibility to the Civil Defence Ambulance Service, which had resources in staff, accommodation and servicing facilities.

RIVER EMERGENCY SERVICE (PORT OF LONDON AUTHORITY)

Although not strictly classed as a unit of the civil defence casualty or general services, mention must be made here of this service. It was designed by the Port of London Authority as a casualty service early in 1939, to co-operate with the Civil Defence Casualty Service on land when its assistance was required. The service had its own fleet of ambulance ships and others for patrol and messenger work, and operated between Hammersmith and Canvey Island, a distance of forty-one miles. The ambulance ships carried doctors, nurses and stretcher bearers, and were in constant communication with civil defence controllers on land. In addition to casualties caused by enemy action, the River Emergency Service dealt with all other types of casualty met with on the river. Equipment and replacement of medical stores were arranged for from Regional stores of the London Region by the Ministry of Health, whose Regional Hospital Officer made frequent inspections of the ambulance ships and attended exercises held to demonstrate their efficiency.

The River Emergency Service did some good work during the raids of the latter part of 1940 and early in 1941, and from the beginning of the year until May 31, 1941, had dealt with 165 casualties from enemy action and 672 others, putting in altogether 1,650 attendances.

CASUALTIES TREATED BY THE CIVIL CASUALTY DEFENCE SERVICES, 1940-41

During these two years 84,808 casualties were treated in first-aid posts and by mobile units, of which number 4,121 occurred before September 1940, the month in which the heavy raids began.

LESSONS LEARNED FROM THE RAIDS

WORK OF CASUALTY SERVICES

The years 1940–41 were eventful ones for the Civil Defence Casualty Service and, as indicated in the foregoing pages, many improvements had been made as the result of experience gained from air raids. All branches of the Casualty Service can be said to have found their feet in 1940 and to have won their spurs in 1941.

The general trend in the evolution of the services was towards smaller units, great mobility and interchangeability. The expected heavy casualties had not occurred, and even where intensive raiding had taken place, the general experience was that casualties were often widely scattered, so that the demand had been for numerous small units rather than for large ones. Seldom had the flow of casualties to first-aid posts been overwhelming, and the posts were on the whole so well organised and managed that few were called upon to operate at full capacity. The call for smaller and more numerous units was met by establishing incident doctors, by the light mobile first-aid units and also perhaps by upgraded first-aid points.

First-aid Parties. During 1940 the shortage of personnel in the first-aid parties continued to engage the attention of the authorities in the Ministry of Home Security. Since August 1939, their strength in the whole country had increased and by the end of March 1940, was 78,251, of which 36,123 were whole-time and 42,128 part-time. The total in England and Wales was 71,396. To this figure must be added a number of part-time volunteers who were not required to do regular turns of duty each week, but were to do duty when called upon. These volunteers were classified as 'other enrolments' and totalled 50,328. The grand total for England and Wales thus became 121,724. The position as regards whole-time and part-time personnel had improved, but it was still far from satisfactory. There was, however, considerable relief that during the heavy raids in the autumn the number of first-aid parties had proved to be adequate and that they had acquitted themselves well in spite of being under strength. The reason for the sufficiency of first-aid parties was that the number of casualties, though heavy, had been much less than the pre-war estimate.

By the end of December 1940, part-time personnel had further increased to 51,990 by absorbing some of the 'other enrolments' but the whole-time figure had remained pretty constant and was 33,746.

By the end of September 1941, part-time personnel had increased to 62,000, partly by absorption of 'other enrolments' and partly by new entrants of a more mature age, who took the place of younger men called to the Forces and to industry. Whole-time personnel had decreased slightly, because the younger men were being called up, and numbered nearly 33,000, making a total of approximately 95,000. Because of the difficulty in recruiting sufficient men for first-aid parties in some areas, it had been agreed in 1940 that in exceptional circumstances a proportion of women could be recruited on a part-time basis only, provided that not more than two women were allowed in any one party, and that they were to be employed primarily on first-aid work and not for lifting casualties or carrying stretchers. At this time there were about 5,800 women in the first-aid party service. In some places local authorities, possibly influenced by zealous persuasion, had permitted the formation of first-aid parties manned entirely by women, under their own leaders, who were ready to carry out all duties performed by men and, in many cases, showed themselves capable of doing so.

The raids demonstrated that the less first-aid party personnel attempted in the way of treatment the better. Measures to prevent death or to prevent further injury and shock must of course be taken, but the principles previously referred to, namely, quick decision on priority of treatment and the despatch of casualties to hospitals or first-aid posts as soon as possible, proved to be well founded.

It was reported generally by hospitals to which casualties had been sent from incidents that the work of classifying injuries, rapid despatch and the distribution of casualties to hospitals and first-aid posts was most efficiently carried out by the leaders and personnel of first-aid parties. In towns where distances which casualties had to travel were short, little or no attempt was made at elaborate splinting, which would in most cases have had to be carried out in the dark. Immobilisation of the injured parts by sandbags, by bandaging limbs together or, in the case of upper limbs, to the trunk was found sufficient, the chief object being to get the casualty to a doctor as quickly as possible. Tourniquets were seldom used, as the application of a pad and bandage over a wound was usually found to be effective in checking even violent haemorrhage. The Trigglift (webbing bands) was extensively used at incidents and found to be extremely useful, although sufficient sets of this equipment had not by then been provided to fulfil the full requirements of the first-aid and rescue party services. The Wanstead and Woodford method of blanketing which was taught to first-aid party personnel was a great advance on former methods, and provided for the efficient wrapping up of casualties so as to minimise shock, using only the two blankets authorised for each stretcher.

Fixed First-aid Posts thoroughly justified their existence and functioned extremely well. Many were damaged, some demolished, but nothing deterred the personnel, including the part-time workers, from reporting for duty at their posts, even though they had to come some distance from their homes during the height of raids. Some idea can be gathered of the amount of work done by the first-aid post (and mobile unit) service from the figures of casualties treated during the last four months of the year. These figures (England and Wales) were:

September 1940	16,628
October 1940	14,408
November 1940	9,422
December 1940	8,962
Total	49,420

As already mentioned, the establishment of fixed first-aid posts had been reduced, as it was found that the country was over-insured in this respect. The work at these posts and the attendance of personnel had, with few exceptions, been consistently good, and on the whole few cases which should have been sent to hospitals were sent to first-aid posts. Occasionally, however, casualties which were found to be hospital cases were sent to first-aid posts, and a certain amount of delay occurred in their transfer by ambulances. The fears which had been expressed earlier that too much might be attempted at first-aid posts were seldom justified. In the early days a few instances of this did occur, but after the heavy raids in 1940 and the early part of 1941 this tendency had practically disappeared and hospitals were satisfied that only first-aid measures were being carried out. In some parts of the country the entrances to first-aid posts would not allow easy access for stretchers, the argument being that stretcher cases should not be sent to first-aid posts. Theoretically, this was correct, but in practice it was unavoidable that stretcher cases were sometimes brought to first-aid posts during the height of raids, especially at night, and that some cases who walked in had to be carried out on stretchers; defects in the construction of entrances undoubtedly caused delays which were detrimental to the wounded and a handicap to their rescuers.

The total number of casualties dealt with by fixed first-aid posts and mobile first-aid units was, from January to May 1941 (inclusive), 27,518 and from June until the end of the year 3,749 making a total of 31,267.

Mobile Units. Contrary to expectation, mobile units were not extensively used and in some places not at all, although they were always ready, fully staffed and standing by. One of the main reasons was that the heaviest raids usually occurred on built-up areas and damage to roads and buildings made it difficult to manoeuvre the large unit vehicles into position near to incidents where they could best be used; consequently they were not called out. Furthermore, in built-up areas there was usually an adequate provision of fixed first-aid posts and hospitals within easy reach of incidents. On occasions, however, they had proved useful in taking over the duties of fixed first-aid posts which had been damaged or demolished (see Plates XXVII and XXVIII).

Another valuable purpose which they fulfilled was to act as the parent for light mobile first-aid units, and to reinforce them at incidents when the doctors of the light units found that they had more than they could cope with and summoned further assistance. Many mobile units were based on hospitals and the personnel of these units assisted the nursing staff of the hospitals, thereby acquiring a useful practical training.

The Ambulance Service deserved the highest praise and carried out its work with great efficiency, even though it was at times handicapped by a shortage of personnel, which meant long hours of duty for drivers and attendants, often under conditions of extreme discomfort and danger during raids which often lasted for several hours. Even when telephone communications had been broken down and messenger services had to be used, very few delays were caused. One criticism which had been made was that casualties which could have been carried in sitting-case cars had frequently to be transported in ambulances as stretcher cases when sitting-case cars were not available. This defect was removed when the adaptation of stretcher fitments in ambulances was completed. Experience had shown how much the success of a casualty service depended upon the efficient organisation and operation of the ambulance service and satisfactory arrangements for mutual support and reinforcement. This was well carried out and largely contributed to the success which the casualty service had achieved.

By December 31, 1940, the number of ambulances in England and Wales was 8,785 whole-time and 6,078 part-time, of which the London Region was responsible for 2,250 whole-time and 141 part-time. The number of sitting-case cars had increased to 3,387 whole-time and 15,087 part-time, of which 1,497 whole-time and 708 part-time were in the London Region. Trailer ambulances which were in use in some parts of England and Wales had not proved their worth and during 1941 the Ministry of Health declined to sanction any further ambulances of this type.

The personnel figures showed 9,348 men as whole-time and 23,519 as part-time; whole-time women as 13,765 and part-time as 29,725, making a total of 76,357.

SECTION III: THE MIDDLE YEARS, 1942–43

CHANGES IN THE ORGANISATION OF THE CASUALTY SERVICES

The year 1942 was not a memorable one for air raids, but for the Civil Defence Casualty Service it was eventful, as several important changes were made in the organisation and equipment of various branches of that service.

EQUIPMENT OF FIRST-AID POSTS, FIRST-AID PARTIES, ETC.

During the year 1942 several important changes were made in the equipment of fixed first-aid posts, mobile first-aid units, etc. These changes were notified in circulars issued by the Ministry of Health from time to time.

Changes in the Treatment of Gas Casualties. Amendments to the prescribed methods of dealing with gas casualties were made from time to time as the result of experience and of experiments made at the Chemical Warfare Research Station at Porton, and local authorities were advised to impress on the civil population by sustained publicity that their best protection against gas was the use of the respirator and shelter indoors to escape contamination by poisonous gases in their liquid or vapour form. If, however, people were unavoidably splashed by liquid gas when at a distance from a cleansing centre, the immediate shedding of contaminated clothing, cleansing with soap and water at their own homes or in the nearest convenient house would in most cases prevent serious harm.

The original instructions for the treatment of the eyes splashed with liquid gas were altered. The instillation of sulphacetamide, which was at first recommended to be used at first-aid posts, was now considered inadvisable at that stage. Immediate flushing of the eyes with warm water at the incident and with warm normal saline at the first-aid post was considered to be the only practical treatment in the early stages. Another amendment brought in later was that the provision of trays of bleach at entrances to cleansing units was discontinued, the Ministry having been advised that if contaminated boots or shoes were removed and put in the bins with other contaminated clothing the risk of the importation of gas to first-aid posts and hospitals was negligible.

Fortunately the policy of the Ministry in providing defence against gas warfare was not tested, and it is a reasonable assumption that the large measure of insurance provided by the Ministry against casualties was one of the chief reasons why gas was not used by the enemy.

DIRECTION OF NEW PART-TIME ENTRANTS INTO THE CIVIL DEFENCE SERVICES

In March 1942, local authorities were asked by the Minister of Home Security, in consultation with the Minister of Health, to notify their requirements for additional part-time members, men and women separately, for each of the general services. They were asked to review the effective strength in relation to the establishment of each service and, if there were surpluses in some and shortages in others, to redress the balance as far as possible by the voluntary transfer of part-time members from one service to another.

If there were deficiencies after this had been done, the numbers of additional part-time members required for each service were to be notified to the office of their Regional Commissioner for transmission to the Ministry of Labour and National Service, who would take action to fill the vacancies by direction under Defence Regulation 29B.A or otherwise.

The Ministry of Labour and National Service would furnish local authorities with particulars of the persons upon whom directions were served, and the date and time at which they should report for duty. Any person failing to report after direction would be reported to the Ministry of Labour and National Service who would be responsible for any further action.[24]

At this time the effective strength of the first-aid party service was approximately 58,000 men and 5,450 women part-time, and 27,000 men and 660 women whole-time in England and Wales. That of the first-aid post service (including mobile units), was approximately 19,000 men and 70,700 women part-time, and 4,220 men and 18,000 women whole-time. That of the ambulance service was approximately 21,000 men and 26,000 women part-time, and 7,600 men and 16,700 women whole-time. Each of these totals showed a decrease from the previous quarter, that of the first-aid party service being approximately 4,400, of the first-aid post service 10,200, and of the ambulance service 4,300. At the end of March 1942, the numbers of ambulances and sitting-case cars in England and Wales were approximately 11,150 and 10,500 respectively.

THE CIVIL DEFENCE RESERVE

The Civil Defence Reserve had been declared to be a civil defence force for the purpose of the National Service Act, 1941, by the National Services (Civil Defence Force) (No. 2) Order, 1941,[25] and came into being from March 1942. This force was to be made up of a series of mobile civil defence units, all members of which were highly trained in rescue, first aid and decontamination. The units would be built up into Regional columns under the direct operational and administrative control of Regional Commissioners. The units would have their own headquarters, in which the members would live, and these were to be situated at convenient places whence services could be deployed at short notice to reinforce local authorities whose own services were overstrained by heavy attacks. This force which has been referred to as 'the corps d'elite' of the Civil Defence was to prove a most valuable asset and fill a long felt want.

REDUCTION OF WHOLE-TIME CIVIL DEFENCE PERSONNEL

In order to enable persons engaged in civil defence work on a whole-time basis to make a more active contribution to the general war effort, steps were taken to reduce by one-third the total number of whole-time personnel of the Civil Defence Services throughout the country. The precise number to be released from each service in the area of each scheme-making authority would be determined by the Regional Commissioner in consultation with the authority.

THE MORTUARY SERVICE

It will be realised that the mortuary service had passed through a very trying time during the heavy raids, and it was not to be wondered that the resources of the service were at times strained to the breaking point, and even beyond it. Many causes contributed to temporary breakdowns which occurred in some places, chief among these being (*a*) local undertakers on whom the local authority were depending for the staffing of a mortuary, failed to take up their duties; in some cases members of the voluntary staff were not available, (*b*) it was found that persons appointed as mortuary superintendents were not always free in an emergency to devote their whole time to running a mortuary, (*c*) the obtaining of adequate clerical assistance gave rise to anxiety; delays occurred and caused congestion in the mortuaries and distress to relatives, (*d*) bodies which had not been properly labelled at incidents before being brought to mortuaries, caused a dislocation of the work of identification.

A circular issued by the Ministry of Health in June, dealt with some of these difficulties, and suggested the further use of mutual aid which had been found useful after heavy raids. The establishment of mobile mortuary teams had been tried with success in some places, especially in university towns, and had been manned by medical students, who carried out the work of mortuary attendants, assisted by female students, who did the clerical work.

In 1942, a useful and instructive booklet entitled *War Deaths* was produced by the Ministry of Health.

TRAINING OF CIVIL DEFENCE PERSONNEL

Intensive training in first aid was being carried out throughout the country, and combined exercises and competitions were held in all Regions. Large numbers of leaders and deputy leaders of first-aid parties had attended the Regional Training Schools and received instruction in first aid and rescue work; on their return to their local authorities they had imparted the knowledge gained to the personnel of their parties. A civil defence staff college had been established in February 1942, by the Minister of Home Security in consultation with the Minister of Health and was, in some respects, a successor to the A.R.P. staff school which had functioned in London up to the outbreak of war. The college, which was located at Stoke D'Abernon, Cobham, Surrey, was organised and administered by the Inspector General's Department of the Ministry of Home Security, and provided courses designed for the general instruction of senior officials concerned with the organisation and administration of the Civil Defence Services (e.g. Controllers, Medical Officers of Health, Regional and Local Authority Training Officers, etc.). The instruction given at the college was based not only on the latest information available from the ministries and departments concerned, but also on practical experience gained under air raid conditions.[26] Lectures on the casualty services were included in the main subjects taught at the staff college and were given regularly.

In June 1942, A.R.P. Training Manual No. 3 (1st Edition), Rescue Service Manual, was produced by the Inspector General's Department of the Ministry of Home Security. This manual dealt fully with all problems of rescue work and was profusely illustrated.

In December 1942, A.R.P. Handbook No. 10 was issued by the Ministry of Home Security in conjunction with the Ministry of Health, as a second edition, and its original title was changed to *Training in First Aid for Civil Defence Purposes*. The handbook brought up to date all the changes that had been made in the civil defence services, and included chapters on mutual aid and reinforcement, and on co-ordination with the civil defence casualty services and the Home Guard medical organisation.

CASUALTIES TREATED BY THE CIVIL DEFENCE CASUALTY SERVICES, 1942

The total number of casualties dealt with at first-aid posts and mobile first-aid units during 1942 was 7,107, a marked contrast to that of the previous year.

TRAINING IN THE RESCUE OF CREWS FROM CRASHED AIRCRAFT

Civil defence personnel had sometimes played a valuable part in the rescue of crews from crashed aircraft, but little instruction had been given to them on the best means of accomplishing this. An important pamphlet was drawn up in January by the Ministry of Home Security in consultation with the Air Ministry, giving the most up-to-date information on the subject, and this was to form the basis of lectures which would be given to civil defence personnel.[27]

AMALGAMATION OF RESCUE AND FIRST-AID PARTY SERVICES

Following the general plan referred to previously for releasing whole-time personnel of the civil defence services to industry, and in order to make the best use of the whole-time and part-time personnel available, specialisation in the services was reduced by amalgamating the rescue and first-aid party services into one service—The Civil Defence Rescue Service. The new service was to combine the functions of the two previous services. There would be no waste or loss of acquired skill in rescue or first-aid work as the personnel would be trained and equipped to perform either duty when the need arose. The disappearance of 'first aid' from the title of the new service caused some concern and dissatisfaction among members of the former first-aid parties and medical officers of health, but when it was understood that 'rescue' in its fullest sense included 'first aid' and that most first-aid parties had already taken a large share in rescue work the objection gradually faded. Standard rescue parties were to consist of seven men each, including the driver of their vehicle, and they would be furnished with a new scale of first-aid equipment.[28]

LABELLING OF CASUALTIES

A circular was issued in April, which dealt with the symbols used on labels for casualties at incidents. It had been pointed out by hospital authorities that unconscious casualties were sometimes received without any labels on them, which made identification difficult. It was therefore decided to label all unconscious casualties and to designate them with the symbol 'X', which denoted priority of removal from an incident and of examination when reaching hospital. Amendments were made accordingly in A.R.P. Handbook 10 (2nd Edition) which contained directions for labelling casualties.

ADAPTATION OF STRETCHER FITMENTS TO TAKE ARMY TYPES OF STRETCHERS

A reference had already been made in the previous year, pointing out that difficulty was sometimes experienced in loading Army pattern stretchers into the standard civil defence ambulance fitments, especially when the stretchers had become strained or worn. This reference was in connexion with the carriage in civil defence ambulances of Home Guard casualties. At that time it was considered that stretcher fitments should be adapted locally by a slight alteration in their tracks, and local authorities were notified accordingly.

In July 1943, it was decided that in order to accommodate satisfactorily all types of stretchers (including Army pattern, American and Canadian), it would be necessary to adapt the existing fitments by the incorporation of stretcher brackets of a new design. Arrangements had been made for the new stretcher brackets to be made and supplied centrally and they would be delivered to local authorities as they become available. This was a most important departure as, apart from the Army pattern wood and canvas stretchers, the runners of the American and Canadian types would usually not fit into the tracks of the civil defence standard fitments. In the event of invasion, which was still considered possible, this defect might have had serious results, if the civil defence ambulances had been required to transport military as well as civil casualties.

INCIDENT CONTROL

A considerable amount of experience had been accumulated on incident control, and all services who dealt with casualties at incidents fully realised the importance of the control exercised by a responsible and properly trained Incident Officer. It was laid down in a circular issued by the Ministry of Home Security in July to local authorities that in each Region there should be a pool of incident officers trained in the principles of incident control. These officers should be police officers, wardens and other persons especially selected for the work. It was notified that a new training manual on the subject of incident control was in course of preparation. This was published in November 1943.[29]

CRUSHING OR CRUSH INJURY

Much experience had been gained of this type of injury as found among casualties pinned down by beams, brickwork or other heavy debris across their limbs in collapsed buildings. A great deal of research work had been and was being carried out to discover the true cause and proper treatment of what was called the 'crush syndrome'. (See Surgery Volume, Chapter 19.) In this condition, which occurred among a proportion of crushed casualties, persons who might possibly have shown little or no signs of injury after release would die within a few days with gradual and finally complete suppression of urine. This syndrome had been described in A.R.P. Handbook No. 10 (2nd Edition). As a form of local treatment for a limb which had been crushed, it was recommended that a rubber bandage should be applied loosely between the part crushed and the body, as a tourniquet; this bandage would be tightened just before removal of the weight compressing the limb in order to prevent poisonous substances in the damaged muscles from entering the blood stream. In August, a memorandum from the Sub-Committee of the Medical Research Council was circulated by the Ministry of Health.[30] This memorandum omitted the local tourniquet treatment as it had not been proved to fulfil a useful purpose, but laid particular stress on giving fluid and alkalis. This amendment necessitated a change in the instructions for the rescue service personnel, who had up till then been taught to use the rubber bandage when necessary.

EVE'S 'ROCKING' METHOD OF RESUSCITATION

During 1943, a new method of artificial respiration devised by Dr. C. F. Eve, of Hull, was introduced into the training of the rescue service, as a supplementary method after artificial respiration had been started by Schafer's method. Eve's method had been tested by naval medical officers and was described in the manual *First Aid in the Royal Navy*, 1943.

FIRST-AID EQUIPMENT FOR THE LONDON HEAVY AND LIGHT RESCUE SERVICES

In November 1943, a circular was issued by the Ministry of Home Security notifying changes in the scales of first-aid equipment for London heavy and light rescue parties. Schedules of equipment with this circular showed the number of pouches and haversacks, with their contents, which would be carried by the parties.

CASUALTIES TREATED BY THE CIVIL DEFENCE CASUALTY SERVICES—1943

The air raids in 1943 were much on the same scale as those of 1942. The total number of casualties dealt with at first-aid posts and mobile first-aid units during 1943 was 5,250, of which 4,091 were in the first half of the year.

LESSONS LEARNED FROM THE RAIDS

WORK OF THE CASUALTY SERVICES

Although raiding was not in any way as severe as in 1940–1, it was nevertheless fairly constant and dispersed over many areas. Many useful lessons were learned and the results of the prolonged and careful training of the casualty services were manifest in every direction. The civil defence services as a whole had become battle hardened and were very much 'on their toes'. This was particularly true in coastal towns where tip-and-run raids by day had been frequent, especially during the first half of 1943. As operational work was mostly carried out by day, these raids had provided wide scope for the casualty services to observe how casualties should be disposed of, and how incidents should be controlled. The work of the casualty services was reported to be uniformly good, and delay in arrival of the rescue parties or ambulances at incidents was very rare. At coastal towns the military and naval forces were often extremely helpful, especially when their members were acting under the immediate direction of rescue party leaders. Measures for safeguarding casualties against shock, and the frequency with which this condition caused a fatal issue amongst casualties, had been so repeatedly taught and stressed to casualty service personnel, that few cases of delay occurred in getting injured persons from incidents to hospitals, after necessary first aid and careful handling. Because of the demolition of buildings, which was perhaps on a larger scale than before owing to the enemy using heavier bombs, the excavation of trapped casualties was a frequent occurrence. At this work the new rescue service proved that it was in no way inferior to the previous service, and the former first-aid party personnel were taking to the work with energy and keenness. A useful piece of equipment, the Remote Breathing Apparatus, was frequently used and the Trigglift (webbing bands) had further justified its inclusion in the equipment of rescue parties. Sound-detector units were tried in some places to locate trapped casualties, but on the whole they were not a success. Incident control had improved out of all recognition, due largely to the instruction given to selected officers in Regions, and also to courses held at the Civil Defence Staff College for controllers and for officers selected as instructors in incident control. It will not be out of place to mention here the excellent work done by the Civil Defence Staff College at Cobham in bringing together at courses held there, not only all classes of officers connected with the civil defence services, but also military and Home Guard officers. By these courses a wider knowledge of civil defence work was imparted and a more active spirit of co-operation obtained. In the London Region, where separate heavy and light rescue parties were still retained, these parties acquitted themselves very well and their standard of co-ordination was high. Ambulances and fixed first-aid posts maintained their reputation for efficiency all over the country, and although mobile first-aid units were not much used, they proved their value as parent units to light mobile first-aid units which were often in action and gave useful service. A word of praise must be given to incident doctors, who were always ready to turn out at a moment's notice and remain at their posts, often in great danger, until all casualties for whom they were responsible had been cleared from incidents.

STANDARDS OF ACCOMMODATION FOR CIVIL DEFENCE PERSONNEL AND VEHICLES

Before the outbreak of war, accommodation had been arranged by most local authorities for part-time volunteers required to stand-by at night in first-aid posts, first-aid party and ambulance depots, and in most cases this was adequate.

After war had broken out, the number of volunteers increased and whole-time paid personnel were authorised and enrolled for duty by day and by night. To cope with this expansion local authorities were faced with a bigger problem. Satisfactory arrangements had to be made for housing, sleeping, protection, feeding, sanitation and recreation facilities for a larger number of first-aid workers who would be on continuous duty, by shifts, throughout every twenty-four hours.

Far-seeing local authorities, with the welfare of their services at heart, tackled the problem with energy and did their best with the means at their disposal. The result was that a number of posts and depots possessed good and sufficient accommodation for their personnel and vehicles, and the personnel were able to spend their hours of stand-by duty in comparative safety and comfort without finding their periods of inactivity irksome. Such places in England and Wales could be called 'happy', and the highest credit is due to the local authorities responsible for them.

Certain local authorities, however, by no means few, whether from a misguided optimism as to the duration of the war, or for other reasons, appeared to consider anything good enough for their casualty services, and made little or no serious effort to provide suitable accommodation for them, in spite of instructions from the Ministries concerned.

On the whole, arrangements for personnel were better at first-aid posts than at first-aid party and ambulance depots. Among the latter there were frequent instances, even as late as the fourth year of the war, where members of first-aid and rescue parties were housed and maintained under conditions of extreme discomfort and even squalor.

The modest standards of amenity laid down by the Ministries of Health and Home Security had but seldom been attained;[31] indeed, the premises occupied by civil defence services were often found lacking in the rudiments of comfort, decency and hygiene. In some cases, in spite of detailed directions and instructions,[32] valuable equipment was stored in damp airless places, where it could be preserved from decay only by constant and laborious attention.

Later in the war, the solid buildings erected for the National Fire Service provided an example of apparent discrimination against the civil defence services, which caused profound dissatisfaction among those associated with their administration.

Although instructions had issued from time to time from the A.R.P. Department of the Home Office and later from the Ministry of Home Security, that civil defence ambulances and sitting-case cars should be kept in garage, as far as possible,[33] it was not uncommon for the fleets of ambulance vehicles of one local authority to be kept standing in the open because no garage accommodation had been found for them, while a few miles away the vehicles of another local authority were housed in excellent garages.

Furthermore, the accommodation provided for women drivers and attendants was often primitive and devoid of any comfort. In some places drivers and attendants were obliged to sleep in their ambulances, even during the winter months, as no satisfactory accommodation had been provided for them. In the absence of any cover or anti-freeze mixture, they were compelled to crank up the engines of their vehicles at intervals throughout the night to ensure that they would start at a moment's notice.

Many of the conditions in these 'bad spots' were brought to light as a result of the frequent visits to Regions by members of the headquarters staff of the casualty services, by members of the staff of the Inspector-General of Civil Defence Services and, in Regions, by Assistant Hospital Officers and by Regional Officers of the Ministry of Home Security.

As a result of these revelations, a circular was sent to local authorities in June 1942, in which the Minister of Home Security said that he had been impressed by the unsatisfactory standards of comfort, sleeping and sanitary accommodation and cleanliness still to be found in some civil defence posts and depots. He stated that the responsibility for such conditions was shared by the Ministry and local authorities, and without attempting to apportion blame, he desired to appeal to all authorities to co-operate with his officers in securing an early improvement wherever standards were low. After this circular some improvements were effected but, as labour and materials became more scarce, little further was done.[34]

One important contributory factor to this state of affairs was that sufficient pressure was seldom brought to bear upon local authorities to make efficient arrangements for their services.

Many of the instructions issued by the Ministries of Health and Home Security contained permissive or persuasive clauses which left local authorities too much discretion in following the instructions or neglecting them. Many local authorities took advantage of this and neglected or modified the instructions, which they could do with impunity. Officers in charge of civil defence services, and sometimes even members of local authorities, often asked why the Ministries did not issue definite orders instead of indefinite instructions, and added that had orders been given they would usually have been carried out without demur.

DISCIPLINE

Lack of discipline among civil defence workers, especially in the early days, tended to encourage slackness in first-aid party and ambulance depots, particularly when there was little incentive for personnel to take a pride in their living quarters and keep them tidy and clean. Depot superintendents as a class were a fine, conscientious body of men, but they were handicapped by a lack of encouragement from higher authorities in the enforcing of discipline, and the absence of any form of disciplinary code. Added to this was the hesitation on the part of Government to appoint non-commissioned officer grades with increased pay and badges of rank for first-aid party and ambulance personnel. Delay in authorising and issuing uniforms was also a source of dissatisfaction, and complaints were made, even in the third and fourth year of war, that some local authorities had received uniforms but had not issued them in full to their personnel.

With the institution of Regional training schools, and the grant of improved uniforms with service badges, and a national system of badges of rank in 1941, discipline improved, as by this time personnel were beginning to realise its importance. A further stimulus was given by the amalgamation of the first-aid party and rescue services, and by the time the Civil Defence Reserve was established the standard of discipline throughout the services had attained a high level.

These defects in organisation could have been avoided if more weight had been given to the need for disciplinary control. It was a striking fact that in local authorities where the Chief Constable was also the A.R.P. Controller, the civil defence services as a rule maintained a higher standard of discipline than in others.

SECTION IV: RENEWED HEAVY RAIDS, FLYING BOMBS AND LONG-RANGE ROCKETS, 1944–1945

The year 1944 was a memorable one as regards air raids, as towards the end of January heavy attacks by piloted aircraft were resumed on various parts of Great Britain, notably London, comparable to those of 1940–41. Flying bombs (V.1) and long-range rockets (V.2) were also used during this year, and caused a great deal of damage and many casualties.

FLYING BOMBS (V.1)

On the night of June 12–13, 1944, the first flying bombs were launched against this country, the areas affected being Southern England and the London area. Attacks by this new weapon lasted for about eighty days, during which time more than 8,000 bombs were sent over, and of these more than 5,000 came overland.

LONG-RANGE ROCKETS (V.2)

On September 8, 1944, the enemy began firing long-range rockets and, as with the flying bombs, London remained the principal target. The direct effect of these rockets on the essential national war effort was about the same as that of the flying bombs. One difference, however, was that an 'alert' signal could be given for flying bombs but was not found practicable for long-range rockets. The result was that the casualty list for the latter was higher as many people were taken unawares and caught in the open.

Long-range rockets continued to be fired throughout the rest of the year, and in 1945 long-range rockets and a certain number of flying-bombs released from aircraft continued to fall on Southern England and the London area, and many extensive incidents occurred with much damage to property and a heavy casualty list. The last long-range rocket incident occurred on March 27, and the last enemy incident of any kind on March 29, when flying bombs were used. (See Chapter 6 for a full account of these attacks.)

BOMBARDMENT OF THE KENT COAST

In September 1944 also, the Kent coast, which had been shelled intermittently throughout the year, was subjected to a heavy bombardment from guns on the French coast in the Calais-Cap Gris Nez area. This continued until September 26, when the enemy gun-sites were over-run by our forces. (See Chapter 6.)

BASIC TRAINING AND OPERATIONAL TRAINING OF THE RESCUE SERVICE

For some time past a new form of training for the rescue service had been considered combining teaching in rescue and first aid. In January 1944, a Ministry of Home Security circular announced details of three training courses: (a) basic training course (all services), (b) operational course No. 1 designed for new entrants into the rescue service, and given to them immediately after the basic training course, and (c) operational course No. 2, to be taken by all members of the rescue service.[35]

These courses were designed to meet the requirements of a large number of part-time members of the new rescue service who had only a limited amount of time at their disposal for instruction, and whom it was necessary to train as quickly as possible. Rescue and first aid were complementary, and the teaching of both was closely related and to be given in simple non-technical language.

ATLAS OF AIR RAID INJURIES

In February 1944, an atlas containing twenty coloured plates designed to show the appearance of casualties likely to be met with in and after air raids, was published by the Inspector-General's Department of the Ministry of Home Security, in conjunction with the Ministry of Health. This publication was primarily intended for the use of instructors in first aid. Only a limited number of copies were printed and those were largely in demand. Most of the plates, all photographs, were of faked casualties, which were deliberately included so that instructors could realise the value of so preparing their casualties for exercises and for instructional purposes generally.

A.R.P. HANDBOOK NO. 10 (2ND EDITION)

In March 1944, an amended reprint of this handbook was published, and in this edition were embodied all changes which had occurred up to that time.

INCIDENT INQUIRY POINTS

In Civil Defence Training Manual No. 4 (Incident Control) a reference had been made to Inquiry Points for assisting members of the public who required information at air raid incidents. These inquiry points were usually in the charge of the Women's Voluntary Service or of responsible wardens, and had been found to be of considerable value. A Ministry of Home Security circular issued in April 1944, furnished guidance on setting up and running these points.

FIRST-AID TREATMENT OF FRACTURES OF THE SPINE

A good deal of discussion had taken place on the correct treatment for cases of fracture of the spine at incidents. Instructions based on a memorandum prepared by the Nerve Injuries Committee of the Medical Research Council were issued to medical officers of scheme-making authorities on a revised treatment for fractures of the spine and instructions contained in A.R.P. Handbook No. 10 were to be amended accordingly.[36] This was later followed by a Ministry of Home Security circular to local authorities.

FIRST-AID TREATMENT OF BURNS

A great deal of research work had been carried out on the first aid and hospital treatment of burns by sulphonamides, and in 1943 the Medical Research Council had published details of a first-aid treatment of burns by a water-soluble cream containing sulphanilamide and acetyl-tri-methyl-ammonium-bromide. This had been used with success in the Burns Unit, Royal Infirmary, Glasgow. In June 1944, a circular was issued by the Ministry of Health to medical officers of health of scheme-making authorities, notifying them that supplies of this cream, known as No. 9 cream, would shortly be available for use at first-aid posts in selected areas. Directions for its use were given in this circular.[37]

NATIONAL CIVIL DEFENCE RESCUE SCHOOL

To achieve a greater degree of uniformity in rescue training where officially recommended methods, based on research and raiding experience, could be taught, a National Civil Defence Rescue School was opened at Sutton Coldfield, Warwickshire, on August 28. The main purpose of this school was to train rescue instructors who would be available to carry out every kind of rescue training required by the civil defence organisation. The certificate obtained at this school was to be known as the R.I.C. (Rescue Instructors Central) Certificate.

REDUCTION IN CIVIL DEFENCE ORGANISATION

In view of the changes in the war situation which made air raids by piloted or pilotless aircraft unlikely over other areas than London and the south and east of England, it was decided in September 1944, to make immediate substantial reductions in the civil defence organisation in all areas other than those (i.e. Regions 4, 5, 6 and 12). The general principles upon which these reductions were based were:

(*a*) A substantial reduction in the unit establishment of all services.

(*b*) The release of the bulk of whole-time personnel in all services without any continuing obligation to undertake part-time service, the number to be retained by each scheme-making authority being communicated to them by their Regional Commissioner. A higher percentage was to be retained in the first-aid post service, and in the ambulance service one whole-time member would be retained for each ambulance in the revised unit establishment.

(c) A substantial reduction in part-time strength; to be achieved primarily by the release of those wishing to leave.

(d) The reduction of the maximum hours of stand-by duty of part-time personnel at posts or depots from 48 to 12 hours per month. The obligation to turn out for duty on an alert was to remain.

(e) The abandonment of continuous manning of posts and depots, by day or by night, subject to certain exceptions, e.g. in the rescue service.

On or before October 15, 1944, whole-time members selected for release were to be given final notice of discharge to take effect from November 15.

Part-time personnel leaving the service voluntarily would be required to surrender their uniforms and personal equipment, but might be allowed to retain certain items (e.g. armlets, shoulder titles, war service chevrons, etc.).

The number of officers and staff of local authorities employed on organising, administrative and training duties was to be reviewed, and proposals made to Regional Commissioners for its reduction.

Redundant buildings, other than those suitable for the storage of equipment, were to be released.[38]

In fixing the new establishments for the reduced civil defence ambulance service, provision was made for continuing (on a scale likely to be required) any assistance to the Emergency Medical Service in detraining or entraining convoys of service patients; or to the military and civil ambulance services.

The number of whole-time sitting-case cars was to be reduced by about 75 per cent.; in general, part-time sitting-case cars and part-time ambulances could be dispensed with.

As regards the first-aid post service, the number of whole-time personnel to be retained was not to exceed about 7 per cent. of the then existing whole-time strength of a Region as a whole.

Light mobile first-aid units would be reduced proportionately with other services. These units should not be retained in areas where all fixed first-aid posts and heavy mobile units were being abolished.

The reduction of first-aid points was left to the discretion of Regions.

The services of doctors in charge of first-aid posts which were being abolished would be terminated after appropriate notice.

The establishments for gas cleansing were to be left undisturbed until further notice.

At the end of May 1944, the strength of the first-aid post and of the ambulance service was as follows:

(a) In the first-aid post service there were approximately 2,100 whole-time men, and 9,000 whole-time women, a total of 11,100; in addition, there were 20,400 part-time men, and 69,700 part-time women, making a grand total of 101,200 in England and Wales.

(*b*) In the ambulance service there were approximately 4,500 whole-time men and 7,900 whole-time women; in addition, there were 21,700 part-time men and 31,100 part-time women, making a grand total of 65,200 in England and Wales.

LESSONS LEARNED FROM THE RAIDS

WORK OF THE CASUALTY SERVICES

The years 1944 and 1945 were of exceptional interest to the casualty as well as to other civil defence services, as they had to deal with three types of attacks, from (*a*) bombs from piloted aircraft, (*b*) flying bombs or pilotless aircraft and (*c*) long-range rockets.

One noticeable feature of raids early in 1944 was, that they produced larger 'incidents', which were known as 'area' incidents, due to an increase in the size and effect of weapons used. Blast damage was a special feature during the whole period.

The Rescue Service. Reports from all districts where bombs fell showed that the rescue service (in London Region—heavy and light rescue service) had worked well and had accomplished some notable rescues. It was generally agreed that the standard of rescue work appeared to be higher than in 1940–1. This was surprising as cuts in Civil Defence during the past few years had lowered the physical standards of the personnel and increased the average age. The inference was that the higher standard of training, and the experience gained, had accounted for the improvement in the work of the services. Co-operation between the Civil Defence Rescue Service and the National Fire Service had obviously improved. Reports from casualty receiving hospitals showed that in most cases only essential first aid had been attempted at incidents, and few delays had occurred before casualties were sent to hospitals. The importance of good leadership of parties and efficient reconnaissance was frequently demonstrated, and in a few extreme cases where parties failed to attain the usual standard of efficiency, it was generally due to lack of appreciation by the party leader of the best way to tackle rescue operations.

The vital importance to the casualty of efficient control at an incident had been frequently stressed in teaching and at exercises, especially the early arrival of the incident officer, and cordoning off the incident to keep unauthorised persons away from it. There was a shortage of police at some incidents and consequently difficulties occurred in preventing unauthorised persons from climbing over debris and attempting to help the services. Much assistance was given during the raids on London by the Home Guard, by fire-guards and by personnel and vehicles of the U.S. Army. The prompt and valuable help had, however, in some instances, been wasted through lack of early direction at incidents. Casualties were sometimes rushed off to hospitals in military transport (e.g. jeeps), or in private cars before the arrival of the civil defence services, without any first aid or labelling, and confusion arose as there was difficulty in tracing the location of such casualties; moreover, many undoubtedly suffered from this too precipitate action. The most useful service was obtained when troops were acting under the direction of rescue party leaders. Great help was given to rescue parties in freeing and treating casualties at night by providing floodlighting, which had first been used in the early raids and was continued throughout the year. Car headlamps were often useful, and hand-lamps plugged into mains gave good lighting to facilitate tunnelling.

Fixed First-aid Posts. The work of the fixed first-aid posts was of a uniformly high standard and the sorting of casualties and their rapid disposal efficiently done. Many posts, especially in the London area, were overcrowded at times and had to call for mobile first-aid units to assist them. The personnel of the posts and mobile units amalgamated and worked as one team. In some places fixed first-aid posts were damaged and the mobile first-aid units took over their functions. The injection of anti-tetanic serum, when required, was scrupulously observed, and the filling up of the casualty forms and labels (M.P.C. 44 and 46) was satisfactorily done, often under very difficult conditions.

Mobile First-aid Units. As recorded above, mobile first-aid units were frequently used, notably during raids on the London area, and did very good work. At night-time the light mobile first-aid units were generally sent out to incidents. The co-operation between the National Fire Service and the doctor of the light mobile first-aid units proved to be of great value, especially to trapped casualties. Instances occurred in which doctors were able to save seriously injured and trapped casualties from being soaked in cold water, and on at least one occasion a number of persons trapped in a cellar and in danger of being flooded out were saved by the fire service personnel, whose assistance was called by a doctor.

The Ambulance Service. The ambulance service had probably never been harder worked than it was during this period of concentrated raids on London, but it responded nobly to all calls, and there were few delays in the arrival of ambulances at incidents; when this happened there was generally a good reason for the delay (e.g. fog). Reinforcements were needed at many incidents, and it was noted at times that there was a tendency to ask for more ambulances than were strictly necessary. With the ambulance service at reduced strength this was frequently unavoidable, and it was necessary, especially in the smaller London boroughs, to call for reinforcements at an early stage. Reports from other parts of the country where there were raids spoke in terms of the highest praise of the work of the ambulance service.

Organisation of Industrial Civil Defence. The recent raids had shown again the need for strict adherence to the principles of industrial civil defence organisation. In a supplement to Civil Defence Industrial Bulletin No. 11—Notes on recent raids (February–March 1944)—the importance of co-operation between the passive air defence officer of industrial and commercial concerns and the local authorities was stressed. Cases had occurred where incidents at industrial premises had not been reported to the local authority's report and control centre. It was pointed out in the supplement that during air attack the factory controller must assume command and advise the local authority's controller of any event, large or small. Any evacuation or movement of personnel should take place only by direction of the controller. A system of messengers should be instantly available for internal and external communications, in case telephones and loud speakers should be rendered inoperative by bombs falling at some distance from the factory premises. The value of well-trained factory incident officers, who should maintain close liaison with local authorities' incident officers, was also referred to in the supplement.

The Flying Bomb Period. As attacks by flying bombs were nearly all made on Southern England and mainly on the London area, from which regular reports of all incidents were furnished, the experience gained and the lessons learned are those of the London area. The flying bomb was designed for maximum blast effect; there was no fragmentation of the type found with thick-cased bombs, and usually little or no crater, except occasionally in soft ground or when the bomb power-dived. One of the principal causes of casualties was from splinters of broken glass, but where a direct hit had demolished or damaged buildings, people in these buildings sustained similar injuries to those caused when buildings had been struck by H.E. bombs or by parachute mines.

The lessons learned from this type of attack were mainly a re-emphasis of old ones, but a few additional points of interest came to light. All reports show that the work of every branch of the Civil Defence Service had never been better. They had been helped by the fact that incidents were single, but it was only by long and intensive training that an almost clock-work precision had been attained. Many incidents were cleared up within an hour. One important variation of normal practice had been introduced in London with success to meet this particular form of attack. The fall of flying bombs was reported direct to the control centre from N.F.S. observation posts, from posts established by local authorities, by individual depots, or sometimes from wardens' posts. On receipt of a report a flying squad or express party was immediately ordered out, consisting of one or two heavy rescue parties, one or two light rescue parties, one or two ambulances and generally a mobile first-aid unit. As it was found that the proportion of injured to dead was considerably higher than before and, generally speaking, that a large proportion of casualties were ready for immediate disposal, the practice of sending only one or two ambulances in an express party was revised and four to six ambulances were immediately sent. Where observation posts were connected with depots, services were sent out direct, and at the same time the controller was notified.

Valuable help was again given to the civil defence services by British and Allied troops, by the Home Guard and by the N.F.S. As the flying bombs caused few fires, the personnel of the National Fire Service were free to assist in the work of rescue and of first aid. As a general rule these services worked under the direction of the civil defence services. The value of the training in first aid and light rescue given to the Home Guard and the N.F.S. had been well proved, especially when they happened to arrive first at incidents. Reinforcing groups from Regional columns of the Civil Defence Reserve were frequently called upon and rendered noteworthy assistance.

Dogs trained by the Ministry of Aircraft Production did very good work, usually in pairs, in locating trapped casualties.

Mobile first-aid units were more largely used during the flying bomb period than in any other, and completely justified their existence, although some still thought that they should have been replaced by light mobile first-aid units. Experience showed that it was frequently better to send one or more of the latter type of unit first to an incident, and to hold the heavy unit until the situation was made clearer by more detailed reports.

As in former types of attacks, severely injured persons were sometimes taken appreciable distances to hospitals and first-aid posts, by unauthorised persons, although ambulances were present at their loading points at the incidents. Casualties were sometimes taken to the wrong hospital by unauthorised persons, and delay was caused by sending them to hospitals selected for receiving casualties. The importance of 'switching' casualties to hospitals, to prevent overcrowding was realised and, on the whole, well carried out, although a few instances were reported of this rule being neglected. Medical officers of health and incident doctors were generally present at every incident, giving valuable advice and help to the services and to casualties.

Incident inquiry points staffed by the Women's Voluntary Services were always on the spot within a short time after the fall of flying bombs, and were of immense value to the incident officers and to the general public. In addition to this work, the W.V.S. staffed information bureaux and visited all houses in the areas damaged by flying bombs to ascertain if any assistance was required. Mobile canteens manned by this devoted service were always at hand at incidents and did much to sustain the morale of bombed-out persons.

Long-range Rocket Period. Experience showed that an even larger civil defence force should be immediately deployed for long-range rocket incidents in built-up areas, than for flying bombs as, since no warning was given, the number of passers-by could seldom be known; consequently, all debris had to be treated as possibly covering casualties. One factor which made the problem easier was that during attacks by flying bombs and by long-range rockets no concentration was achieved, consequently the bulk of resources could safely be deployed to work at single incidents. The long-range rocket differed from the flying bomb as, on exploding, it broke up into numerous small and large fragments capable of causing severe injuries.

At no time during the war had the London casualty services experienced more trying ordeals than in the period from June 12, 1944, to March 29, 1945, and never had they acquitted themselves better. Depleted in numbers as they were, they had to be continually on the alert to go to incidents, many of which had occurred suddenly and without any warning, but they cheerfully and willingly obeyed all calls for assistance and gave useful and noble service with complete disregard of personal danger. No invidious distinction can be made between the work of the various branches of the casualty services in Great Britain. Every man and woman in them, in common with those of the National Fire Service and the Police Force, aided by members of the Armed Forces, gave of their best throughout the war with one object in view—to do all in their power to help the casualty. The casualty figures which follow indicate how much their help had been needed.

CASUALTIES TREATED BY THE CIVIL DEFENCE CASUALTY SERVICES, 1944-5

During the year 1944 and the first three months of 1945, 48,316 casualties were treated by the first-aid posts, first-aid points and mobile first-aid units. Of these, 13,105 occurred in the first six months of 1944, 26,449 in the next six months and 8,762 in the first three months of 1945.

The total civilian casualties recorded as having been treated by first-aid posts, first-aid points and mobile first-aid units in England and Wales during the whole period of the enemy attacks were 145,481 from September 1, 1940 to March 29, 1945.

The actual number treated must have been considerably more than this number, as many cases were treated at posts which were bombed and in which the records were destroyed. In addition cases were often treated and not recorded at times of stress under heavy attack in partially demolished posts, and in adjacent buildings. In addition to those treated at posts it is known that considerable numbers of lightly injured persons did not present themselves for treatment, especially during the early raids, but went either to their own doctor or to chemists' shops for first-aid treatment. No record of the numbers thus treated is available.

CASUALTIES AMONG CIVIL DEFENCE CASUALTY SERVICE UNITS

From September 3, 1939, until March 31, 1945, the following casualties occurred among units of the Civil Defence Casualty Services:

Casualties in Civil Defence Casualty Services

	Killed			Seriously injured			Slightly injured		
	Males	Females	Total	Males	Females	Total	Males	Females	Total
First-aid and stretcher parties	143	5	148	317	11	328	937	52	989
First-aid Post Service	23	69	92	56	119	175	122	253	375
Ambulance Service	58	31	89	51	83	134	192	382	574
	224	105	329	424	213	637	1,251	687	1,938
Rescue Parties	126		126	460	3	463	1,469	3	1,472

NOTE. The figures for the Rescue Party Service are given separately, as before the amalgamation of the Rescue and First-aid Party Services in January 1943, the Rescue Party Service was not part of the Casualty Service organisation.

STRENGTH OF THE CASUALTY SERVICES AT THE CLOSE OF ENEMY ATTACKS ON BRITAIN

First-aid Posts. At the end of March 1945, first-aid posts numbered 1,089, of which 528 were fixed and 561 mobile. Of the fixed posts 465 were active, the remainder being on 'care and maintenance'. Of the mobile units 333 were heavy and 228 light. In addition there were 5,708 first-aid points, 786 of which were 'upgraded'.

Whole-time personnel employed in this service numbered approximately 750 men and 3,200 women, in addition to which some 11,000 men and 36,000 women were giving part-time service, making a total of 50,950, this being about half the number employed in May 1944.

Ambulances. Ambulances numbered 5,166 (of which 4,922 were whole-time and 244 part-time) and sitting-case cars 1,594 (1,201 whole-time, 393 part-time). In the ambulance service there were approximately 2,500 men and 4,200 women whole-time, and 14,600 men and 20,500 women part-time, a total of 41,800, this being a reduction of more than one-third since May 1944.

The diminution in first-aid post and ambulance personnel was wholly due to reductions carried out in six Regions during the autumn and winter of 1944–5.

AWARDS TO MEMBERS OF THE CIVIL DEFENCE CASUALTY SERVICE

The following awards were gained by members of the Civil Defence Casualty Services for gallantry and devotion to duty up to the end of hostilities in Europe:

O.B.E.	1
M.B.E.	22
George Medal	34
B.E.M.	53
Commendation	147

THE WORK OF THE MEDICAL OFFICERS OF HEALTH

No history of the Civil Defence Casualty Service would be complete without a reference to the work of the medical officers of health. While still engaged upon their full-time normal duties, and other heavy duties imposed upon them by the war, such as measures to safeguard the health of the enormous shelter population, especially in London and other large towns and cities, these officers were called upon to assist, without extra remuneration, in the organising of the casualty services of their local authorities, and later, to assume responsibility for the administration and operational control of these services, subject to general directions from A.R.P. controllers, to whom they looked for broad decision.

A few, a very small minority, were inclined to regard this additional work as onerous, and to show little enthusiasm for it. The vast majority, however, responded nobly to the call and, by their untiring zeal and energy formed the back-bone of a casualty service organisation which, from small beginnings, developed into a model of efficiency second to none.

Their work for this organisation, arduous, often unrecognised and frequently adversely criticised, was carried on unceasingly, with little or no substantial help in the early days, but many of them found time to take a keen personal interest in the various units under their control, and on very many occasions shared their lot under most dangerous conditions. Not only did they earn the respect and gratitude of their staff and of the injured, but also the appreciation of a grateful country and many an award was given for gallantry in action and devotion to duty. Their war-time record is one of which they may justly be proud.

REFERENCES

[1] A.R.P. Dept. Circular 700,216/14 dated July 9, 1935.
[2] *A.R.P. Memorandum No.* 1 (2nd Edition) and *A.R.P. Memorandum No.* 7.
[3] Home Office A.R.P. Dept. Circular 703,189/19 of August 26, 1938.
[4] Min. of Health Circular 1764 of January 10, 1939.
[5] Min. of Health Circular 1789 of March 24, 1939.
[6] Min. of Health Circular 1764 of January 10, 1939.

[7] A.R.P. Dept. Circulars 701,593/106 and 701,593/95 of April, 1939.
[8] *A.R.P. Memorandum No.* 1 (2nd Edition) 1936.
[9] Min. of Health Circular 1764 of January 10, 1939.
[10] Min. of Health Circular 1789 of March 24, 1939.
[11] Min. of Health Circular 1893 of October 20, 1939.
[12] A.R.P. Dept. Circular 288/1939 of October 28, 1939.
[13] E.M.S.I No. 13 of January 7, 1939: Ministry of Health Circulars No. 1764 of January 10, 1939 and 1794 of April 3, 1939.
[14] Home Office (A.R.P. Dept.) Circular 1/1939 of January 4, 1939.
[15] Welfare Pamphlet No. 4 (3rd Edition). *First Aid and Ambulance for Factories and Workshops.*
[16] *A.R.P. Handbook No.* 6 (1st Edition) 1937.
[17] Min. of Health Circular 1779 and Memorandum 222 under Defence Regulations—Section 30(a).
[18] E.M.S.I. 144 of May 8, 1940.
[19] GROGONO, E. B. (1940), *Brit. med. J.*, 2, 638.
[20] Min. of Health Circular 2148 of September 17, 1940.
[21] The Stretcher Patient Secured, *Lancet* (1941), 1, 289.
[22] Min. of Home Security Circular 49/1941 with enclosure of February 20, 1941.
[23] *A.R.P. Training Bulletin No.* 6. Appendices A and B.
[24] Min. of Home Security Circular No. 63/1942 of March 21, 1942.
[25] S.R. & O., 1941, No. 1567.
[26] Min. of Home Security Circular No. 27/1942 of February 11, 1942.
[27] Min. of Home Security Circular No. 1/1943 of January 4, 1943, and Civil Defence Training Pamphlet No. 6.
[28] Min. of Home Security Circulars No. 16/1943 and 36/1943 of January 27 and February 25, 1943.
[29] *Training Manual No.* 4 (1st Edition), *Incident Control.*
[30] Emergency Medical Service Instruction 427 of August 21, 1943.
[31] Home Office (A.R.P. Dept.) Memorandum No. 1 (2nd Edition) of 1939; Ministry of Health Circular 1789, Para. 3, of March 24, 1939; Home Office (A.R.P. Dept.) Circular 134/1939 of July 7, 1939; Ministry of Home Security Circular 262/1941 of November 22, 1941; Ministry of Home Security Circular 117/1942 of June 6, 1942; as relevant examples.
[32] Home Office (A.R.P. Dept.) Circular No. 100/1939 of May 4, 1939; *A.R.P. Memorandum No.* 15 (four editions) *Care and custody of Equipment*, first published April, 1940, and many others.
[33] Min. of Home Security (A.R.P. Dept.) Circular No. 288/1939 of October 28, 1939. Min. of Home Security Circular H.S.R. 235/1940 of December 20, 1940. Min. of Home Security Circular H.S.R. 233/1941 of September 12, 1941, etc.
[34] Min. of Home Security Circular No. 122/1942 of June 15, 1942.
[35] Min. of Home Security Circular No. 10/1944 of January 10, 1944.
[36] Emergency Medical Service Instruction 459 of May 22, 1944.
[37] Emergency Medical Service Instruction 479 of June 27, 1944.
[38] Min. of Home Security Circular No. 115/1944 of September 19, 1944.

CHAPTER 8

THE AMBULANCE SERVICES

AMBULANCE transport formed so intimate and vital a part of the Emergency Medical Services that it has not been found practicable completely to segregate the subject from the general history of these Services. This chapter, therefore, which deals with the work of inter-hospital transport and of the ambulance trains, with the American ambulances and to a small extent with river ambulances, does not contain the complete history of the Ambulance Services. It could not do so without repeating information given in earlier chapters which recorded the development and work of the Emergency Medical Services as a whole. It does not deal with civil defence ambulances, which formed part of the local civil defence machine and were not, like the inter-hospital transport, directly administered by the Ministry of Health and its regional organisations. Their history is inseparable from that of the civil defence casualty services and is therefore more appropriately dealt with in Chapter 7 (Civil Defence Casualty Services). Nor does it deal with the evacuation of battle casualties by air—a development of special interest and value. After the Allied invasion of Europe a large proportion of casualties were brought back by air, and their reception and distribution, being an E.M.S. responsibility, are referred to in Chapter 6. The actual work of the air ambulances, however, was the responsibility of the Air Ministry and not of the Ministry of Health, and is described in the R.A.F. volumes.

AMBULANCE TRAINS

The following account of the organisation and work of the ambulance trains is a contribution (abridged) by Dr. Philip D. Oakley, C.B.E., Medical Officer in Charge of Casualty Evacuation Trains, on the staff of the Director-General, Emergency Medical Services.

When, in September 1938, it was considered necessary to prepare for the evacuation of the London hospitals, a representative meeting was held at the Ministry of Transport to draw up plans for conveying patients by train to towns approximately fifty miles distant from London. This meeting was the precursor of the Ambulance Trains Committee, afterwards renamed the Casualty Evacuation Trains Committee, which dealt with all matters relative to the casualty evacuation trains from the date of its first meeting on July 6, 1939. This committee, of which a representative of the Ministry of War Transport was chairman, consisted of representatives also of the Ministry of Health and the Department of Health for Scotland, and of the Admiralty, War Office,

THE AMBULANCE SERVICES

Air Ministry, the Railway Executive Committee and the four main railway companies.

PLANS FOR THE EVACUATION OF HOSPITAL PATIENTS

At the meeting in September 1938, it was agreed that twenty-one trains would be required for the evacuation of London hospitals, each to be made up of ten parcel vans (adapted to accommodate approximately thirty stretcher-cases per van) and two brake vans. In addition to fitting removable brackets for carrying stretchers, certain other improvisations had to be made. At the request of the Ministry of Health the War Office agreed to lend 4,000 G.S. stretchers and pillows, to be sent to the hospitals from which patients were to be evacuated. The supply of certain other equipment, such as bedpans, urinals, mugs, bowls, bandages, drugs and first-aid satchels, was arranged by the London County Council, who also undertook to provide a medical officer and five nurses for each train. Forty stretcher bearers were to be provided by the St. John Ambulance Brigade at each of the selected entraining points. A clerical officer from the Ministry of Health was to be appointed to each train to act as transport officer in charge of entraining and equipment.

A programme was worked out with the London Passenger Transport Board for the buses which would be required and within a fortnight the Board were ready at twelve hours' notice to bring the necessary number of buses to the entraining points, which were not the London termini.

PLANS FOR TRANSPORT OF CASUALTIES

The above plans, made under the threat of war, were for the first emergency clearance of hospitals. Fortunately, the political situation eased considerably and the Ministry of Health were then in a position to work out long-term plans for the subsequent transport of casualties. In March 1939, the Ministry of Transport were informed that, in the event of war, in addition to the 21 ambulance trains required for the initial transfer of patients the Ministry of Health would require ambulance trains throughout the war in London and other large centres of populations, such as Birmingham, Liverpool, Manchester, Sheffield, Leeds, Newcastle, Southampton and possibly Hull. It was estimated that as many as 50 trains on any one day might be necessary. The matter was further discussed at a meeting held at the Ministry of Transport on April 3, 1939, when it was agreed that 34 trains would be sufficient, 28 in England, 2 in Scotland and 4 on loan to the War Office. The railways' representatives undertook to explore the possibility of releasing and adapting the necessary rolling stock, and by the end of June a sample van fitted with brackets for carrying the stretchers in tiers was inspected and accepted as a suitable type (see Plate XXIX). These brackets could be easily removed and placed in receptacles under the van so that it could be put back into operation and remain earmarked for recall if necessary. Orders were then given by the Ministry of Transport to provide 34 casualty evacuation trains.

As these trains were constructed for the transport of patients who had already received treatment and who were to travel only the comparatively short journeys required to remove them from target areas, they were of a much simpler design than the Home Ambulance Trains provided for the War Office, which were necessarily equipped for greater travelling comfort, including the provision of cooked meals en route for both patients and staff.

NUMBERS AND LOCATION OF TRAINS

It was decided that of the 30 evacuation trains for civilians, 1 each should be allocated to Newcastle, Leeds, Bristol, Exeter, Manchester, Liverpool, Birmingham and Scotland, leaving 22 to be distributed around the outskirts of London. Most of these trains were in position at their berthing sites on September 3, 1939, and all the London trains were safely berthed by September 5.

Of the four trains lent to the War Office, two were handed back to the Ministry of Health in October 1939. One of these was allocated to Scotland and the other was disbanded and returned to the railway company.

This was the position until December 1939, when because the war had not followed its expected course and in view of the acute shortage of rolling stock, it was decided to disband ten of the twenty-two trains berthed near London and hand them back to the railway companies for general service, earmarked for recall if necessary. The companies had stated that trains could be reconstructed and placed in position at seventy-two hours' notice.

In June 1940, owing to the collapse of France it was considered advisable to recall the 10 trains which had been disbanded in December, 1939. The War Office also handed back the 2 remaining trains on loan, 1 of which was allocated to Scotland, so that 30 trains were available in England and 3 in Scotland. Further, the War Office announced that they would release 2 trains which had been prepared for overseas. After necessary alterations had been made these were handed over to Scotland, making 5 in Scotland.

The trains, which had been recalled plus the two handed back by the War Office, were all in position in seventy-two hours and fully staffed and equipped in three weeks.

In October 1941, the position was reviewed once more. After discussions with the three Services and the Home Defence Executive, it was agreed that the number of casualty evacuation trains could be reduced with safety and it was decided to release twelve trains. Scotland had also reduced the number of trains from five to three.

DESCRIPTION OF TRAIN

Each train consisted of 12 coaches whose final marshalled order was 1 brake third van, 4 stretcher vans, 1 staff and kitchen car, five stretcher vans, and 1 brake third van (see Plate XXX).

The brake third vans each consisted of a third-class corridor coach with a guard's van at the end. There was some difference in size between the rolling stock of the four companies, but they were all fitted similarly. The guard's van was fitted with two water tanks, one 200-gallon cold water and one 100-gallon hot water, the latter being heated by means of a copper worm connected with the steam heating from the engine. In one brake third van an oil drum and stillage was fitted for storing paraffin. Two of the compartments were stripped and cupboards and shelves fitted for storing drugs, dressings and provisions. The remaining compartments were for the train crew to put their outdoor clothes and personal belongings in when they came on the train, the nurses being at one end and the orderlies at the other. One compartment was fitted up as a general office and one as a personal office for the Medical Officer of the train. The Sister-in-Charge had a compartment to herself.

The staff and kitchen cars provided rest rooms for the train crews and kitchens for preparing meals for the patients and crews. The type of car varied according to the company providing the rolling stock. The Great Western and Southern Railways provided their own kitchen and dining cars. The cooking range had been taken out and a 'dixie' stove, burning solid fuel, installed. This stove had a 50-gallon hot water tank over it. The seating accommodation on this type was Great Western 30; Southern Railway 28. The London and North Eastern and London, Midland and Scottish Railways provided a third vestibule car with a guard's compartment at the end, fitted out as a kitchen with the dixie stove and the necessary sinks, cupboards, etc. The seating accommodation in the London and North Eastern Railway was 32, and in the London, Midland and Scottish 40 (see Plates XXXI, XXXII).

Stretcher vans consisted of bogie brake vans fitted with removal brackets on which two tiers of stretchers were carried in addition to one row on the floor of the van (see Plate XXXIII). The number of stretcher cases carried varied according to the stock released by the four companies, that of the Great Western, London and North Eastern and Southern Railways being able to take more than the London Midland and Scottish. The average accommodation per train was 300 stretcher cases, or 345 in emergency. In practice, however, it was not found advisable to bring into use the emergency accommodation for 45 stretchers, which had been allowed for, on the floors of the stretcher vans, because this would have made it extremely difficult for the train crew to carry out their duties.

Each van was heated by a steam pipe running along the roof and connected with the engine. When the vans were not connected with the engine, heating was by Aladdin stoves burning paraffin. These stoves could be carried from van to van as required for airing blankets, linen, etc., and keeping the equipment in good condition. Electric lighting was installed, supplied from batteries carried under the floor of the coach. The batteries were charged from time to time to keep them in good condition, but when the train was stationary lighting was supplied by hurricane lamps and A.R.P. torches. Holes and sluices were cut in the floors of vans for the disposal of excreta. A Louvre ventilator was placed at either end of each van to maintain adequate ventilation when the windows were shut. All windows were blacked out to conform to A.R.P. regulations and were covered with anti-splinter mesh fabric. Two chemical fire extinguishers, supplied by the railway companies, were placed in each van and scoops and sand buckets were carried to deal with incendiary bombs.

MAINTENANCE

The Ministry of Health were responsible for the upkeep and cleansing of the interior of the trains and their equipment; and the railway companies were responsible for the exterior and all repairs, additions and alterations, mechanical overhaul and the general supervision of the trains in order to keep them in condition for operation at a moment's notice.

CONTROL

The control of the casualty evacuation trains was undertaken by the Ministry of Health and placed under the direct supervision of the Director-General, Emergency Medical Services, who appointed one of his staff, Dr. P. D. Oakley, to assume the duties of Medical Officer-in-Charge and to be responsible to him for the general upkeep and operation of the trains. Personnel matters were dealt with by the Establishment Division of the Ministry of Health; the financial duties were undertaken by the Regional Finance Officers; equipment, stores, etc., were under the Supplies Division and the Regional Equipment Officers.

PERSONNEL

Before the state of emergency, preparation had been made to provide crews for the casualty trains. The crew of each train was to consist of 1 medical officer in charge, 1 hospital train officer to act as staff officer, 3 trained nurses, 10 auxiliary nurses and 8 orderlies. The medical officers were provided by the Central Medical War Committee; the hospital train officers were clerical officers of the Equipment Division of the Ministry of Health, and the nursing staff were appointed from the Civil Nursing Reserve. Two superintending sisters were also appointed, whose duties were to supervise the welfare of the nurses. The orderlies were recruited from the St. John Ambulance Brigade, through the good offices of the Commissioner, Captain Goodly, O.B.E., M.C.

In November 1939, the hospital train officer attached to each train was withdrawn and four executive officers were appointed from the Regional Finance Officer's staff for the financial work in connexion with the trains.

In August 1940, the senior trained nurse in each train was made responsible to the train medical officer for staff and equipment and given the title of Charge Sister, the appointment being comparable to that of Sister-in-Charge of a ward in a hospital.

When the train crews were called upon to provide meals for patients it was found that the staffs were not sufficient to deal with the kitchen work and at the same time serve the meal. It was therefore decided to carry three extra nurses when the train was fully loaded. These nurses were supplied on application to the Sector Matrons in the London area and the Regional Nursing Officers in the Provinces.

Since the trains were not constructed for the continued residence of the crews it was necessary to have recourse to billets. The train medical officer received an allowance in lieu of quarters and was required to find his own lodging.

EQUIPMENT

The original equipment had been worked out by the Ministry of Health on the basis that the patients to be carried would in all probability have received treatment in hospital and would therefore require little attention on the journey. Owing, however, to the extremely heavy demand made on manufacturers before the outbreak of hostilities it was only possible to place a skeleton equipment on board each train. After the trains had been in operation for a short time it was found that the original equipment was inadequate and as supplies became available various items were increased and others added until medical supplies, instruments, drugs and dressings, linen, domestic utensils and stores were carried in adequate quantities, the utmost use being made of limited storage space permitted. Eventually domestic equipment was increased to enable a knife and fork meal to be given on the longer journeys, e.g. to oversea casualties on trains running from port or transit hospitals to base hospitals.

FOOD SUPPLIES

The original intention was that patients admitted to the casualty evacuation trains should bring with them rations for one day, supplied by the discharging hospitals. Supplies of tea, coffee, cocoa, sugar, milk, Horlick's malted milk, Benger's food, etc., were carried to augment these rations. When, during the heavy air attacks on the larger cities, it was found that the discharging hospitals were not always able to supply rations, it was considered expedient to increase the amount of food carried on the trains so as to enable a simple meal of stew, potatoes, rice pudding, etc., to be prepared and served on the trains. This proved satisfactory and further stocks of foodstuffs were added to enable each train to cater for its crew and 300 patients for one week. This was thought sufficient to meet any contingency.

OPERATIONS

All operations were directed from headquarters at Whitehall and were under the supervision of the Director-General, Emergency Medical Services (Movements). The actual movement of the trains was under the control of the Railway Executive Committee, and the train medical officers were not permitted to interfere with the running of the trains unless exceptional circumstances necessitated a change of movement, in which case the guard was notified and requested to take the necessary action.

Departmental instructions were issued from time to time on the general management of trains, including crews, equipment, stores and operations.

Lists of entraining and detraining stations were compiled and special medical officers appointed to undertake the duties of entraining and detraining. Instructions were issued setting forth the various duties these officers might be called upon to perform. Close liaison with the movements of Home Ambulance Trains (War Office) was maintained through the Railway Executive Committee and also with the responsible department of the War Office.

Entraining and Detraining. The patients were brought to the trains in ambulances and buses adapted for stretchers. Loading was from the platform or ground level according to site. Steps were provided for the walking cases when loading from the ground.

The stretchers with patients were placed on the floors of the stretcher vans and were then lifted on to the brackets by the train orderlies. Green metal stretchers were generally used, but the brackets could also take the canvas Service stretchers. When a patient was put into a train on a stretcher with blankets an orderly handed out one stretcher and the same number of blankets. The same procedure was adopted at the detraining point so that there was a system of replacement along the line. It was found to be essential at both entraining and detraining stations to exclude the public and all unnecessary personnel.

The medical officer in charge assumed complete control, but the assistance of the police was always sought in order to keep the station and its approaches as clear as possible and to regulate traffic. When entraining or detraining was carried out during the black-out special lighting was used to conform with police regulations. This lighting was installed and controlled by the station authorities. When detraining, walking cases left first, so as to leave the platform or the siding clear for the stretcher cases. Time taken to load varied according to site, suitability of the approaches and the skill of the stretcher bearers. If the patients arrived in a continual stream 120 stretcher cases could be loaded in one hour. This was done by loading two stretcher vans at a time, but if a sufficient number of stretcher bearers was available more coaches could be loaded at the same time and the rate of loading increased accordingly.

Stretcher Bearers. There was great difficulty in the early days of the war in obtaining suitable bearers. In London it had been arranged that members of the St. John Ambulance Brigade should hold themselves in readiness to report at a central collecting station, whence they were to be transported to the entraining point. This method proved impracticable. Arrangements were then made whereby members of the civil defence first-aid parties could be used if they were not required at an incident. As the trains did not come into operation until the day after an air raid this method was tried and proved satisfactory. A supply of trained stretcher bearers was always forthcoming. In the North West Region, military stretcher bearers from the infantry training centres were supplied, by the courtesy of the G.O.C. Western Command, to all ambulance trains arriving in the area, whether Home Ambulance trains or Casualty Evacuation trains. Refreshments for the stretcher bearers such as tea, coffee, cocoa, etc., were usually supplied through the good offices of the Women's Voluntary Services. This proved a great boon on cold days and nights especially if the train was running late.

Movements. The actual movements of the trains up to the end of 1940 were divided into four main phases :

Phase 1 : Initial clearance of the London hospitals on September 1, 1939. The numbers carried were: 2,902 patients in 18 of the original 21 trains. All the patients arrived safely at their destinations.

Phase 2: Clearing the Public Assistance Institutions on the East Coast between July 5 and 11, 1940;

9 trains carried 1,727 patients, an average of 191·8 per train.

Phase 3: Clearing the coastal belt from the Wash to Bournemouth on September 10, 1940;

15 trains carried 2,352 patients, an average of 156·7 per train.

This move was completed in 24 hours and all trains were back at their berthing stations by 18·00 hours on September 11, 1940.

Phase 4: Clearing the aged and infirm from London County Council hospitals between October 10 and November 14, 1940;

34 trains carried 7,612 patients, an average of 223·8 per train.

The cases carried included many homeless from the shelters.

In addition to these main phases casualty evacuation trains were called upon to clear reception hospitals during the evacuation from Dunkirk.

The following Service convoys were operated:

Naval: 88 trains carried 8,913 patients: 101·2 per train.

Military: 29 trains carried 5,619 patients: 193·6 per train.

French Wounded Repatriation: 3 trains carried 536 patients: 178·6 per train.

In addition to these moves stretcher vans were attached to ordinary passenger trains in order to accommodate stretcher cases from the Navy and R.A.F. which required medical attention on the journey.

THREAT OF INVASION

Special arrangements were made in order to cope with exceptional circumstances which might arise in an invasion of this country.

The hospitals in the twenty-mile coastal belt extending from the Wash to Weymouth were to be partially cleared. The War Office required this movement to be completed in seventy-two hours. The patients from these hospitals were to be transported to hospitals in Regions 2, 3, 8, 9 and 10; both home ambulance trains (War Office) and casualty evacuation trains were to be used and a schedule was drawn up showing the entraining and detraining point for each train and submitted to the Railway Executive Committee for timing. In due course the Railway Executive Committee submitted an agreed time-table by which the hospitals could be cleared in forty-eight hours.

A weekly list of numbers to be cleared from each entraining point was submitted by the Hospital Officer of the Region to be cleared, and reception areas were informed of the number of cases to be expected at each detraining point.

Movement instructions were drawn up and sent to the train medical officers and all other officers concerned in the clearance, so that it could be carried out at very short notice.

It was decided that if after this move any particular Region was cut off from communication with Whitehall, four regulating points should be fixed round which certain trains would be berthed, ready to proceed forward as required. These trains would be requisitioned by the Hospital Officers of the Regions through the Movement Control Officers of the Command who would take the necessary action to bring the trains forward.

Each train carried sufficient rations to feed 300 patients and 22 crew for one week. Reserve dumps of food containing one week's supply for each train were made at each regulating point. This procedure was necessary because of the difficulty of reprovisioning the trains if they were side-tracked at small sidings in out-of-the-way places. The dumps and the rations carried on board were arranged with the Ministry of Food.

TYPES OF CASES CARRIED

During the early months of the war the trains were used principally to transport naval cases, usually from Chatham and Haslar to Barrow Gurney, Bristol and Newton Abbot. Later they were used to evacuate hospitals on the south and south-east coast and to clear the old and infirm from London after the heavy air raids.

All classes of cases were carried, from babies to one old lady of 94 who stood the journey from London to Manchester quite well and was genuinely grateful for all that had been done for her. Only one death on the trains was recorded, that of an old man who had an attack of coronary thrombosis on Paddington station and who decided to continue the journey. Unfortunately, he had another attack on the train which proved fatal.

PREPARATIONS FOR 'D' DAY AND SUBSEQUENT OPERATIONS

From the autumn of 1940 until the spring of 1944 there had been very little movement of complete ambulance trains, as transfers of cases had usually been made in small numbers in one or more coaches from a casualty evacuation train attached to an ordinary passenger train. There was more activity in May 1944, when casualty evacuation trains were used to clear the hospitals that would be needed for the reception of battle casualties.

The Ministry of Health had been informed by the War Office that they would require the use of all casualty trains in addition to their home ambulance trains. At this time the War Office had seven home ambulance trains, the Ministry of Health eighteen casualty evacuation trains and the Department of Health for Scotland three casualty evacuation trains. The Department of Health for Scotland handed over their three trains for operations in England. All trains were placed under Q.(M) 4, War Office, for operations, but the staff of the casualty trains remained under the control of the Ministry of Health.

Staff. The staff of each casualty evacuation train was increased by 3 nurses and by 2 fourth-year medical students who would assist the Train Medical Officer. The staff therefore was brought up to 27, consisting of 1 medical officer, 2 fourth-year medical students, 3 trained nurses, 13 auxiliary nurses and 8 orderlies. Replacement of the nursing staff in case of sickness was made by arrangement with the British Red Cross Society, Southampton, who undertook to supply reliefs at very short notice. Reliefs for the orderlies were supplied by the R.A.M.C., on application to the A.D.M.S. covering the South Coast ports or A.D.M.S. Command as occasion arose.

As all trains were to be ready to move at a moment's notice, it was necessary for the crews to leave their billets and to live on board. As casualty evacuation trains were not constructed for continuous residence, living accommodation had to be improvised. Each train was inspected and the crews informed of the discomforts in store. All members of the train crews willingly accepted the conditions and it is to their credit that no serious complaints were received. When the first rush was over, one stretcher van was given up for the exclusive use of the nurses, and added to their comfort considerably. During the winter casualty evacuation trains not connected with steam heating were given additional warmth at berthing sites by attaching an engine for so many hours a day, as the Aladdin stoves already installed were not sufficient to keep the vans suitably heated.

Supplies. Since all casualty evacuation trains were expected to be moving frequently, the War Office undertook the complete servicing of laundry and other services on lines similar to those for the home ambulance trains. The existing method, including the replenishment of food from dumps which had been arranged in conjunction with the Ministry of Food in case of the invasion of England, was no longer appropriate and the War Office supplied all food for both train crews and casualties. The train medical officer indented on Command Supply depots for his requirements. On November 22, 1944, four trains were returned to their permanent berthing points, and the crews put in billets which had been retained for them. These crews ceased to draw Army rations except for the period during which the trains were in actual operation.

Hard and fresh rations for the train crews were replenished at the permanent berthing points. To provide complete replenishment, including linen and fresh rations for the casualties, depots were established at Chichester, Cosham, Winchester, Basingstoke, Woking, Guildford, Epsom Downs and Tattenham Corner. All trains visited one of these stations during each journey and stores were replenished during entrainment or detrainment. Supplies were ordered and issued as follows:

(a) *Linen*: Ordered by O.C. train on arrival at the station, whether for entrainment or detrainment. N.C.O.s in charge of supplies were issued with clean linen at once in exchange for soiled linen.

(b) *Bread*: Immediately a hospital knew that entrainment was to take place, the military registrar informed the N.C.O. in charge of supplies who ordered the necessary quantity of bread to be delivered to the station.

(c) *Other supplies and rations* were issued at the berthing point.

The stocks of drugs and dressings were increased and new drugs issued. Oxygen apparatus was supplied to each train. Penicillin was issued to each train on application to the embarkation medical officer by the train medical officer; any surplus of penicillin at the end of the journey was handed over to the detraining medical officer on arrival. Sedatives consisting of barbitone, phenobarbitone and paraldehyde were supplied for the treatment of exhaustion cases. Replenishment of drugs and dressings was made by the Supplies Division of the Ministry of Health.

Provision of Meals. During the run from port to transit hospital time did not permit of a hot meal being prepared. Casualties were given as many sandwiches as they desired and were supplied with hot tea, coffee, cocoa, Horlick's, Benger's, lime-juice, etc. On the longer runs from port to base hospital and from transit hospital to base hospital it was possible to serve a cooked meal. No train chefs were employed, the cooking being carried out by an orderly and three nurses. The stoves supplied were not large enough to cook hot meals for 240 people and in a few instances there was a delay in serving some of the patients. The installation of larger cooking units, and qualified chefs for each train, would have been advisable.

Method of Conveying Patients to Hospitals. The convoy receiving hospitals were placed in two categories: (*a*) transit and (*b*) base.

Casualties arriving at the ports of entry or 'hards' were examined by a surgical specialist who decided whether they required immediate treatment or were able to continue their journey. Those requiring immediate treatment were taken by ambulance to the nearest designated hospital and those who were able to undertake a journey of not more than three hours were transported to a casualty train and taken to a transit hospital where they were admitted and classified. A schedule of pre-determined detraining points which would serve the transit and base hospitals was prepared. A list was made out giving the detraining points for the transit and base hospitals, and as trains were called forward from their berthing sites they were automatically despatched to the first railhead on the list, which was then cancelled. Detraining points were so arranged that the transit hospitals which were served by each point would be able to deal with two or three convoys in the twenty-four hours according to the number of beds available. Bedstate figures were supplied twice daily so that any necessary alteration could be made in the roster of detraining points. Similarly convoys proceeding from transit to base were despatched to the first detraining point on the list. A strict watch was kept on all bedstates so as to switch convoys if necessary. All routes and timings had been worked out by the railway companies beforehand and the whole operation worked well.

Positioning of Trains. Prior to D-day it had been agreed with A.M.D.12, War Office, that the casualty evacuation trains, which had a stretcher-carrying capacity of 270 stretchers against 126 of the home ambulance trains, should undertake the transport of casualties from port to transit hospitals. Eight casualty evacuation trains were earmarked for this run and were fitted with Army type stretchers, the metal stretchers being removed and stored in a small van which was attached to the train for this purpose. These eight casualty trains were placed at strategic points covering the South Coast ports and hards. The journeys from port to transit hospital were so arranged that it would be possible for each train to make two trips a day. This gave a total lift of 4,320 stretchers. Fortunately the casualties were very much fewer than expected. The greatest number ever carried on one day was 1,761 on June 12, 1944. The remaining casualty evacuation trains were placed at convenient points from which they could be called forward to convey casualties from the transit hospitals to base hospitals. In July, ten trains were allotted wholly for oversea cases, leaving eleven for civilian transport. In November one C.E.T. was handed over to the U.S. Army.

Interchange of Stretchers and Blankets. As in the evacuation of hospitals in the earlier days of the war, the supply of stretchers and blankets was maintained by a system of replacement at all points of transfer.

Operation of Trains. The actual movement of trains was carried out by Q.(M.)4. War Office in conjunction with the Railway Executive Committee. Procedure was as follows:

(1) From Port to Transit Hospital: Movement Control in conjunction with Q. Movements Southern Command called forward and despatched trains as required. Immediately on the departure of a loaded train, M.C. Port despatched an 'Immediate' teleprinter message to Movement Control in the receiving district giving name of detraining station, time of arrival and the numbers of stretcher and sitting cases. District Movement Control at once notified the Sector or Regional Hospital Officer. The Hospital Officer was responsible for making all arrangements for stretcher bearers, transport and the admission of cases to hospital. Macintosh sheeting was supplied to protect the patients from rain during transfer from train to ambulance.

(2) From transit hospital to base hospital: Movement was initiated by the Regional or Sector Hospital Officer who telephoned direct to Q.(M.)4, War Office, giving entraining station and the numbers of lying and sitting cases. Q.(M.)4 selected the train and nominated the detraining point to be used, asked the Railway Executive Committee to arrange the move and informed District Movement Control by 'Immediate' teleprinter. Thereafter the procedure was the same as that from port to transit hospital.

To enable Regional and Sector Hospital Officers to communicate with Q.(M.)4 and Headquarters, Whitehall, with the least possible delay, direct lines were installed between the War Office and the Ministry of Health and between the Ministry of Health and the Hospital Officers of Sectors 8 and 9 and of Region 6 at Reading and 12 at Tunbridge Wells.

DOCUMENTATION

Each casualty admitted to a train at the port or hard wore the casualty evacuation label bearing his name and other Service particulars and showing the diagnosis, whether a lying or a sitting case, and whether a battle casualty or not. The name of the evacuating unit and name of ship (or, in airborne cases, aircraft number and type), were also given. This label, which was used for all oversea casualties, was made out in triplicate before evacuation and detached in three stages—the first on embarkation (or emplaning), the second on disembarkation and the third at the receiving hospital. There was no documentation until the patient arrived at the transit hospital. Categories of patients were listed for the transport from transit to base hospital and the lists were handed in duplicate to the train medical officer who retained one copy and gave the other to the detraining medical officer. It was the duty of the train medical officer to sort out special cases, such as head, chest and joint injuries and compound fractured femurs, so that these cases could be handed over to the detraining medical officer for immediate despatch to the special centres.

CLOSING OF TRANSIT HOSPITALS

In the autumn of 1944, when casualties were held longer in North-West Europe, it was decided to close the transit hospitals as such and to transport casualties from port to base hospitals. The change-over was made on October 24, 1944, up to which date, 63,292 casualties had been transported by casualty evacuation trains from ports and hards to transit hospitals.

OPENING OF TILBURY

Tilbury was opened as a port of entry on October 24, 1944, and four casualty evacuation trains were moved to cover this port, two stationed at Tilbury and two at Shoeburyness.

AIRBORNE CASUALTIES

Early in June 1944, preparations were made to transport airborne cases arriving at airfields near Swindon. Shrivenham was the entraining point chosen and came into operation on June 17, 1944. As these casualties were more recent than those now arriving by sea, it was considered advisable to make the train journey as short as possible and comparable to that between port and transit hospital. For this purpose, certain railheads were deleted from the main priority list and formed into an inner circle of convoy-receiving railheads strictly reserved for convoys from Shrivenham.

EVACUATION OF LONDON HOSPITALS

At the end of July 1944, instructions were issued to evacuate the London hospitals as a precaution against expected attacks by long-range rockets. The move was made in August and between the 3rd and the 30th, 68 trains carried 13,152 patients, an average of 193·4 per train. Although this move placed a great strain on the casualty evacuation trains, it was carried out according to plan without any hitch. Two entraining points were used, Addison Road and Marylebone. Stretcher bearers were supplied by 348 Coy. Pioneer Corps for Addison Road and 381 Coy. Pioneer Corps for Marylebone. Working parties for trains entraining at Gravesend West were supplied by courtesy of the Commander, Chatham Naval Barracks.

DISBANDMENT OF THE CASUALTY EVACUATION TRAINS

In May 1945, the War Office informed the Ministry of Health that they no longer required the Casualty Evacuation trains and by July, eight trains had been disbanded, leaving two berthed at Reading to bring home the London hospital patients.

RETURN OF HOSPITAL PATIENTS TO LONDON

In June 1945, it was decided to bring back to the London hospitals as many as possible of the evacuated patients and, as stated above, two casualty evacuation trains were retained for this purpose. Between August and October, 2,721 patients were brought back to London, the last train running on October 16, 1945. All these patients were detrained at Addison Road and sent to the Western Hospital, which acted as a clearing station. Stretcher bearers for these moves were supplied by the Officer-in-Charge of Italian prisoners-of-war, 100 of whom were quartered at the Western Hospital. When the hospitals were unable to admit any more evacuated patients this operation had to close down and the last casualty evacuation train was disbanded and handed back to the railways on November 2, 1945.

NUMBER OF PATIENTS CARRIED

The total number of patients carried from D-day to the disbandment of the casualty evacuation trains was 192,551, of whom 152,492 were Service cases. Of these 101,900 were British, 47,319 were American and 3,273 were Canadian. The total number of patients carried in the casualty evacuation trains, including those carried in stretcher vans attached to passenger trains, from September 3, 1939, to final disbandment, was 223,737.

INTER-HOSPITAL AMBULANCE TRANSPORT

This service formed part of the Emergency Medical Services and, in London, with which this account mainly deals, was initiated primarily to evacuate air raid casualties from casualty receiving hospitals in the target area to base hospitals on the periphery or outside the Region. Its main work was done in daylight, hospitals usually being cleared either in anticipation of or after nights of bombing during which the more spectacular and exciting work of collecting casualties and conveying them to first-aid post or hospital had been performed by the civil defence ambulances, to the courage and devotion of whose drivers and attendants tribute is paid in the chapter on the Civil Defence Casualty Services. But inter-hospital transport was by no means confined to daylight operations between the raids; its Green Line ambulance coaches were manned day and night and their drivers and attendants, drawn from the ranks of the intrepid transport workers who kept London's buses on the streets throughout the war, were ready to go anywhere, at any time. 'Their reputation of always going wherever they were needed, whatever the conditions', wrote Mr. A. G. Naldrett, the Chief Ambulance Officer 'was more than justified'. Confirmation of this will be found in the several extracts given in this chapter from his Report on the Civil Defence Ambulance Service and E.M.S. Inter-Hospital Transport in the London Civil Defence Region, 1939–45, on which the following account of the work of inter-hospital transport in London is based.

LONDON REGION

The London inter-hospital ambulance fleet, which was supplied, manned and maintained by the London Passenger Transport Board for the Ministry of Health, consisted of some 250 Green Line coaches, converted to carry from eight to ten stretchers each and known as ambulance coaches. In addition to these, buses for sitting cases were hired from the Board as and when required.

As recorded in Chapter 1, stretcher fitments sufficient for 320 coaches were prepared in advance for installation at short notice, and the coach-ambulances, which were first used in the evacuation of the London hospitals in September 1939, immediately before the outbreak of war, were ready a year earlier for use in the hospital clearance which had been planned for the autumn of 1938 but did not then take place. In the hospital clearance of September 1–3, 1939, referred to in Chapter 3 and in the section of this chapter on Ambulance Trains, these ambulances were used under the direction of the Hospital Officer to carry some 3,000 patients from London hospitals to the ambulance trains by which they travelled to their destinations in distant towns. In the evacuation of children's hospitals in the inner zone, the coach-ambulances carried between 1,800 and 1,900 patients direct to the receiving hospitals in the outer areas.

At this time some 18,000 cases were also evacuated from hospitals in large provincial towns, nearly all by bus-ambulances.

When war was declared and the Regional organisation came into operation, the London Inter-hospital Transport Service was operated by Regional Communications. Ambulance coaches were stationed at twenty-one L.P.T.B. garages spread over the Region and were placed under the direct operational control of the group ambulance officers in whose groups they were situated. To these ambulance coaches were added, in July 1940, some 45–50 smaller American ambulance vehicles, which were garaged at depots in each of the five inner groups and placed under the same operational control.

Ambulances and cars belonging to local authorities (in London, the London County Council) and various other vehicles were also used, especially in the transportation of small numbers of cases, for which they were more suitable and economical than the larger bus-ambulances. The Home Ambulance Service of the Joint Council of the Order of St. John and the British Red Cross Society, consisting of some 400 ambulances throughout England and Wales, was made available in May 1940, for the movement of individual cases.

Although all coaches chosen for ambulance work were adapted for the conveyance of stretcher cases, sitting cases also were carried in them and for this purpose some of the seats were restored to twenty coaches in 1942, providing in each coach for eighteen sitting cases and four stretcher cases. This followed the decision early in that year to use the inter-hospital transport to assist in the evacuation of expectant mothers from hospitals and clinics in London to emergency maternity hostels in the country.

The size of the London ambulance-coach fleet varied during the years 1940–5 between 219 and 269. In the spring of 1940, 200 were always immediately available, with 19 in reserve. In July 1940, the total was brought up to 269 by the addition of 50 immediately available coaches; but, because of the demands of the Services for man-power, the London Passenger Transport Board found it difficult to continue to reserve sufficient drivers and maintenance personnel to hold 250 coaches available for immediate use. The number was therefore reduced to 129, the remaining 121 being available at two hours' notice, manned by staff withdrawn as required from other bus services. In 1942, by the release of 30 coaches for the use of the American Forces, the total number was reduced to 239, of which 125 were available immediately and 95 at two hours' notice, 19 being held, as before, as spares.

The numbers available immediately and at short notice varied from time to time. In the spring of 1944, when it became apparent that the invasion of Europe could not be very far ahead, special arrangements had to be made to meet possible contingencies. Ambulance personnel were instructed in detraining casualties and efforts were made to have more coaches staffed ready for immediate use. Drivers who had returned from the coaches to public services vehicles were no longer available, and the only source of supply was a pool of heavy vehicle drivers who had volunteered for special duty in connexion with the invasion. Many of these drivers were taken on by the L.P.T.B., given a week's training on coaches and then detailed to garages. Gradually the number of ambulance coaches available increased and by 'D' day, 188 were staffed day and night, the drivers working 12-hour shifts.

During the previous year further fitments had been ordered, and these were now installed, so that all ambulance-coaches, as well as Civil Defence ambulances, were adapted to take the various types of stretchers in use, including those in the British and American Forces, thus considerably increasing their usefulness and, since the nearest available ambulances could be used as required, effecting economies in time and mileage (see Plate XXXIV).

Shortly afterwards, it was agreed that inter-hospital transport should assist in the conveyance, between their billets and working sites, large numbers of workmen who had been brought into the London Region from various parts of the country to repair houses damaged in the flying bomb attacks. In November, 123 of London's coach-ambulances were diverted to this work, leaving 116 for inter-hospital work. At that time 101 of these were continuously staffed, but by the end of the year the number of drivers available at night was reduced from 101 to 59. Further economies in the numbers and manning of night ambulances followed in 1945. After 'V.E.' day the number of staffed coach-ambulances was reduced to 72, in addition to which there were 24 held (not staffed) as spares. Including the 123 coaches used for transport of war workers the total remained at 219 until after 'V.J.' day (August 15, 1945). By that date the coach-ambulances had made 38,834 journeys covering 1,737,750 miles in the transport of hospital cases.

Inter-hospital transport in the London Region was operated as follows: a hospital with patients to evacuate applied to the Sector, who arranged for their reception at base or advanced base hospitals, generally within the same Sector as the evacuating hospital. Application for transport was then made by Sector or hospital to the Group Ambulance Officer, who instructed garages in his group to send the required number of vehicles. If a Group Ambulance Officer had not enough vehicles to meet the demands made upon him he applied to the Chief Ambulance Officer, London Region, for reinforcements from other groups.

Originally it was intended that ambulance drivers should be told the destination at the evacuating hospitals, but in practice it was usually found possible to give this information when the initial instructions were passed to the garages.

INTER-HOSPITAL TRANSPORT IN ACTION

Reference has already been made to the initial evacuation of London hospitals on the eve of the war with Germany. Thereafter, until the onset of air attacks nine months later, inter-hospital transport was used for the transfer of hospital cases from inner to outer hospitals so as to keep the casualty wards of the former cleared ready to receive air raid casualties should attacks begin. In addition, a considerable number of wounded and sick Service cases, principally those that were evacuated from Dunkirk, were conveyed from detraining stations to hospitals. By the end of August 1940, inter-hospital transport had carried 16,347 stretcher cases and 15,500 sitting cases. This was a task well within its capacity; ample time was left for organisation and training under war conditions, and the coach-ambulance fleet joined in combined exercises at which the various Civil Defence Services practised their duties in local and Regional co-operation. The value of this training was soon to be shown.

It was in the first week of September 1940, that the heavy assault on London began in earnest. A heavy attack on the dock area at Silvertown during the afternoon of September 7, was followed by a still heavier attack after nightfall which lasted most of the night; large areas were burning fiercely and communications broke down. It was apparent, however, that casualties must be far more numerous than the local services could possibly cope with, so reinforcements were sent not only from other areas in the same group but also from other groups.

During the night an S.O.S. was received by Group 7 from Albert Dock Hospital and ambulance coaches were despatched. They were not heard of again for over twenty-four hours, and some anxiety was felt as to their fate, but later it was discovered that they had maintained a continuous evacuation service from Albert Dock Hospital to hospitals outside the area under attack, and there is no doubt the drivers of these vehicles made a most valuable contribution to combat what was one of the worst attacks of the war.

In the intense night attack of December 29, 1940, made mainly with incendiary bombs, large areas of the City of London and surrounding districts were quickly set ablaze, and four hospitals had to be evacuated while the raid was in progress. St. Peter's (Whitechapel) and Mile End Hospitals both received direct hits and were evacuated under the supervision of Mr. C. H. Cunningham, the Ambulance Officer of Group 3. Mr. Naldrett writes:

> 'In Group 5, Guy's Hospital had been damaged and was seriously threatened by nearby fires. Mr. J. B. Cunningham, the Group 5 Ambulance Officer, had kept in close touch by telephone with Guy's Hospital but when the telephone failed, knowing the situation, he sent some ambulance coaches along to stand by and proceeded there himself. The coaches arrived fifteen minutes before the decision was made to evacuate the hospital.
>
> In the meantime an S.O.S. was received from St. Bartholomew's Hospital, situated in Group 3, saying that owing to spreading fires they must be evacuated.
>
> As Mr. C. H. Cunningham was already engaged on the evacuation of St. Peter's and Mile End Hospitals, Mr. T. Fowler of Group 1 with his assistants, superintended the evacuation of St. Bartholomew's. Just before the evacuation was completed the Fire Service got the fires in the vicinity under control and this operation was stopped.

It was an impressive sight to see the Green Line Ambulance Coaches threading their way to hospital past fire pumps, fire hoses and blazing buildings, then out again with their patients conveying them to safety.'

For inter-hospital transport the heaviest raid of the war was that which occurred on the night of April 16–17, 1941.

'Fourteen hospitals were damaged during this raid but it was not necessary to evacuate any of these while the raid was in progress.

Of the 250 ambulance coaches held by the Ministry 125 were staffed day and night and 125 could be staffed at two hours' notice.

In the early hours it was evident that the evacuation of casualties from the inner hospitals would reach larger proportions than ever before and L.P.T.B. garages were warned that some staff in addition to that normally standing by would be required.

With daybreak the evacuation commenced and continued all day. It was completed by nightfall when 1,996 casualties were conveyed, nearly all of which were stretcher cases. The hospitals were then ready for the reception of further casualties.

178 ambulance coaches and 41 other vehicles were used for this evacuation.'

Hospitals again suffered damage on the night of May 10–11, 1941, and Poplar Hospital was evacuated while the raid was in progress. The evacuation of other hospitals, some of which had been filled to capacity with casualties, began in the early hours of May 11 and was completed by nightfall, 1,782 cases (of which less than 300 were sitting cases) being conveyed by inter-hospital transport in 164 ambulance coaches and 56 other vehicles.

The large number of hospitals that were damaged was a feature of the attacks during the first year of the raids (July 1940—July 1941). 'During the whole of this period of raids', wrote Mr. Naldrett, 'the Inter-hospital Transport Service worked with remarkable smoothness and high praise must be given to the L.P.T.B. coach drivers and staff of the American Ambulance (Great Britain) for the way they carried out their duties under all sorts of conditions'.

From July 1940, to July 1941, inter-hospital transport conveyed over 100,000 patients, the majority of whom were stretcher cases.

The next twelve months were free from air raids but the normal work of the inter-hospital transport continued steadily. Transfers of sick patients to the outer hospitals, to annexes which, as a war-time measure, some hospitals had set up in the country, and to special centres kept the coach-ambulance fleet usefully employed. A total of 73,234 persons were conveyed during the period July 1941, to July 1942, the total number conveyed to the latter date being 196,731.

Meanwhile the lessons of the previous year's raids had been incorporated in the training programme, which aimed at keeping all branches of the Ambulance Service ready for and efficient to cope with air raids when they should be resumed. They were in fact resumed in July 1942, with attacks that presented no new problems till January 1943, when enemy activity increased by both day and night and raids were made by one or two aircraft at a time, flying low and diving out of the clouds to drop their bombs and make a quick get-away. These tactics were obviously designed to beat the warning system and were sometimes successful.

A raid on Sunday, November 7 of this year, provided another opportunity for inter-hospital ambulance coaches to engage in the actual collection of casualties at an incident. These coaches, from their size, were generally unsuitable for use at an incident but 'on this occasion' wrote the Chief Ambulance Officer in his report on the incident, 'their large capacity was just what was wanted'. At approximately 20.55 hours a bomb had penetrated the roof of a dance hall at Putney and exploded in the room while the dance was in progress. There were many casualties among the dancers, a bus queue outside and persons in a public-house on the other side of the street. The incident occurred close to an L.P.T.B. garage where Green Line ambulance coaches were stationed and the part they played is described in the following extracts from the report by A. J. Mott, Group Ambulance Officer, to Chief Ambulance Officer, London Civil Defence Region, November 12, 1943 :

> 'A police inspector arrived at the incident immediately after the bomb had dropped and his part in the proceedings is of extreme interest. It was immediately evident to him that there were many scores of casualties—more than a few were injured and killed in the street. He did not see an ambulance on the scene and as he knew that some L.P.T.B. ambulance coaches were parked a few yards away in Putney Garage, he proceeded immediately to the garage and called out three vehicles. The ambulance coaches were on the scene of the incident and were being loaded (this work being done by the drivers and by members of the public and of the fighting forces) within fifteen minutes of the bomb having dropped. Altogether nine ambulance coaches were engaged on the work and the last coach left the incident with casualties before 22.15 hours. The services of regular omnibus drivers were used to supplement the ambulance coach drivers.
>
> The drivers of the ambulance coaches worked with enthusiasm and efficiency and it was chiefly due to their untiring efforts that casualties were so quickly loaded and conveyed to hospital. It is no adverse criticism of the ambulance service to suggest that if only Civil Defence ambulances had been used, it would have taken much longer to get so many injured persons to hospital.
>
> It is probably true to say, however, that with the better equipment (ambulance coaches do not carry hot water bottles) and trained staff on Civil Defence ambulances the casualties would have had better care during the transit to hospital. I am told that the injuries from the

incident were particularly severe and many of the injured died on the journey and shortly after admission to hospital. It must be a fact that with untrained persons loading the casualties into the ambulance coaches, with many of the casualties not blanketed and with no provision for hot water bottles or proper first-aid treatment, the condition of the casualties during transit was definitely worsened.'

In addition to the nine coaches, eighteen ambulances were sent to the incident and 143 casualties were suitably distributed among nine different hospitals. In the Chief Ambulance Officer's report on this incident the fact that some casualties were conveyed on stretchers without blankets was attributed to ambulances being unable to replenish their stocks by interchange at the hospitals: in some of the hospitals the 'interchange of blankets and stretchers quickly broke down'. First aid to casualties was in the main scanty and it was 'probable that many casualties were loaded into ambulances by members of the public before it was possible to give them any first-aid treatment'. (C.A.O.'s report.)

The Putney incident is mentioned as an instance of resource and common-sense in the use of ambulance transport. Though not intended for incident work, 'it was providential that the Green Line Ambulance Coaches were so near and available. It would have taken an appreciable time to send sufficient Civil Defence ambulances to the incident. There is little doubt that the sight of the ambulance coaches with the sign 'AMBULANCE' on them being so quickly on the spot greatly reassured the public, who regard an ambulance as the outward and visible sign that help for the injured is at hand', (see Plate X, page 146).

Continuing with the evacuation of air raid casualties and sick persons, inter-hospital transport had by the end of 1943 conveyed over 329,000 persons since the commencement of the war.

1944

Early in 1944, in anticipation of the opening of the Second Front, instructions were received that the inter-hospital transport would be required to deal with casualties from oversea.

The first emergency call made on the Service in connexion with impending military operations was for the conveyance of nurses, etc., for the complete staffing of the casualty evacuation trains of the Ministry of Health. This was quickly followed by orders to take staff from E.M.S. hospitals in London and the Home Counties to their emergency stations in preparation for 'D' day operations. In one day a total of over 1,100 staff, consisting of medical officers, medical students, nurses, radiographers and complete surgical teams were collected and transported to their hitherto secret destinations in Surrey, Sussex and Hampshire. Over 50 ambulance coaches and 12 American Ambulance (Great Britain) vehicles were used for this operation, which was completed without mishap.

Twenty-four hours after the 'D' day landings in Normandy, the arrival of oversea casualties, including many prisoners-of-war, was notified and inter-hospital transport began to convey them between railway stations and the transit hospitals which had been specially prepared to receive them. During the period June 7 to December 31, 1944, 86 convoys of wounded were dealt with, involving the conveyance of over 16,000 casualties of which over 10,000 were stretcher cases.

FLYING BOMB ATTACKS

On June 13, a new type of aerial weapon—the V.1 flying bomb—was employed, in attacks which lasted with little respite for two and a half months during which the Ambulance Service underwent its greatest strain of the war. (These attacks and the V.2—long-range rocket—attacks which followed, are dealt with in Chapter 6 and in the chapter on Civil Defence Casualty Services.) Hospitals suffered particularly heavily during this period, no fewer than twenty requiring immediate evacuation after severe damage by flying bombs.

In addition to the normal transfer, in increasing numbers, of cases between hospitals, London's inter-hospital transport was called upon to undertake many onerous duties during this period. Until July 15, when hospital trains were diverted away from London, casualties from oversea continued to arrive at Epsom and over 6,000 were conveyed. On August 2, the evacuation of chronic cases from hospitals in the target area began and by August 28, sixty-five ambulance trains had been loaded with some 12,000 patients and staff at various railway stations in or near the London Region: thousands of persons made homeless by the flying bombs' widespread destruction of property, and thousands of workers imported from all parts of the country to carry out first-aid repairs to damaged buildings were carried in ambulance coaches, over one hundred of which were engaged solely in carrying workmen between their hostels and the working sites. During the period June 13 to August 31, 1944, approximately 78,200 persons were conveyed, of whom 21,000 were first-aid repair workers.

By the end of the year the number of workers carried increased by some 147,000 to 168,000, the number carried during the latter half of that year averaging 28,000 per month and exceeding by 19,000 the number of patients carried (149,000) during the whole of 1944. Compared with an average of 6,300 per month during the period September, 1939—December, 1943, patients carried in 1944 averaged 12,400 per month. In addition, over 15,000 nurses and others were conveyed during the year, an average of over 1,250 per month.

1945

'V.E.' day and the subsequent disbandment of the Civil Defence Ambulance Service brought no corresponding relief to inter-hospital transport. Convoys of wounded continued to arrive, and on July 9—a week after the Civil Defence Ambulance Service had ceased to exist—many of the chronic sick patients who had been evacuated during the previous August began to return to London. These patients were usually detrained at Addison Road Station, conveyed to the Western Hospital for a night and transferred to their destinations the following day.

The dissolution of the Civil Defence Services affected the inter-hospital transport service in various ways. As the ambulances went out of commission and the ambulance stations and group centres closed down, the administration and operational direction of inter-hospital transport was increasingly centralised in Regional Headquarters, to which some of the assistant group ambulance officers were transferred for the purpose.

One of the difficulties which arose from the disbandment of the Civil Defence Services was that of providing stretcher bearers and other helpers at entraining and detraining points. Hitherto reliance had been placed on the Light Rescue Service for the provision of stretcher bearers at the railway stations. 'This Service', wrote the Chief Ambulance Officer, 'had done magnificent work, often sending parties to assist in these operations at a time when they could ill be spared, and had perhaps been working at incidents for many hours just before the arrival of a convoy. The willingness with which the personnel of this Service undertook these duties at all times of the day and night . . . was to a large extent responsible for the satisfactory working of the detraining operations'.

Other arrangements therefore had to be made. For loading and unloading Service convoys the D.D.M.S. London District provided Army stretcher bearers on demand, and for the convoys of civilian sick some hundred Italian collaborators, billeted at the Western Hospital, were used as stretcher bearers both at detraining stations and at receiving hospitals.

Valuable help was also given by volunteers from the Civil Defence Ambulance Service, teams from which had hitherto been used by group ambulance officers to assist in supervising the work of detraining. In continuing this work after the Service was disbanded, these volunteers showed admirable public spirit and remarkable keenness: they 'never failed to report for duty when required, whether by day or night'.

The work of inter-hospital transport was not without risk to life and limb, nor was courage lacking in performing it; but casualties among ambulance personnel were, fortunately, remarkably few.

The numbers of patients carried and of vehicle journeys made by inter-hospital transport of the London Civil Defence Region are shown in the following table:

TABLE I
London Civil Defence Region: Return of Work carried out by Inter-Hospital Transport

	L.P.T.B. Ambulance coaches			American ambulances			American cars			L.C.C. ambulances			Others			Totals		
	Vehicles	Str.	Sit.	Vehicles	Str.	Sit.	Vehicles	Str.	Sit.	Vehicles	Str.	Sit.	Vehicles	Str.	Sit.	Vehicles	Str.	Sit.
1939 (September–December)	676	?	?	—	—	—	—	—	—	119	?	?	74	?	?	869	4,707	2,594
1940 (January–April)	973	?	?	—	—	—	—	—	1,066	108	?	?	122	?	?	1,203	6,939	4,228
„ (May–December)	4,755	29,260	24,097	1,203	2,330	1,124	557	221	1,449	417	221	1,449	126	130	128	7,058	31,941	27,864
1941	5,192	29,672	25,362	3,567	6,563	2,698	2,315	4,182	4,182	475	370	2,434	830	271	1,206	12,379	36,876	35,882
1942	4,749	23,125	38,909	3,554	6,263	4,231	2,250	4,476	4,476	234	119	1,406	1,072	248	1,462	11,859	29,755	50,484
1943	5,115	25,666	48,540	4,596	7,997	7,292	2,240	4,789	4,789	138	42	740	1,752	543	2,226	13,841	34,248	63,587
1944	9,485	46,666	74,982	5,569	9,363	5,936	3,104	5,791	5,791	259	132	407	2,783	1,998	3,770	21,200	58,159	90,886
1945 (to August 15)	4,604	14,568	68,935	3,203	4,425	3,646	2,891	5,080	5,080	459	78	677	2,299	751	2,794	13,456	19,822	81,132
	35,549	168,957	280,825	21,692	36,941	24,927	13,357	25,384	25,384	2,209	962	7,113	9,058	3,941	11,586	81,865	222,447	356,557
1945 (August 16 to Dec. 31)	3,150	6,827	65,252	1,004	1,293	1,501	951	1,718	1,718	1,787	745	2,111	224	59	859	7,116	8,924	71,441
Totals	38,699	175,784	346,077	22,696	38,234	26,428	14,308	27,102	27,102	3,996	1,707	9,224	9,282	4,000	12,445	88,981	231,371	428,098

In addition, the following are the numbers of nurses and others, and also of repair workmen conveyed during 1944 and 1945 (to August 15):*

	Nurses, etc. Vehicles	Persons	Repair workers Vehicles	Persons
1944	1,128	15,327	4,489	167,167 (from July)
1945 (To August)	365	6,019	17,369	810,478

* Particulars are not available for years prior to 1944.

It will be noted that from September 1939, to April 1940, there is no record of the numbers of patients carried by L.P.T.B., L.C.C. and other vehicles respectively; the totals shown under these headings are therefore only of cases carried from May 1940. Of the total cases carried by all forms of inter-hospital transport approximately 35 per cent. were stretcher cases and 65 per cent. sitting cases.

INTER-HOSPITAL TRANSPORT IN THE PROVINCES

The foregoing account deals with inter-hospital transport in the London Region. Similar work was organised and carried out under the Hospital Officers in other Regions, and bus ambulances were available in large centres of population for carrying transferred sick from vulnerable areas to outer hospitals, and later to carry Service casualties to hospitals, either direct from ports of disembarkation or from detraining points to which they were brought by ambulance trains.

The burden of the 'transferred sick' (see Chapter 3) was lighter in the provinces than in London, where they formed a high proportion of the cases carried. In the London Region transfers of patients from inner to outer zone hospitals, to keep the former clear for air raid casualties, was a daily routine which continued throughout the raid-free periods as well as during the raids. For example, over 73,000 persons were conveyed by inter-hospital transport during the year 1941-2, in which London was almost entirely free from raids, this number being approximately 70 per cent. of the yearly average of all cases carried during the war. Returns from the provinces indicate that transferred sick formed approximately 32 per cent. of their total cases carried. In these Regions the grouping of hospitals in inner and outer zones respectively was not so extensive as in the London Region, although in large centres of population and industry, such as the Liverpool and Manchester areas, hospital grouping was carefully planned to meet local conditions and needs. The working of the hospital system and the inter-hospital transport provided in these Regions is described in the accounts of the night raids in Volume II, Part III.

Certain other demands were made on provincial transport to which London was not subjected in the same way. The arrangements, described in Chapter 4, to evacuate the coastal belt under threat of invasion, for instance, involved the evacuation of sick from all E.M.S. hospitals in the areas in which an attempt at invasion seemed probable, extending first from Great Yarmouth to Southend, and from Margate to Hythe on the coast and including later certain inland towns, such as Colchester, Ipswich, Canterbury and Ashford, and further stretches of coast to the Wash in the north-east and to Plymouth in the south-west. The disembarkation of overseas casualties at the southern ports and later at Tilbury, was a frequent operation in which the provincial inter-hospital transport played an important part. The plans for the reception of overseas casualties and the work of the port and transit hospitals to which casualties were conveyed by road and rail are recorded in Chapter 6.

The Regions differed considerably in their need of inter-hospital transport. Of the 974 ambulances standing by or on call in the provinces in December, 1939, nearly half (45 per cent.) were in Regions 4 (Eastern) and 10 (North-Western), and nearly one-third (32 per cent.) in Regions 6 (Southern), 9 (Midland) and 12 (South-Eastern). Regions 2 (North-Eastern) and 7 (South-Western) each had approximately 7 per cent., the remaining 9 per cent. being spread over Regions 1 (Northern), 3 (North-Midland) and 8 (Wales). During the following year the proportion of total provincial ambulances held in Regions 4 and 10 was reduced to roughly one-third, at which it remained fairly steady throughout the war. The numbers of ambulances held by the various Regions (excluding London) and the numbers of patients carried by ambulances and sitting-case cars are shown in Tables II and III.

AMERICAN AMBULANCE (GREAT BRITAIN)

Table I shows that approximately 17 per cent. of stretcher cases and 14 per cent. of sitting cases in the London Region were carried by American ambulances and cars which, from July 1940, thus took an important share in the work of inter-hospital transport.

These American ambulance vehicles were seen and appreciated as evidence of interest and goodwill at a time when we valued and were encouraged by American friendship and sympathy, but were still awaiting the United States' entry into the war as the most powerful of our Allies.

The American vehicles were used for various purposes and, as mentioned in the following account of the formation and work of the fleet, operated in Scotland as well as in England and Wales. The figures in the appended table are those for England and Wales:

'Early in 1940 a group of members of the American Society in London, with the approval and under the presidency of His Excellency the American Ambassador, initiated a plan to aid Britain by providing, maintaining and operating a fleet of vehicles in connexion with the emergency hospital and casualty services for the benefit of the civil population. The funds for this service were to be contributed entirely by American donors, (whether individuals, business firms or other bodies, in Britain and America) and the organisation was to be known as the American Ambulance (Great Britain), with headquarters in London.

'Representatives of the group responsible for this project approached the Ministry of Health to ascertain how the American ambulances could best be of service, expressing the wish that they should retain their

Table II
Inter-Hospital Ambulances in each Provincial Region as at December 31

Region	1939 A	1939 B	1940 A	1940 B	1941 A	1941 B	1942 A	1942 B	1943 A	1943 B	1944 A	1944 B	1945 A	1945 B
1	25	—	35	—	35	—	35	—	35	—	35	—	—	—
2	69	—	69	—	69	—	68	—	68	—	31	—	10	—
3	30	—	30	—	37	—	37	—	37	—	14	—	—	—
4	188	—	103	—	97	—	98	25	101	25	59	14	11	—
6	101	—	93	6	78	12	73	18	75	18	33	21	9	—
7	68	—	31	35	37	29	37	14	36	35	16	10	2	—
8	32	—	13	17	13	17	13	14	13	14	2	46	—	—
9	107	—	65	32	56	27	56	41	56	41	51	35	8	—
10	118	136	68	123	66	123	66	70	66	35	91	—	41	—
11	100	—	112	—	112	—	104	—	109	—	80	—	4	—
Totals	838	136	619	213	600	208	587	182	596	168	412	126	85	—
	974		832		808		769		764		538			

A = Standing by.
B = On call for conversion at short notice.

Table III

Numbers of Patients carried in Inter-Hospital Ambulances and Sitting-Case Cars

A = Stretcher cases.   B = Sitting cases.

Region	1939 A	1939 B	1940 A	1940 B	1941 A	1941 B	1942 A	1942 B
1	<—————————————— 898‡	4,764‡ ——————————————>						
2	850‡	40‡	5,990‡	2,984‡	2,692‡	518‡	562‡	123‡
3	<—————————— 'Practically negligible' § ——————————>						817*	218*
4	346	226	816	487	1,315	822	839	829
6	2,129		9,738		6,320		2,215	
7	No record		No record		No record		80	2,327
8	Nil	Nil	170‡	2,759‡	—	58‡	292‡	1,079‡
9	74	—	4,199	4,151	5,928	745	6,058	145
10	267	86	4,527	5,328	8,979	4,860	11,709	
12	1,543	277	5,506	4,336	1,062	1,223	180	26

Region	1943 A	1943 B	1944 A	1944 B	1945 A	1945 B	Totals A	Totals B	Cases
1	14	Nil	682	6,073	1,101	2,456	2,695‡	13,293‡	15,988‡
2	516	499	13,243	12,716	5,008	9,439	28,861‡	26,319‡	55,180‡
3	2,788	1,323	3,030	4,083	1,370	4,468	8,005‡	10,092‡	18,097‡
4	933	1,705	2,333	2,143	1,470	1,694	8,052	7,906	15,958
							20,402†		
6	562	332	24,265	10,656	1,739	1,395	26,566	12,383	59,351
7	54	5,181	3,148	4,602	77	4,870	3,359‡	16,980‡	20,339‡
8	438‡	1,825‡	10,337‡	10,675‡	7,377	10,061	18,614‡	26,457‡	45,071‡
9	5,216	240	2,084	7,367	3,285	4,854	26,844	17,502	44,346
							48,810†		
10	2,005		27,459		7,637		13,773	10,274	72,857
12	120	258	22,160	15,635	976	1,264	31,547	23,019	54,566
							69,212†		
							168,316‡	164,225‡	401,753‡

† Total cases for years in which no distinction made between ambulances and sitting-case cars.
* August to December only.
‡ Approximate.
§ Hospital Officer, Region 3, letter dated February 28, 1945.
(In Region 12, 83% of total cases carried in 1944, and 62% in 1945 were battle casualties).

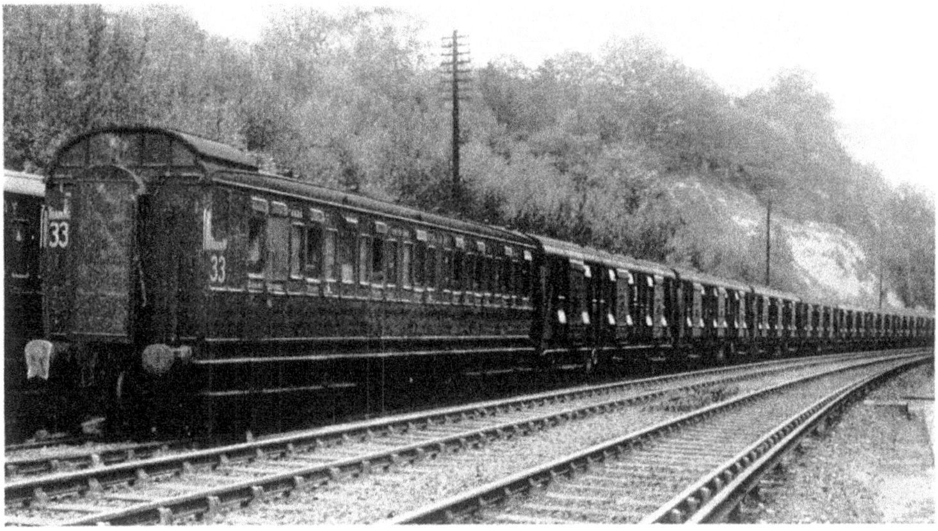

PLATE XXX. Exterior of casualty evacuation train—S.R.

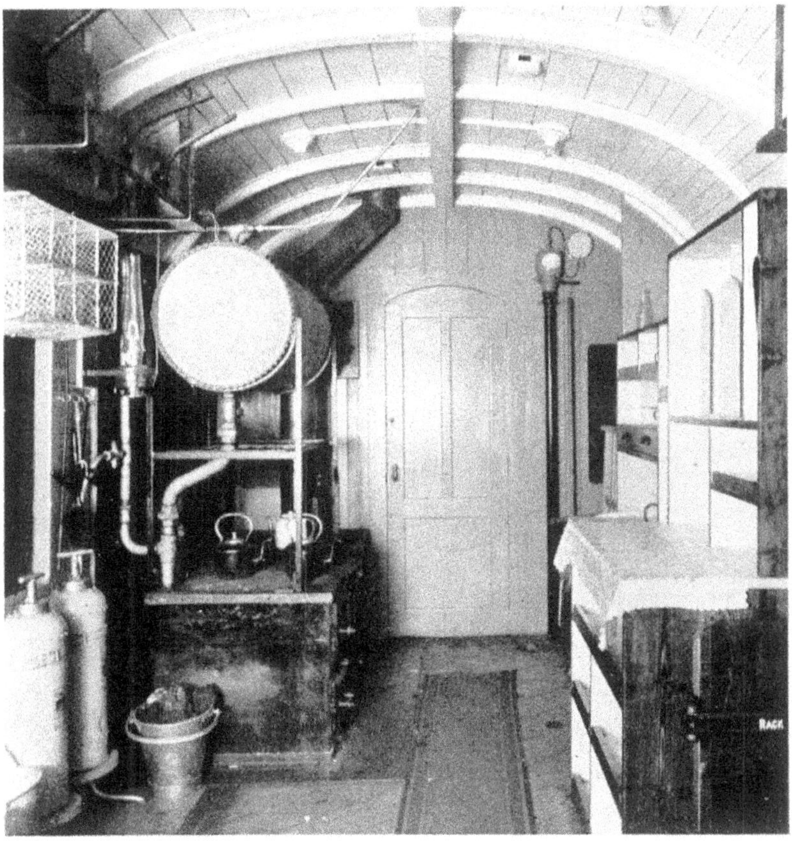

PLATE XXXI. Kitchen compartment—L.M.S.

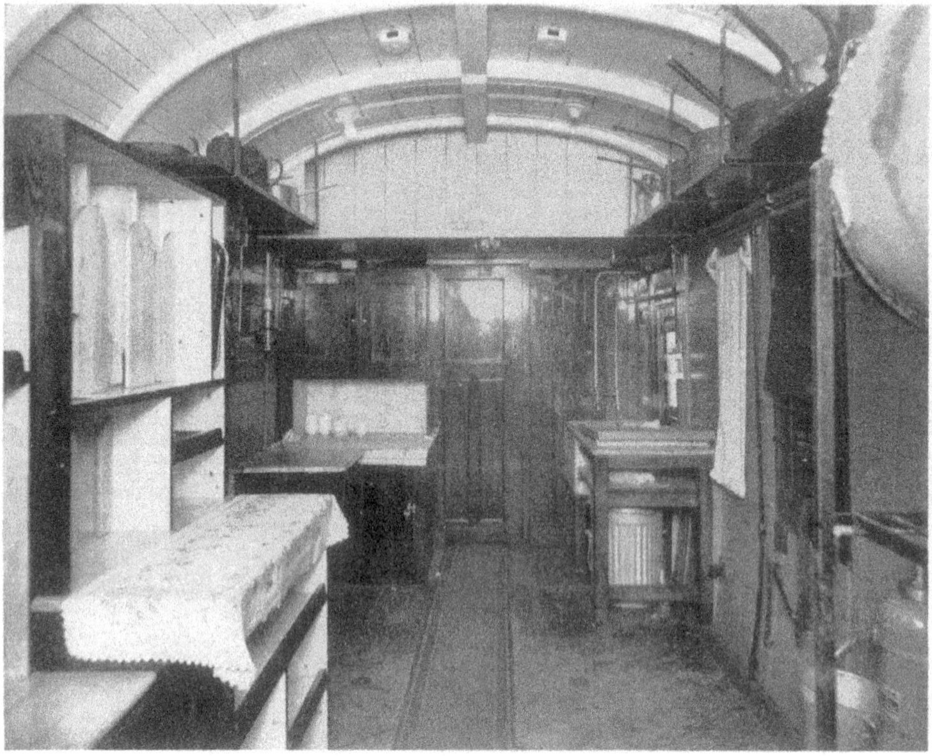

PLATE XXXII. Kitchen compartment—L.M.S.

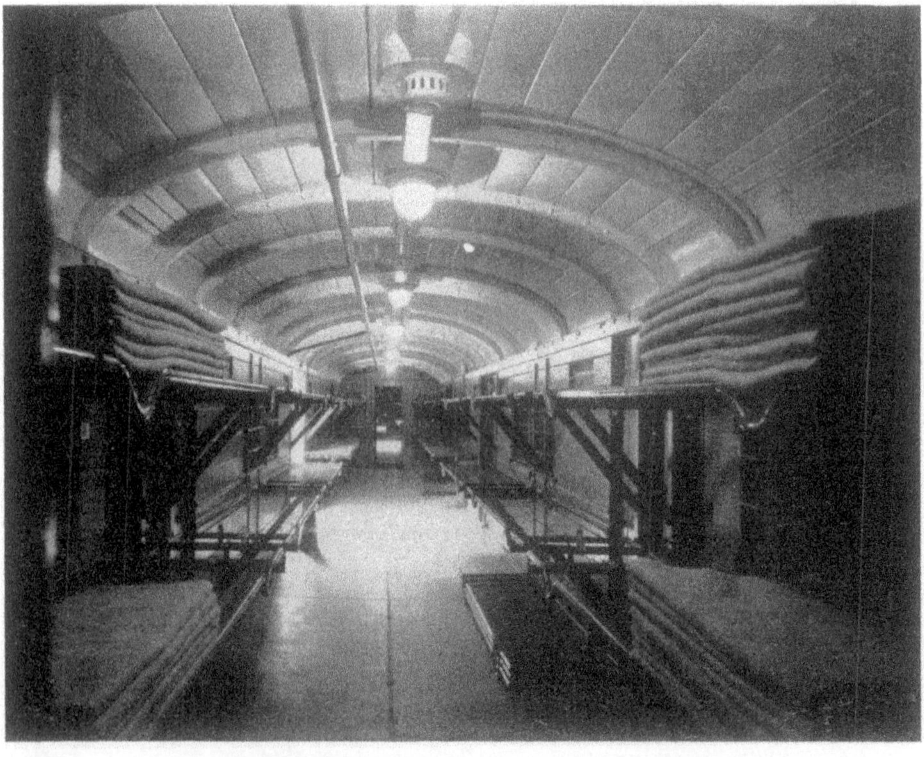

PLATE XXXIII. Stretcher van with stretchers fitted—S.R.

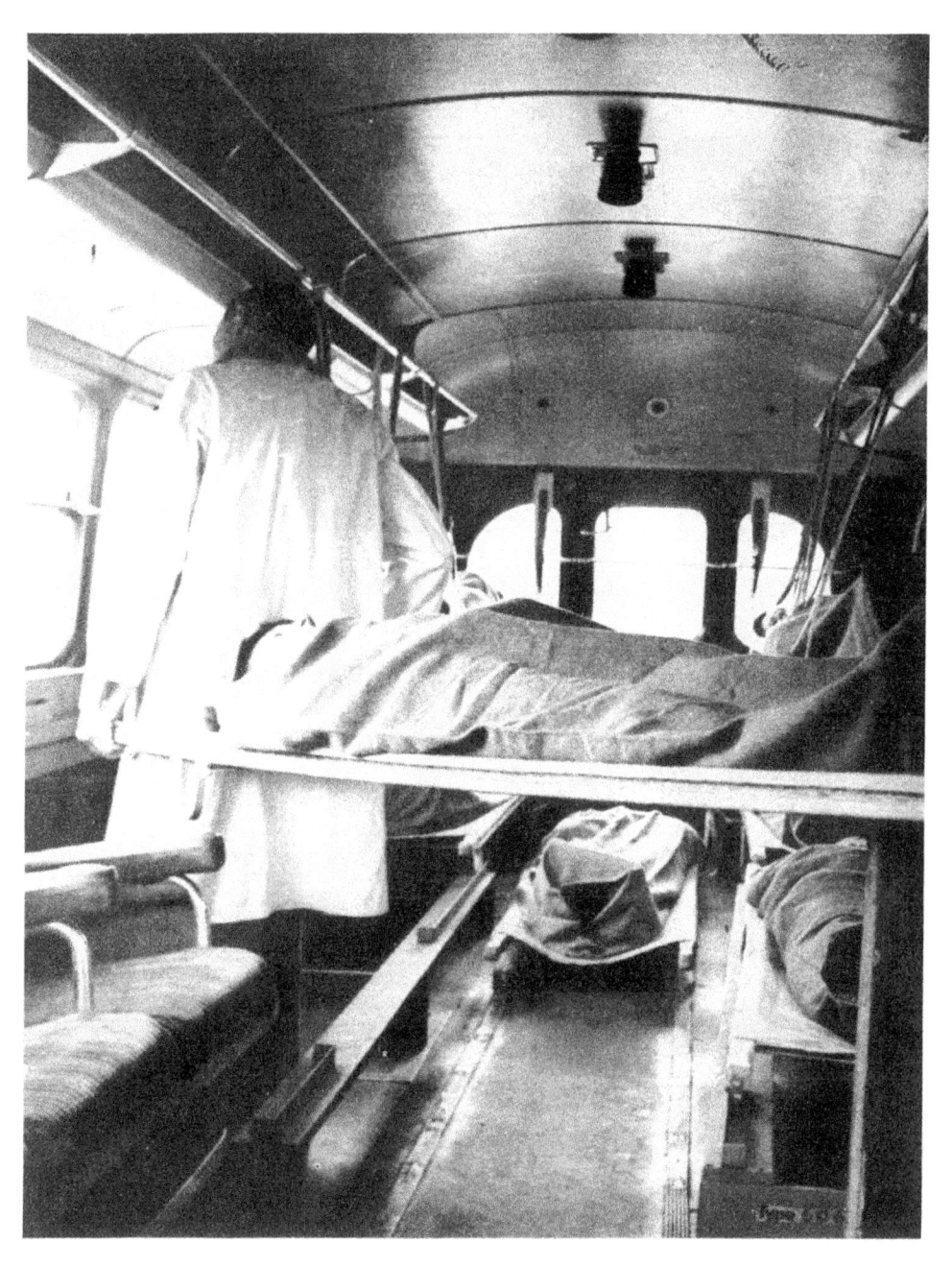

PLATE XXXIV. Loading bus ambulances with Service cases—L.P.T.B.

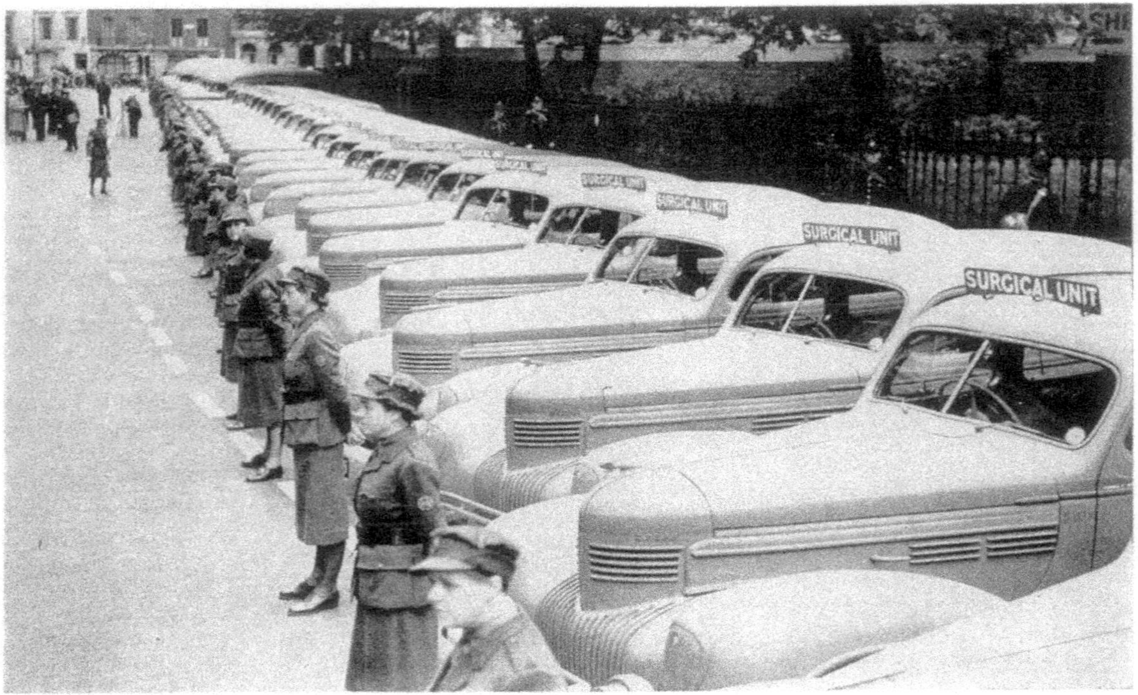

PLATE XXXV. Over sixteen million miles were covered by American Ambulance Great Britain with this fleet which transported more than eight hundred thousand patients

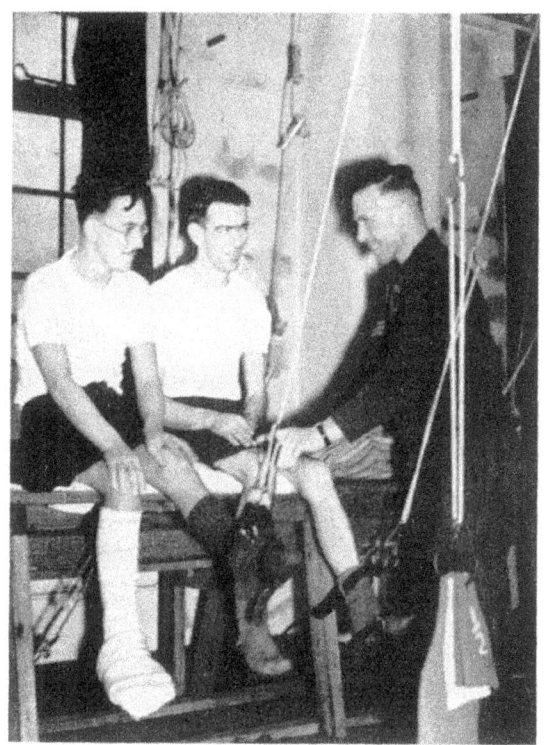

Pictorial Press
PLATE XXXVI. Redeveloping thigh muscles

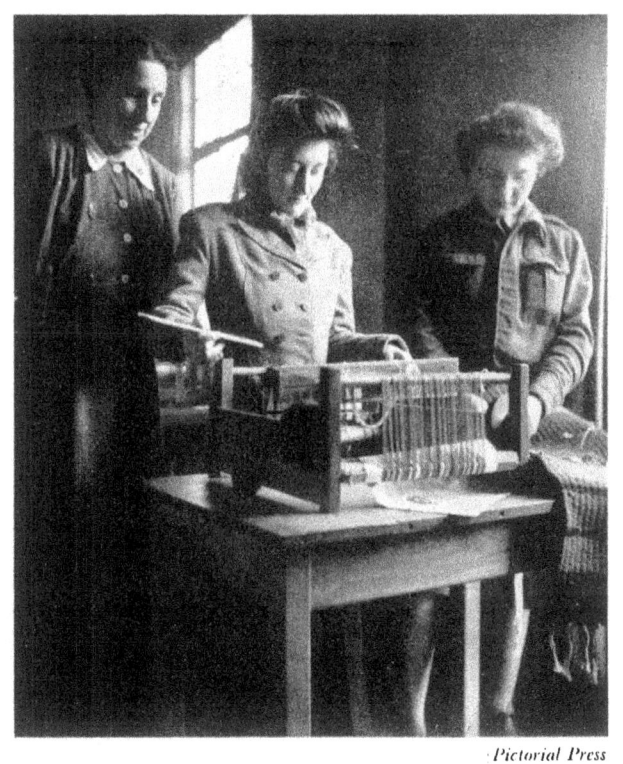

Pictorial Press
PLATE XXXVII. Infantile paralysis—both arms.
Recovery of muscles by using loom

[Pictorial Press

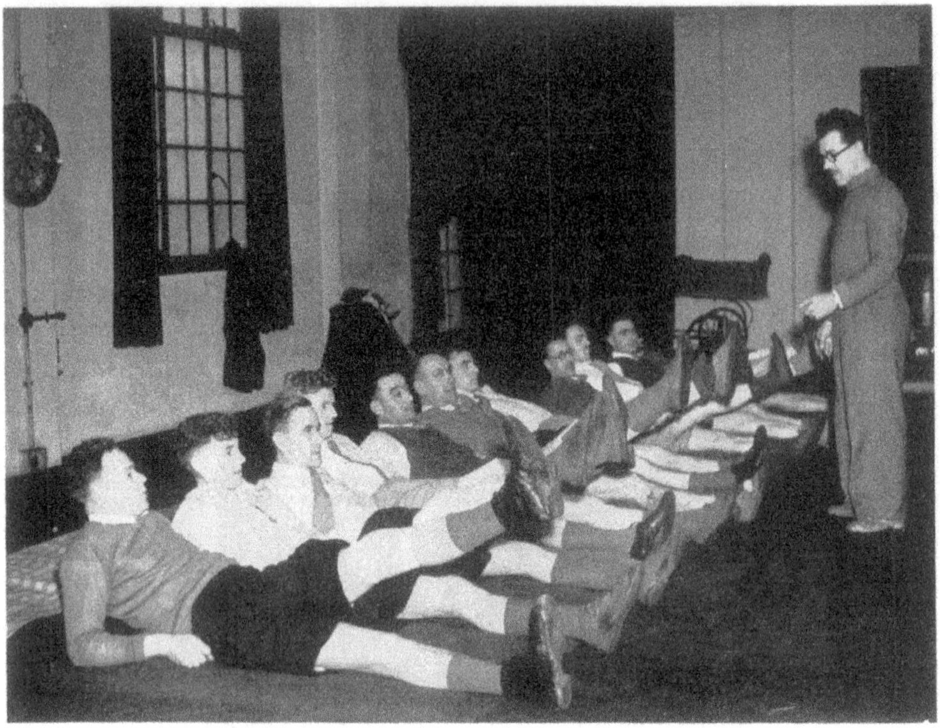

PLATE XXXVIII. Knee injuries. Restoring strength of thigh muscles

[Pictorial Press

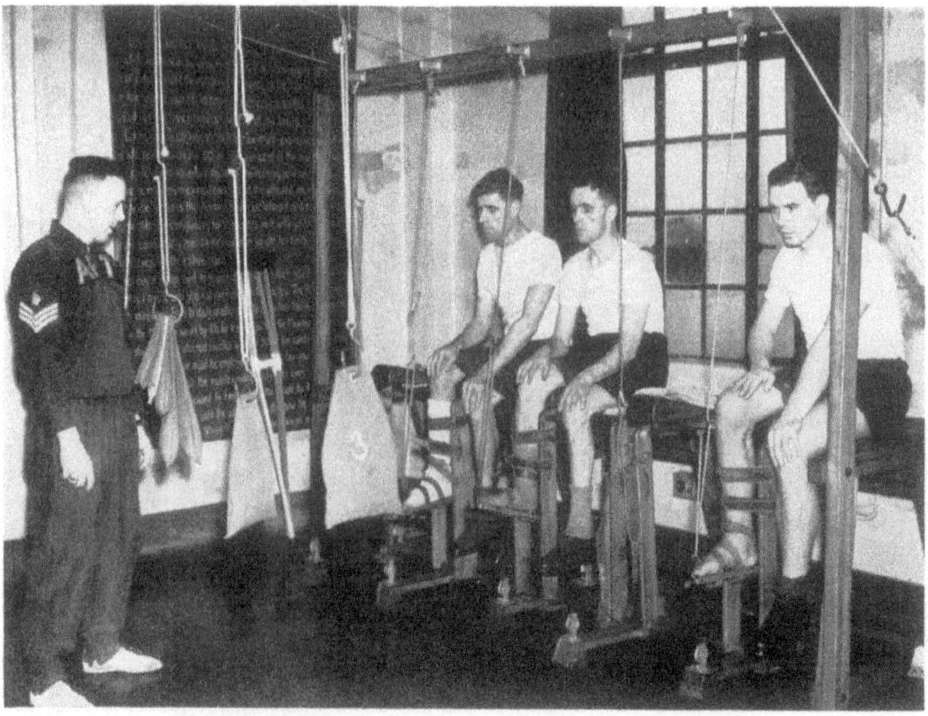

PLATE XXXIX. Restoring strength of calf muscles

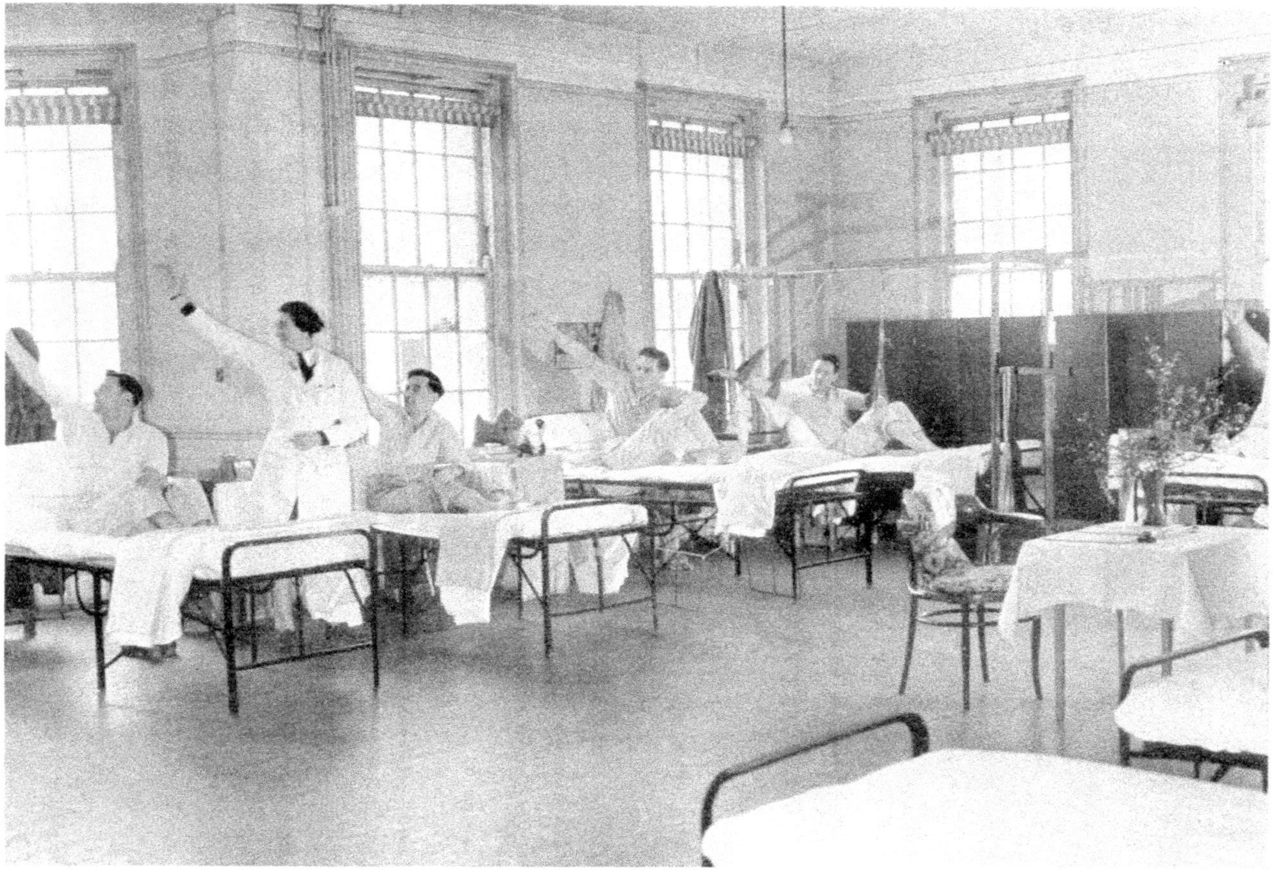

PLATE XL. These men, who are suffering from various injuries, carry out daily exercises in bed

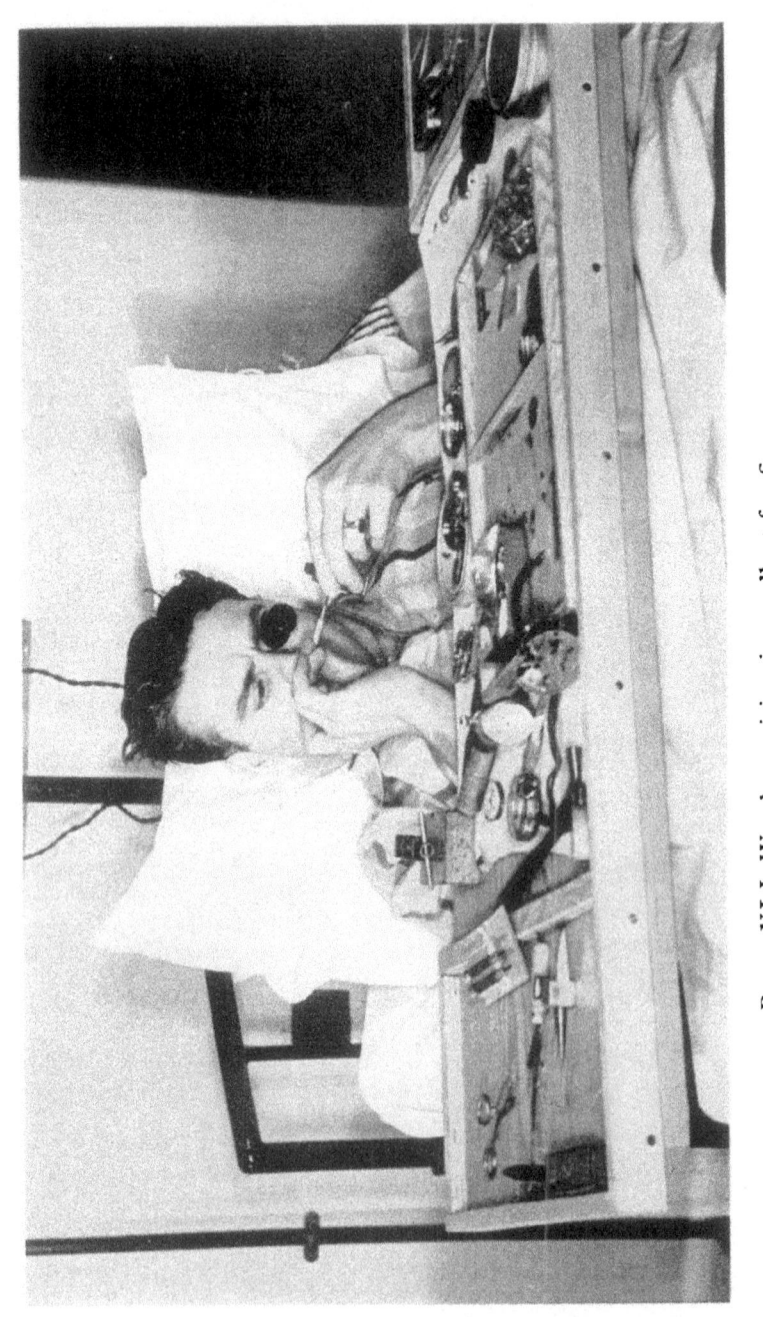

PLATE XLI. Watch-repairing is excellent for fingers

independence and individuality, working in association with and under the direct operational control of the Ministry and the Department of Health for Scotland. In response to this unique and generous offer, the American Ambulance organisation was informed that it could give valuable assistance to the Health Departments, while remaining independent of the civil defence casualty organisation of local authorities, by providing ambulances for those needs of inter-hospital transport for which large converted-bus ambulances were inappropriate: cars for the transport of mobile surgical teams from one hospital to another and a number of mobile first-aid posts to be used, in effect, as regional reserves to supplement local units provided for the same purpose as part of the local authority casualty services.

'The American Ambulance organisation agreed at the outset to provide 50 ambulances, 50 cars and 50 mobile aid posts, the last each comprising two vehicles, one specially designed and fitted to carry the operational equipment and the other to transport the necessary personnel to the scene of action. The number of ambulances was subsequently more than doubled, and eventually the American Ambulance Fleet amounted in all to some 260 vehicles, including a reserve to enable the service to be maintained at full strength in case of loss of units or temporary withdrawal of vehicles for repair and overhaul. With the exception of a few ambulances brought over from the United States, all the vehicles were obtained in this country, and a uniform colour-design was adopted of grey and red, with the organisation's distinctive emblem combining the British and U.S.A. national flags. So energetically was the project developed that the first units were put into service in London within a few weeks after the formulation of the scheme.

'The plans for the organisation were formed before large-scale air attacks on this country had begun, and when the situation to be met in dealing with air raid casualties was largely conjectural. From this standpoint the request which was made to the organisation to provide 50 mobile aid posts was therefore based on the view that local authority resources in this particular part of the casualty services were not as strong as could be wished. As events proved, however, actual experience of heavy air raids showed less need for mobile aid posts than had been expected: and it became apparent that there was likely to be little or no necessity to call on the American ambulance units of this type. It was, therefore, arranged that its vehicles originally provided for this purpose should be adapted for other uses that could keep them in more active employment. They were accordingly reconstructed or suitably fitted to serve as supplementary ambulances for stretcher or sitting cases, and as utility vans for general transport work in connexion with the emergency medical services (e.g. the blood transfusion service).

'It was arranged that the American Ambulance organisation should have its own depots in the headquarters town of each Region in England

and Wales, and in certain towns in Scotland selected by the Department of Health for Scotland. As its operations developed certain sub-stations also came to be set up in some Regions, one or two of which were only temporarily maintained. In London five stations were established, each associated with a "group control centre" of the Civil Defence Service. The American ambulances thus operated in and from London (five stations), Newcastle, Darlington, Scarborough, Leeds, Sheffield, Nottingham, Cambridge, Reading, Oxford, Bristol, Exeter, Cardiff, Swansea, Wrexham, Birmingham, Stoke-on-Trent, Manchester, Liverpool, Maidstone, Tunbridge Wells, Edinburgh, Glasgow and Aberdeen. At each of its stations it made its own arrangements and assumed full financial responsibility for garaging and maintaining its vehicles and for providing accommodation for its personnel. It appointed its own officer-in-charge of each main station, who took responsibility for carrying out operational instructions received from the Regional Hospital Officer of the Ministry.

'The whole of the officers and driving staff of the American ambulances were uniformed women (see Plate XXXV). To begin with this Staff was drawn in about equal proportion from two women's transport organisations in this country—the transport division of the First Air Nursing Yeomanry and the Mechanised Transport Corps respectively. Subsequently, the association with the first of these bodies was terminated and thereafter the American Ambulance organisation assumed direct responsibility for its own corps of drivers over and above those which members of the Mechanised Transport Corps continued to provide.

'The duties performed by these ambulances took many forms. Its main function was to provide, from day to day, ambulance transport for patients requiring to be moved from one hospital to another under the war-time working of the hospital system which the Ministry of Health and Department of Health for Scotland were responsible for directing. In addition, it undertook such duties as providing urgent transport for medical consultants; conveying to hospitals from detraining points military sick convoys and persons from evacuation areas requiring hospital care on arrival in reception areas; transporting hospital cases from coastal areas to inland places; taking hospital patients requiring special treatment to the centres for such treatment, and generally providing ambulance transport in various circumstances, including long journeys where conveyance by train was not practicable or expedient. General transport duties associated with the blood transfusion service were also performed by the American ambulances on a considerable scale. Operations in these categories constituted their constant day-to-day work, and were irrespective of the occurrence or absence of air attack. When there were air raids the American ambulances played their own active part by assisting and supplementing the local Civil Defence Ambulance Service, removing patients from hospitals bombed or set on fire in the course of the attack, and helping to meet the various transport needs of the community in the period immediately after heavy raids on particular areas. In all these ways the American ambulances not only proved of the greatest value to the Ministry of Health and Department of Health for Scotland in the discharge of their responsibility for the emergency hospital and medical services, but also won high repute and grateful recognition among the population to whom its service was devoted in the name of the American people. The closest collaboration was maintained throughout between the American Ambulance headquarters and the Ministry on matters of general policy and administration, and between officers-in-charge of stations and the Ministry's regional officers on operations. The service of the American ambulances indeed, carried out with the utmost devotion and efficiency, finds a notable place in the medical history of Great Britain at war, the more significant as a unique and generous expression of American aid and goodwill in the earlier part of the struggle, and of united purpose in the later development of allied effort.'

The following table summarises the work done in England and Wales by the American ambulances:

TABLE IV

Year	Total mileage	Number of journeys	Numbers carried
1940 (July to December)	499,136	7,377	10,456
1941	2,432,996	36,622	57,256
1942	2,398,678	42,829	89,283
1943	2,744,550	51,170	153,407
1944	3,832,266	65,088	186,437
1945 (to date of disbandment, November 3, 1945)	2,903,045	48,688	214,133
Totals	14,810,671	251,774	710,972

RIVER AMBULANCES

In the section of this chapter which deals with inter-hospital transport in action, reference is made to an attack on the London Docks during which coach-ambulances were called out to work in co-operation with ambulance craft on the Thames. These river ambulances, which formed part of the Port of London Authority's River Emergency Service, were in constant touch with civil defence controllers on land and carried doctors, nurses and orderlies, who not only dealt with all types of casualty met with on the river, but also landed occasionally to assist in dealing with casualties in the various riverside boroughs.

The main work of the river ambulances was done during the heavy raids on London in 1940-1 and is briefly described in the story of those raids contained in Chapter 7, and in Volume II, Part III, Chapter 1.

CHAPTER 9
MEDICAL SUPPLIES

POLICY AND ORGANISATION

THE problem of finding sufficient bed accommodation for the thousands of air raid casualties which were to be expected had, as a corollary, that of providing adequate medical, surgical and domestic equipment as well as the beds and bedding. The principles followed in supplying these needs were the same as in finding the accommodation; every advantage was taken of existing equipment, and the Government undertook the general responsibility of providing on free loan all the extra equipment that would be needed to enable hospitals to carry out the additional services to be required of them under the Emergency Hospital Scheme. One exception to the supply of the required equipment from central sources was that hospitals were authorised to acquire and maintain necessary stocks of crockery.

The responsibility for dealing with casualties under the Air Raid Precautions Act, 1937, had been imposed on local authorities, with a percentage grant from the Government. Under the Civil Defence Act, 1939, however, the Government assumed full financial responsibility in this matter, but local authorities were required, by Section 51 of the Act, in return for the relief of any charge on the local rates, to provide a quantity of equipment for the extra accommodation needed for the Emergency Hospital Service in their peace-time hospitals, excluding public assistance institutions, mental hospitals, etc. This equipment was estimated to be the reserve which such hospitals were normally expected to hold, viz. a month's supply of drugs and dressings, an excess of one-tenth of the normal capacity of beds and mattresses and of one-fifth of the bedding and ward equipment.

As the extra hospital accommodation was to be administered as an integral part of the existing hospitals and any attempt to segregate the emergency functions from the ordinary functions of the hospital would create all manner of obstacles to smooth and efficient running, the arrangements were that, once the extra initial equipment had been provided, the maintenance of these stocks should be undertaken by the hospital authority in precisely the same way as it secured its normal requirements, the Government's financial responsibility being discharged by suitable accounting arrangements.

In addition to supplies for hospitals, the Ministry of Health, conjointly with the Home Office (later the Ministry of Home Security), had to supply scheme-making authorities (broadly speaking, the councils of counties and county boroughs) with the equipment required for the

A.R.P. services which were designed to collect casualties, to deal on the spot or in first-aid posts with the slightly injured and to transport the seriously injured to hospitals. As this was a totally new and national service, the cost of all medical and surgical equipment, including the replenishment of consumable supplies, was met by the Government.

HEADQUARTERS ORGANISATION

The first step towards securing the medical supplies necessary for the Emergency Hospital Scheme was taken in September 1938, when Dr. J. G. Johnstone was seconded from the London County Council to advise on medical requirements and on specifications. He retained this post until August 1944, when he was appointed to a similar post in U.N.R.R.A. Dr. S. Cochrane Shanks was appointed after the outbreak of war to deal specially with X-ray equipment, and in June 1940, Dr. J. W. G. Steell was appointed to assist Dr. Johnstone and took over his duties on his departure. A Physical Medicine Committee was appointed to advise on electro-medical apparatus and allied matters, but generally it was to the Minister's consultant advisers that Dr. Johnstone and Dr. Steell looked for advice on the more specialised items of equipment.

The general duties, other than medical and advisory, were undertaken by the staff of the Ministry working first as a branch of the Division dealing with the organisation of the emergency hospitals; first aid, and related services. Later, it became desirable to give to this branch the status of an independent Division of the Ministry (the Supplies Division) and its work was organised into three principal sections dealing in the main with (1) the ordering and distribution of medical and surgical apparatus, (2) the ordering and distribution of ward equipment (beds, bedding, lockers, trolleys, etc.), and similar types of equipment for other emergency services as well as for the Hospital Service, and (3) records and storage. At a later date, when regional offices were established by the Ministry, the distribution of the less specialised types of equipment under the general guidance of Headquarters was one of the functions transferred to the Regional Officers.

Assistance was also rendered by the Engineering Division of the Ministry of Works, in regard particularly to electrical specifications and maintenance.

THE BASIS OF SUPPLY

The supply of equipment was based on a schedule system. For each unit, a schedule of equipment was drawn up, and as the Emergency Medical Services developed and new types of centres were established, fresh schedules of equipment were prepared. By this means fairly accurate estimates of requirements could be made and production programmes framed. The basic schedule was that comprising the equipment for a hospital of 200 beds (five wards of 40 beds, based on the projected hutments designed to hold from 36 to 42 beds, with one operating theatre). The schedule included some 320 different types of apparatus, instruments and general equipment; it provided a full range of theatre and ward equipment, ranging from the operating table to the thermometer, from the ward tables to the nurses' caps and, in addition, certain theatre, orthopaedic, genito-urinary, thoracic, E.N.T. and eye instruments. Complete issues on the bases of these schedules were made to new hutment hospitals, 'upgraded' institutions and so forth. As, however, much of this equipment was already held by general hospitals, the formidable task was undertaken of obtaining from all general hospitals a fairly comprehensive return of the equipment they already had and, on the basis of these returns, additional equipment was, as necessary, issued from central supplies to bring them up to approved scheduled standards. In the course of time, many different schedules were prepared—drug schedules for 'upgraded' P.A.I.s and similar institutions whose peace-time function did not necessitate a complete range of drugs, schedules for maxillo-facial centres, thoracic centres, the various types of fracture hospitals, X-ray departments, pathological laboratories, blood transfusion centres, casualty evacuation trains, inter-hospital ambulances and other ancillary services.

A similar procedure was followed in equipping the A.R.P. services. First-aid post and first-aid point schedules were drawn up in the first instance and, as the services developed, schedules were prepared for light mobile first-aid units, nurses' haversacks, gas cleansing centres, mobile gas cleansing centres, mobile gas cleansing units, etc.

The schedule system was considered the only means by which the provision of vast quantities of equipment could be planned in advance, but it was realised that such a system must be operated with a considerable measure of latitude which, nevertheless, must not be allowed to develop into licence.

First, schedules had to be reviewed from time to time. This was particularly necessary as regards the first-aid services, for which there were no comparable precedents and in which estimates of quantities particularly were based on little or no experience. As raw materials became more difficult to obtain, substitutes had to be provided, and when the A.R.P. services actually went into action fresh needs were revealed. The hospital schedules were, of course, framed in the light of wide experience and little basic alteration proved to be necessary.

Secondly, a measure of flexibility was necessary in order to enable surgeons to use the instruments they preferred in their particular specialty. In many E.M.S. hospitals, such as the general hospitals in cities and large towns, the full range of equipment normally used in peace-time was still available, and upgraded or purely emergency hospitals in the outer zone, notably in the London area, were supplied with much of the specialised equipment distributed from the inner hospitals. As the surgeons from the inner hospitals had also been distributed among those of the outer zone, they had the advantage of using the specialised instruments to which they were accustomed. The arrival after a year or so of very considerable gifts, from America in particular, enabled the Ministry to supply a wider range of specialised equipment, which in a measure met needs of this kind. In addition, hospitals at all times were given a reasonable degree of latitude in obtaining, by direct purchase upon reimbursement terms, instruments, etc., which were not included in the standard equipment schedule.

METHOD OF ACQUISITION OF SUPPLIES

Beds and bedding, stretchers, furniture and domestic equipment of types in general use were obtained from the Ministry of Works, and the first order for the bare necessities of such equipment for E.M.S. hospitals and the casualty services was placed with them in 1938. Uniforms for the Civil Nursing Reserve, etc., were purchased on behalf of the Ministry by the General Post Office.

The department which would, in accordance with accepted departmental arrangements, have undertaken to purchase medical and surgical equipment for the Emergency Medical Services was the Contracts Branch of the War Office, but when in January 1939, the first lengthy list of medical and surgical instruments was prepared (although it proved before the end of the scheme to cover only a fraction of the list of equipment ultimately provided), it was found that that department was so heavily engaged in providing for the expansion of the Army Medical Service that they could not undertake this extra work; and in these circumstances the Ministry of Health, with the approval of all departments concerned, turned to the London County Council. This innovation of turning to a local authority to obtain Government requirements, surprising though it may seem, was a measure much more of prudence than of adventure, for in their Medical Supplies Branch the L.C.C. had an unrivalled fund of knowledge and experience acquired during the ten years since the passing of the Local Government Act, 1929, by which they had become the largest hospital authority in the country. They pictured very quickly the size of the task they had undertaken and made provision to meet all demands upon them with the utmost promptitude.

DIFFICULTIES OF SUPPLY

The wide knowledge of the whole subject possessed by the officers of the Medical Supplies Branch of the London County Council proved its value, particularly when it became apparent that the requirements of the Emergency Medical Services would far exceed the available capacity of the recognised suppliers of medical equipment after meeting the demands of the Fighting Services, which received much higher priority. The resource and inventiveness of these officers resulted in numerous improvisations. Working in very close touch with the medical advisers and other officers of the Ministry of Health, all possible sources of supply were considered and it was generally accepted that to cope with a problem of such magnitude and urgency, quality might have to be subordinated to quantity. The methods adopted can be best illustrated by one or two examples:

> The quantity of Spencer Wells forceps required was many times greater than the existing annual output of the country; arrangements were accordingly made for mass production so that, though the articles thus provided were of a lower standard than the well-finished hand-produced forceps the medical profession were accustomed to use, there was in fact a sufficiency of forceps good enough for the job, if not of the highest quality. One of the firms engaged in this work had specialised in the manufacture of a proprietary brand of foot supports; they were encouraged to manufacture various types of artery forceps from drop stampings supplied by a London firm of cutlers; the War Office subsequently became customers as well, so that before long the firm became the largest single firm in the country producing satisfactory surgical instruments from drop stampings.
>
> Again, the number of ward screens required presented a difficult problem but, the medical advisers being prepared to accept an American-cloth covered wooden screen, a large firm of motor body builders turned out large numbers in a very short time. It was a time when the emphasis was on the production of vast quantities of the more general instruments, appliances and equipment.

The London County Council continued to act as purchasing agents for the Ministry of Health, the Ministry of Home Security and the Department of Health for Scotland until November 1941. By then the Directorate of Medical Supplies had been established in the Ministry of Supply and was able to combine the purchasing of medical and surgical supplies for Emergency Hospital and A.R.P. Services with those required by the Fighting Services. But approximately 80 per cent. of the medical and surgical supplies required by the Ministry of Health throughout the period of the war was obtained through the London County Council.

ESTABLISHMENT OF CENTRAL STORES

At first the arrangements with the London County Council provided for delivery of goods direct from the manufacturer to the hospital and scheme-making authorities, but it quickly became apparent that for a number of reasons, there must be adequate stocks under the control of the Ministry of Health, from which the supplies could be issued to authorities. This need was met in the first instance by using part of each of the Regional stores of the Ministry of Home Security to store medical supplies; later, the Ministry of Works provided and staffed stores in each of the Civil Defence Regions for this purpose. With the establishment of the Regional stores, the normal procedure was that all purchases of medical and surgical equipment made on behalf of the Ministry of Health were delivered to these stores, where they were held on behalf of the Ministry and from which issues were made on the strength of authorised indents from the Ministry.

Similar stores were maintained by the Ministry of Works for goods supplied by them; but the goods formed part of a common pool to meet the demands of all departments for the class of goods which the Ministry of Works supplied, so that stocks drawn for the purposes of the Health departments did not become their property until issued for their use.

SPECIAL SUPPLY ARRANGEMENTS

Generally, of course, the medical, surgical and domestic equipment for E.M.S. hospitals was supplied to the hospitals where it was to be used but, additionally, a number of reserve arrangements were made. Thirteen petrol-generated field service X-ray sets, ordered by the Rumanian Government, were requisitioned and distributed throughout the country, so that they could be rapidly transported to any hospitals whose apparatus might be put out of action. Some 70 emergency surgical kits comprising 65 types of instrument were held in Regional offices for the use of doctors who might be required at short notice to supplement overworked staff dealing with an abnormal influx of casualties.

The War Organisation of the British Red Cross Society and Order of St. John of Jerusalem lent to the Ministry of Health twenty mobile X-ray vans and supplied drivers; these were distributed throughout the country so that they could be quickly sent to any hospital requiring extra X-ray facilities. The War Organisation also lent to the Ministry two fully-equipped vans for the treatment of head and chest injuries. It was intended that these should be available, with a team of specialists, to go to any hospital in need, but actually they were stationed at two of the major hospitals.

Four mobile 'Haab' magnets were supplied at central points for the treatment of patients suffering from intra-ocular foreign bodies, and so seriously injured that they could not be moved to a hospital equipped with a giant magnet.

Arrangements were also made with a firm of specialists to provide services (a) for treating cases of detachment of the retina by a mobile diathermy apparatus and (b) to meet the cases of patients suffering from facial burns, as a result of which the cornea of the eye might become perforated by ulceration owing to exposure caused by cicatricial ectropion.

In the active stage of the burn nothing could be done to overcome this tendency to eversion of the lids and exposure of the eye, but when cicatrisation was completed, a plastic operation could be performed upon the lids so that they could regain the function of covering the eyes. This service could supply a contact lens to protect the cornea during the period of cicatrisation of the lids.

DEVELOPMENTS IN SCOPE OF SUPPLY ARRANGEMENTS

The gradual evolution of the Emergency Medical Service from one with emphasis on the emergency rather than on the medical aspect, into a highly organised and complete hospital service at the accepted levels of peace-time efficiency, called for a complementary extension of the equipment to be provided. The various types of special centres were supplied with their peculiar specialities, often with considerable difficulty, since the capacity of the manufacturers was taxed to the utmost. Much assistance in this direction was given later by gifts from the U.S.A. and by equipment provided under lend/lease. But, in addition, a general improvement was made as occasion offered in the type of equipment provided. For instance, the standard X-ray unit at the outbreak of war was a mobile X-ray unit designed primarily for the diagnosis of fractures and the localisation of foreign bodies; fixed X-ray sets of greater output were provided in due course for only the largest hospitals, as a general rule only to hospitals with at least 500 beds. As, however, the beds of the E.M.S. became filled with large numbers of civilian patients suffering from all manner of complaints, this type of set was developed into a good quality medium-powered set and was supplied to any hospital which required a set to enable it to play its part in the Emergency Hospital Scheme.

SPECIAL MAINTENANCE ARRANGEMENTS

In the main, the problem of the supply side of the Emergency Hospital Scheme was to equip an expansion of existing facilities commensurate with the expected flow of casualties. Three services were, however, in a very undeveloped state at the outbreak of war and special measures, both administrative and in relation to the supply of equipment, were found necessary to the rapid expansion that the needs of war demanded. These were pathological laboratories, the blood transfusion service and rehabilitation.

Pathological Laboratories. Measures were taken to ensure that adequate laboratory facilities were available within the Emergency Hospital Scheme. The principal hospitals in the inner London area had large and well equipped pathological laboratories which, under the arrangements for moving staff and equipment from the centre outwards, were resited in the Emergency Hospitals in the Sectors. No substantial addition to the equipment of these was found necessary.

After a survey of the facilities for pathological work in the provinces, it was found necessary, in certain areas, to establish and equip new laboratories or to extend existing ones. These provincial laboratories were classified according to function, and equipment for them was provided from central purchases on the basis of a standard schedule for each type.

Under the normal arrangements for providing equipment for the Emergency Hospital Scheme, the owning authorities of the hospitals in which the laboratories were situated would have been responsible for maintenance. It was feared however, that owing to production difficulties, laboratories would not in all cases be assured of regular supplies, and it was arranged that those in the more important provincial centres, whose costs were met in full by the Exchequer, should obtain replacements of consumable apparatus, etc. free of charge from central stocks. Supplies were also made available, on payment, to certain smaller laboratories working under the supervision of the pathologists in charge of the larger ones. In the London Sectors, it was found more convenient for laboratories to obtain their supplies through the Southern Group Laboratory of the London County Council. To secure uniformity of material, the services of that laboratory in providing culture media, reagents, etc., were also made available to all, whether in London or the provinces.

Blood Transfusion Service. Shortly before the outbreak of the war, arrangements were made with the Medical Research Council for the establishment of four blood transfusion depots in the London area. These depots were equipped by the Council, which made its own arrangements for equipment. In 1940, a blood transfusion centre was set up by the Ministry in each Civil Defence Region, with the exception of Regions 5 and 12 which continued to be served by the Medical Research Council, and Region 7 which was served by the Army Blood Transfusion Service. The equipment purchased for these centres was of the type already in use by the Medical Research Council. Maintenance supplies for these depots were provided through Regional Stores, and arrangements were made under which the requirements of the Council (and to some extent of the Navy) were included in the orders placed for the maintenance of this service.

Rehabilitation. The special centres and fracture departments set up to rehabilitate patients and to restore them to full health and working capacity, were provided by the Ministry with considerable quantities of apparatus and equipment covering the whole period of treatment from the time when the patient while still in bed required relaxation to take his mind off his illness, up to the completion of his cure by remedial exercises of varying degrees of strenuousness. Particulars of some of the many and varied items of equipment provided are shown in Appendix IV. The department also provided prefabricated huts in which remedial exercises and occupational therapy might be pursued, the terms being normally that the hospitals should pay for erection, but that such part of the shell as was obtainable through the Ministry of Works was issued free as the department's Emergency Medical Service contribution.

MEDICAL SUPPLIES FOR THE EVACUATION SCHEME

With the development of the Emergency Medical Services there proceeded, side by side, a steady expansion of the services provided under the Evacuation Scheme and most of these, such as emergency maternity homes and sick bays in hostels, carried with them a measure of medical provision. Provision was also made for medical attention and hygiene in public air raid shelters and in rest centres for those made homeless by enemy action.

Particular attention was directed to the danger caused to public health by the aggregation of large numbers of people in air raid shelters. Local authorities whose existing facilities were inadequate were provided with portable hot air disinfestors for verminous bedding, and a powder insecticide was available in the shelters for the use of the shelterers themselves. In order to counter airborne infection (particularly in ill-ventilated shelters) a dilute solution of hypochlorite disinfectant was sprayed into the air in the form of a fine mist, by means of a simple hand spray, or in the larger shelters by a portable spray driven by an electric motor compressor. Celluloid and muslin face masks were also provided.

For all these services, the necessary equipment was provided, generally by the same procedure as equipment for the Emergency Hospital Service and casualty services. No segregation of supplies for special purposes was made; central stocks were supplied indifferently for all approved purposes and this principle was extended to the equipment supplied to local authorities, who were encouraged to regard their stocks as a central pool to be used for any emergency service as occasion demanded.

ASSISTANCE FROM AMERICA AND OTHER SOURCES

The acquisition of the vast stock of equipment required for the Emergency Medical Services was fraught with many difficulties. In priorities, their needs were subordinated to those of the Fighting Services, whose large demands often absorbed most of the available productive capacity, so that much of the equipment was obtained only after a long delay. Considerable relief was given in the earlier years of the war by the generosity of friends in many parts of the world, particularly in the U.S.A. and Canada. The channel through which gifts of medical and surgical equipment were received was, on the other side of the Atlantic, the American and Canadian Red Cross Societies, and on this side the War Organisation of the B.R.C.S. and Order of St. John. The gifts covered a very wide field, ranging from ambulances, the most modern types of X-ray apparatus and operating tables, and steam sterilisers to vast quantities of dressings, artery forceps, aspirin tablets and syringe needles. The total value of those supplied to the Health Departments alone was of the order of £350,000.

With the passing of the First American Lend-Lease Act, it became possible to utilise a further means of procuring surgical and medical apparatus from the U.S.A. Much apparatus that was scarce, or superior in quality to that which it had been considered proper to demand in view of the heavy pressure upon the manufacturing capacity of this country, was obtained on lend-lease terms, and so another step was taken towards bringing the Emergency Medical Services up to the level of modern ideas as to how good hospitals should be equipped.

REFLECTIONS

It is possible that too much will be read into the various references to improvements that were made by different methods throughout the war years. The original equipment was by no means of a poor standard ; the first type of collapsible bed did perhaps collapse on too little provocation, but the hypothesis on which the Ministry was instructed to work was that casualties would be numerous at the outbreak of war after which they would rapidly decrease, and consequently, that the reserve stock of beds would for the most part only need to be used for a short time and that it was unnecessary to provide beds strong enough for prolonged use. But, apart from a few items, the equipment provided was of good serviceable quality, and proved itself by the way it stood up to the work required of it.

The outbreak of war occurred before all the goods ordered in the first lists of equipment were received, and it was necessary to take special measures to improve the supply of certain items. There were shortages, particularly of beds, mattresses, bedding, sterilising bags, fish kettles and artery forceps, and various devices were adopted to accelerate production. A type of wooden bedstead with an iron platform was approved and camp beds were issued for the use of staff so that their beds could be released for patients. On September 4, 1939, local authorities were authorised to make up any substantial deficiencies in their first-aid post equipment by purchasing through their normal machinery. In the result, however, because of the high number of casualties for which supplies had been ordered and the period which elapsed between the outbreak of war and the occurrence of substantial casualties, the medical service was at no time seriously handicapped by the shortage of supplies.

STOCK RECORDS

Throughout the operation of the scheme, hospitals and scheme-making authorities were required to keep up-to-date records of the equipment held on charge and to undertake periodic stocktakings: in view of the acute shortage of staff, both in the central department and with local authorities, this was confined to the more important non-consumable items.

DETERIORATION PROBLEMS

The vast stocks held gave rise to a number of deterioration problems, but steps were taken to minimise losses. When the first issue of drugs and dressings were made to hospital authorities, they were instructed to take into use for their ordinary purposes such goods as were liable to deteriorate and to replace them with fresh supplies: by continuing this process of turn-over, the augmented stocks of such items were in general retained in good condition. Certain items were, however, in such large quantities, (based, of course, on the very considerable number of casualties for which provision was made) that they could not be used within the requisite period; those items were removed from the schedule of equipment and if possible replaced by more stable preparations. Ethyl chloride is an example of a scheduled supply which was soon removed from the schedules. Ether needed special attention in view of its short life, the difficulty of safe storage, and the large quantity that had to be in readiness for the numerous casualties which would require anaesthesia. Many of the expanded hospitals needed very little for their normal functions, and the quantity allotted far exceeded their requirements. It was estimated that a total stock of approximately 45,000 lb. of ether should be held available for hospitals as soon as hostilities began, and this quantity was distributed among the large general hospitals, their average holding being supplemented to bring their stocks up to a six months' supply at their normal rate of consumption. These 'ether depots' held the stocks from which the expanded public assistance institutions, etc., could draw emergency stocks in the event of a sudden rush of casualties.

Dressings generally provided little difficulty in this respect, but special measures were necessary to dispose of the vast stocks of absorbent cotton wool which had been acquired and were held in the central stores. A number of Government demands were met from these stocks, issues were made for the ordinary maintenance supplies of a number of hospitals which treated E.M.S. patients only, and sales were made to other hospitals. At one period the stocks of surgeons' rubber gloves presented a similar problem, but losses were avoided by resorting to the same methods.

PROBLEMS ARISING THROUGH WAR-TIME RESTRICTIONS

The above is a short record of the activities of the Ministry of Health in connexion with the equipment required for the operation of the

Emergency Medical Services. The department exercised a number of other functions related to medical supplies of all kinds, particularly in regard to restrictions necessitated on security grounds or through shortage of supplies. The department also undertook the distribution of penicillin when stocks of British manufacture became available for civilian purposes. It had been estimated that some 10,000 mega-units per annum would be required to treat all 'life and death' cases, and supplies at this rate (850 mega-units per month) became available in August 1944. In order to ensure that the best use was made of these limited quantities, the department invoked the aid of the universities and medical teaching schools throughout the country and short courses for pathologists were arranged. Supplies of penicillin were sent to these centres, and its use, either at the teaching hospital or in an approved hospital in the area, was left to the discretion of a committee consisting generally of the surgeon, physician and pathologist. 'Life and death' cases, of course, had prior claim, but subject to this and to a ban on its use, owing to the restricted supply, for venereal diseases and bacterial endocarditis, (a ban which was lifted in less than a year from the inauguration of the scheme), these committees could authorise the use of penicillin for any case in which it was likely to prove of value, within the limit of the quantity available. As the supply of penicillin expanded, the quantities allocated for civilian purposes increased, until in April 1945, it was possible to make a wider distribution to some 200 hospitals. The quantity supplied in that month was 3,185 mega-units, and enabled all cases likely to benefit from it to be treated with penicillin. In view of the limitation placed on the use of the drug, issues were supplied free of charge.

The Board of Trade and the Ministry of Supply (Directorate of Medical Supplies) looked to the Ministry of Health for advice on many of the questions relating to goods in short supply. The Ministry made recommendations on problems arising under the Limitation of Supplies Orders, such as applications for X-ray apparatus, electro-medical equipment, surgical corsets, aseptic hospital furniture, sterilisers, refrigerators, etc. In such cases, where war conditions made it impossible for the supply to meet the demand, it fell to the Ministry in fact to discriminate between applicants, so that goods which became available went to those in the greatest need, or who could make the best and fullest use of them. In addition, the two departments sought the advice of the Ministry on restrictions to be placed on the manufacture of surgical supplies. In particular, the shortage of rubber demanded that it should be used only for such essential articles as could not be made from other material or from synthetic rubber. Again, manufacturers were restricted, on the advice of the Ministry, in the number of types of beds that they could manufacture, the number of sizes of such things as bowls and other hollow-ware, and so forth.

The Ministry was also concerned with the supply departments, to ensure that adequate quantities should be available of such items as liquid paraffin, ascorbic acid, insulin for diabetes, liver extract, benzyl benzoate for the treatment of scabies, essential rubber requirements for the manufacture of rubber prophylactics, many types of surgical apparatus, leather and rubber for surgical boots.

THE NATIONAL RESERVE OF DRUGS AND THE VEGETABLE DRUGS COMMITTEE

There remain to be recorded two supplementary supply activities of the Ministry of Health:

(a) The requirements of the Service departments and of the civil population for medical stores under war conditions were considered before the outbreak of war by Supply Committee No. VIII, which was set up in June 1938, on the recommendation of the Committee of Imperial Defence; two representatives of the Ministry of Health were members of the committee. Investigations on behalf of this committee were conducted by the Admiralty, War Office and the Ministry of Health, to whom, and to the committee itself, the valuable assistance of the Association of British Chemical Manufacturers and of the Wholesale Drug Trade Association was given in connexion, in particular, with the capacity of the trade to produce essential medicines and drugs, and in ascertaining the stocks of raw materials and basic drugs normally available. Special consideration was given to essential manufactured drugs and raw materials normally imported from abroad. Lists were prepared of the essential drugs, etc., of which the supply might be regarded as satisfactory, and those of which the available stock needed to be increased. Arrangements were made to increase the production of essential drugs that could be grown in this country.

On the recommendation of this committee, a national reserve was built up of those essential medical requirements which could not be produced here in sufficient quantity, viz.:

Agar agar .	. 3	tons
Belladonna	. 13½	,,
Digitalis fol.	. 12	,,
Ergot .	. 35	,,
Hyoscyamus	. 15·5	,,
Ipecacuanha	. 13	,,
Opium .	. 43·5	,,
Quinine .	. 20	,,
Catgut	14,400 gross tubes	

These stocks were held by the Ministry of Health, and eventually passed to the Ministry of Supply when they became responsible for the supply of medical requirements.

A further list of chemicals of which the industrial use was of far greater importance than their medicinal use, was referred to the Director of Industrial Planning, in order to ensure an adequate supply for medicinal use.

On the recommendation of this committee, the initial orders for drugs and dressings for the Emergency Medical Services were substantially increased before the outbreak of war.

(*b*) In March 1941, there was set up, on the initiative of the Ministry of Health, the Vegetable Drug Committee, with the following terms of reference: 'To review the present and future requirements of vegetable drugs in the light of Empire consumption and trade, and facilities for cultivation within the Empire; to consider the steps which should be taken to secure organisation of cultivation and collection; and to make recommendations to Ministers'.

The committee quickly decided that it was impossible to embark on any long-term policy in view of the economic and political problems involved. It served to some extent as a clearing house for related questions with the Dominions and Colonies, but its main work proved to be the organisation of the collection of home grown medicinal herbs. In the light of the experience gained in the first year, the committee, which was transferred in 1942 to the Ministry of Supply, recommended the formation of County Herb Committees which in each county organised the collection of a wide range of medicinal herbs: foxglove leaf, belladonna, dandelion root, male fern, nettles, rose hips, etc. Following further recommendations of the committee the Ministry of Supply sponsored a survey of the coasts of Great Britain to ascertain where the red seaweeds could be found in quantities that were worth gathering. This work proved of the utmost importance and much valuable information was obtained which facilitated the manufacture of agar agar from British seaweed.

VOLUME OF SUPPLIES

Some idea of the vast quantities of medical and surgical supplies acquired and distributed may be obtained from the four appendices to this Chapter, in which it will be noted that only selected items are included.

APPENDIX I

QUANTITIES OF SELECTED ITEMS BOUGHT CENTRALLY FOR EMERGENCY MEDICAL SERVICES

Bandages, 2 in. and 3 in.	212,040	gross
,, domette	23,705	dozen
,, plaster-of-Paris	12,363	gross
,, triangular	109,735	gross
Gauze, absorbent	21,718,340	yards
Lint	988,477	lb.
Burn dressing	15,457,359	
Plaster, adhesive	784,728	spools
Wool, cotton, absorbent	1,154	tons
,, unbleached	475	tons
Chloroform	35,206	lb.
Ether	61,296	lb.
Morphia	3,830	ozs.
Morphia tablets	11,777,980	
Pituitary extract	342,726	ampoules
Anaesthetic apparatus, Boyles	995	
Balkan beams for orthopaedic work	15,196	
Forceps, artery, Spencer Wells'	207,523	
Gloves, surgeons'	56,655	dozen
,, rubber, other types (excluding X-ray protection gloves)	8,360	dozen
Scissors	412,477	pairs
Splints for fractures	3,431,777	
Sterilisers	19,526	
Syringes for all types of surgical purposes	77,204	
Tables, instrument and dressing	13,858	
,, operation	1,072	
Tourniquets	838,930	
X-ray apparatus fixed sets	113	
,, ,, mobile sets	167	
,, ,, portable	105	
,, ,, dental	22	
,, ,, field service	13	
X-ray photographic films	64,998	dozen
Thermometers, clinical	89,785	
Blankets	6,000,000	approx.
Sheets	1,725,000	,,
Pallets	733,000	,,
Mattresses	250,000	,,
Beds	250,000	,,

APPENDIX II

QUANTITIES OF SELECTED ITEMS OBTAINED UNDER LEND-LEASE FOR THE EMERGENCY HOSPITAL SERVICE

(a) *Expensive Items*

Auriscope, electric	100 Table, operation, Scanlon Balfour	68
Cardiograph, electric, portable	33 " fracture and orthopaedic, Hawley Scanlon	30
Lamp, transillumination	49 Sterilisers, electric	720
Bone, operating sets, electric	48 " gas	185
Pump, suction, electric portable	50 " steam	138
Refraction equipment	124	

(b) *Large quantities*

Blood pressure apparatus (Baumanometer)	250 Forceps, hysterectomy, Pesin, straight, 8¼ in.	499
Clamps, intestinal, curved, Doyen	248 " sponge holding, 9¼ in.	500
Forceps, artery, large, Mayo Ochsner	3,000 Oxygen masks, male, nasal, B.L.B.1A	1,500
" peritoneal, Allis	7,035 " " female, nasal, B.L.B.2A	1,000
" tongue or towel, Mayo	1,997 " " female, oro-nasal, B.L.B.5A	339
Syringes, all glass, Luer mount	17,987 Re-breathing bags for B.L.B. masks	1,000
Forceps, artery, Moynihan's type 6¼ in.	4,997 Oxygen masks O.E.M. nasal	100
" hysterectomy, Pesin, curved, 8¼ in.	500	

APPENDIX III

QUANTITIES OF SELECTED ITEMS RECEIVED AS GIFTS, CHIEFLY FROM U.S.A.

Basic sets of instruments	18 sets Diagnostic sets	18
Blood-pressure apparatus (Baumanometers)	240 Radiant heat baths, 6-lamp	200
Chevalier Jackson's bronchoscopic sets with batteries	25 " " " 12-lamp	300
Roosevelt's twin stomach clamps	258 Refrigerators (Kelvinators)	50
Cystoscopes and batteries	170 Albee's electric bone sets	42
Padgett's dermatomes	50 Sigmoidoscopes and batteries, electric	112

APPENDIX III—(continued)

Theatre spotlights	90
Dressing sterilisers, gas and steam heated	72
Cooking stoves	1,500
Heating stoves	1,000
Hawley Scanlon fracture and orthopaedic tables	56
Hawley portable fracture tables	50
Operation tables, oil pump	50
Blackburn skull tractors	50
X-ray apparatus	87
Pathological laboratory, vertical autoclaves	15
,, ,, Sartorius balances	15
Pathological laboratory, electric centrifuges	15
,, ,, electric incubators	15
,, ,, microscopes	50
,, ,, Spencer rotary microtomes	15
,, ,, Harvard trip balances	15
,, ,, Arnold sterilisers	15
,, ,, hot air sterilisers	15
Forceps, various	28,221
Injection syringes, various	34,527
Surgical injection needles	200,581
Inhalation masks	14,406

APPENDIX IV

QUANTITIES OF SELECTED ITEMS SUPPLIED FOR OCCUPATIONAL THERAPY AND REMEDIAL EXERCISES

OCCUPATIONAL THERAPY

Weaving looms	876
Rug looms	113
Rug frames	349

CARPENTRY

Wood turning lathes	79
Benches	411
Sets of tools for instructors and general use	86
Sets of tools for each man	623
Treadle and bicycle fret-saws	223

REMEDIAL EXERCISE EQUIPMENT

Balance benches	935
Gymnastic mats	1,720
Medicine balls	1,358
Mirrors, full length	484
Skipping ropes	2,146
Steps with risers	315
Walking chairs	218
Wall bars	975
Weight and pulley exercisers	783
Wrist machines and wrist rollers	314
Dartboards and darts	561
Deck quoits	283
Deck tennis	266
Footballs (Association)	731
Netballs	226
Skittles (indoor)	256

CHAPTER 10

THE EMERGENCY HOSPITAL PATHOLOGICAL SERVICES

by

SIR PHILIP PANTON

M.B., Ch.B.

Consultant Adviser on Pathology to the Ministry of Health

INCEPTION OF THE SCHEME IN THE LONDON AREA

WHEN it had been decided that, in the event of war, the hospital services in the London area would be distributed over a considerable part of the home counties, a meeting of pathologists was held at the Medical Research Council to discuss the position of the hospital laboratories. A committee was then formed, consisting of medical representatives of the Medical Research Council, the London County Council, the British Medical Association, the Association of Clinical Pathologists, and the senior London pathologists subsequently appointed as 'Sector Pathologists'. This committee was primarily concerned with the re-distribution of London laboratories and the formation of a national register of laboratory staffs.

Each Sector pathologist in the London area surveyed possible hospital laboratory sites, and plans were drawn up for the allocation of staff and apparatus. The situation of the public health laboratories in the London area had been previously decided by the Medical Research Council, and the staffing was entrusted to the Sector pathologists. The sites chosen for laboratories had to be those of the main hospital services intended for the Emergency Hospital Scheme, and in many cases were in public assistance institutions unprovided with any laboratory accommodation. Premises which could be converted into laboratories had to be selected and plans prepared for their adaptation in consultation with the owning authorities. All equipment was listed and allocated to the different laboratories, and packing and transport were arranged.

The register was compiled under the direction of the Medical Research Council and formed a complete survey of all medical pathologists, scientific workers, and laboratory technicians in Great Britain and Northern Ireland. The British Medical Association register had not attempted to give the detailed information now required for pathologists, but additional questionnaires were sent out by the Association and copies of the replies forwarded to the Medical Research Council. Duplicate copies of the complete register were subsequently kept at the Ministry of Health and the Medical Research Council, and proved essential to the primary allocation of staff and in particular for the subsequent release to the Services of pathologists, scientists and technicians. All male laboratory technicians with two or more years' experience were placed on the register of the Medical Research Council and granted a block deferment by the Ministry of Labour. Female technicians, if engaged in that occupation before registration, could be reserved on application by the employer to the local labour exchange.

The reservation of pathologists came for decision to the Services Committee of the Central Medical War Committee and the supply, both for civil needs and the Services, was maintained to a limited extent by appointing 'trainees'. These trainees were strictly limited in number and were selected by the professors of their medical schools from recently qualified practitioners who intended to take up pathology as a career, showed an aptitude for the subject, and had held clinical house appointments for at least six months. By the beginning of 1944, permission could only be obtained for the training of non-recruitable practitioners.

PROGRESS OF THE SCHEME

A small executive committee was appointed from the members of the original committee to deal with more urgent problems of allocation, which became more acute as the war progressed and more laboratories were opened.

On the outbreak of war, arrangements were so far advanced that the distribution of staff and equipment was made smoothly and rapidly. The necessary laboratory conversions were completed, for the most part by the works departments of the local institutions, and most laboratories in the London Sectors were in working order within forty-eight hours of the start of hostilities. Altogether sixty-eight laboratories were either newly set up or completely reorganised to form part of the general Emergency Hospital Service in the London Sectors. These were staffed and equipped out of the resources of the Central London laboratories sufficiently well to function for some years, with little addition of equipment, other than the normal replacements, and, as staff was released to the Services, with considerable reduction in establishment.

A notable result of this dispersal of laboratory staffs and facilities from the centre to the periphery was to make modern diagnostic methods available to many of the smaller hospitals, which had previously lacked them, and to upgraded public assistance institutions, which had scarcely needed them and which now had to provide for cases of acute illness. In particular, the Hospital Sector covering Essex, acting for the Emergency Medical Service and in collaboration with the Medical Officer of Health for Essex, eventually set up a complete hospital and public health laboratory service throughout the county, replacing the previous system which had been mainly postal.

All the preliminary arrangements for pathology in the London area had been carried out on the initiative of the Committee of Pathologists meeting at the office of the Medical Research Council, but in association with the Sector Hospital Officers and with the knowledge of medical representatives of the Ministry of Health. By the beginning of 1940, these services had become more completely merged into the general Emergency Hospital Scheme and for professional purposes were administered by a committee of the Sector pathologists meeting monthly at the Ministry of Health. These meetings continued and provided an essential link between the pathologists responsible for the work of their laboratories and the department concerned with the administration.

The relations between the dispersed laboratories and the local authorities owning the institutions in which they were located were at first confused, but by October 1940, it was made clear that these laboratories were under the administrative and disciplinary control of the governing body of the hospitals and under the professional direction of the Sector pathologists. Two classes of laboratories became recognised: 'designated' laboratories were those in which Emergency Medical Service interests were thought to be predominant, and the whole costs of the laboratory were borne by the department, the hospital being charged a standard rate of 3s. a 'specimen' for its ordinary peace-time work. The 'non-designated' laboratories were under a different financial arrangement, and the Sector pathologists had a purely advisory and consultative interest in their management. The 'specimen' standard of recording work was subsequently agreed to be unsatisfactory, both as a measure of the work done in a laboratory and as an estimate of cost. It was replaced by the 'unit' standard in 1943, the number of units allotted to each investigation being reckoned from a schedule which assessed the number according to the cost in estimated laboratory time.

The central laboratories of the parent hospitals in London were, in most cases, almost denuded of staff and equipment, but, in the absence of air raids, skeleton staffs were returned. When air raids became severe, in the autumn of 1940, the skeleton staffs were still retained, and by the end of 1942 the parent hospital laboratories were functioning on scales similar to those of the larger sector laboratories, though with relatively small staffs and at a standard much below that of the teaching hospitals in peace-time. Research work and research staffs were almost entirely confined to problems directly concerned with the war, and many of the research workers and much of their equipment were diverted to essential routine. The Emergency Public Health Laboratories in the Home Counties became a part of the Sector laboratory service early in the war, but the Regional Public Health laboratories remained under the immediate jurisdiction of the Medical Research Council.

THE TEACHING OF PATHOLOGY

The teaching of pathology in the medical schools was mainly directed, following the staffs and equipment, to selected laboratories in the Sector hospitals. Classrooms were often makeshift, but served their purpose, so that, on the whole, the dislocation of teaching in pathology, except in special advanced courses, was less than that of other branches of medicine. By the end of 1942 and the beginning of 1943, there was a distinct move towards bringing back the professorial and teaching staffs with their classes to the parent hospitals. The distribution of students for teaching purposes varied considerably at the different schools, some classes being held in London throughout the war and other hospitals retaining their classes in the peripheral laboratories, but the general trend followed the degree of reopening of the wards in the central London hospitals.

THE SCHEME IN THE PROVINCIAL REGIONS

The re-distribution of laboratories among the new general hospitals set up under the Emergency Hospital Scheme was at first mainly concerned with London and the home counties, and all that had been done in the provinces amounted to the provisional appointment of an Adviser in Pathology for each Region. Some additional laboratory provision was made in the Leeds area, but for the most part the advisers had no definite duties and no powers to institute laboratories. In September 1940, it was decided to make some further investigation of the needs of hospitals for laboratory services in the Regions and to draw up a scheme to provide laboratories, where this was considered essential, for the Emergency Medical Services in England and Wales. A complete survey of the country was not possible, but the Regional offices and the university centres in each Region were visited and subsequently an investigation of the existing services of pathology was made in over 100 of the larger towns in England and Wales. This survey disclosed that adequate services of hospital pathology had been established in some areas, but in others such services only existed because of the initiative and ability of local pathologists to whom little financial encouragement was given by the hospitals. The pay of technicians and other staff could often be met only out of the fees for laboratory examinations received from local authorities and from private practitioners. The professional status and terms of employment of pathologists varied greatly in different institutions and were often most unsatisfactory. Some of the larger provincial universities, for lack of existing facilities, had provided pathological services where none had previously existed; but these services had been extended by a regrettable system of postal pathology.

In many other large towns and areas, the service of hospital pathology was found to be either non-existent, except by postal service to distant parts of the country, or provided by laboratories staffed by technicians and supervised in a most perfunctory manner by members of the clinical staff. Before the war, there was not one qualified pathologist in the whole County of Lincolnshire, and many large towns throughout the country were in a similar position.

The first step taken to remedy this state of affairs was to obtain the consent of the provincial Professors of Pathology, through their respective universities, to act as Honorary Regional Advisers in Pathology. It was then possible to make a regional distribution of pathological services based on university teaching schools, similar to that set up in the London area, but, owing to the limitation of trained staff and building facilities, little more than a skeleton service could be provided. This was made up from laboratories already in existence and judged to be efficient, by strengthening the staff, equipment and premises of less efficient laboratories, and by setting up entirely new laboratories. The Emergency Medical Service accepted full financial responsibility for some of these laboratories, as with the designated laboratories of the London area.

The combination of new and pre-existing laboratories was made up of three types:

(i) Area laboratories, serving other institutions in addition to the hospitals in which they were situated;

(ii) subsidiary laboratories, with as a rule only one pathologist, serving a single hospital and looking to the area laboratory for assistance;

(iii) side-room laboratories, staffed by technicians only, but with regular visits from neighbouring pathologists.

Altogether in the regions, 29 designated area laboratories, two subsidiary laboratories and nine side-rooms were set up and financed under the Emergency Medical Service. Help and close co-operation were given to nineteen pre-existing laboratories, and seven towns were persuaded to set up their own services.

The area laboratories were affiliated to the central regional University Department of Pathology. In the scheme for this affiliation, the Civil Defence Regional areas were followed, except in the cases of Regions 2, 3, 4 and 10.

Region 10, on account of its size, the density of the population and the presence of two university medical schools, was divided into a Western Region centred on Liverpool, and an Eastern Region, centred on Manchester. Region 3 contained no medical school, and Region 2, both Leeds and Sheffield; the greater part of Region 2 was allocated to Leeds and the remainder to Sheffield, which also became responsible for the greater part of Region 3, the remainder of Region 3 and Region 4 being allocated to Cambridge. The whole of Wales was centred upon Cardiff, but because of the greater ease of communication between North Wales and Liverpool, a liaison was also effected between North Wales and Liverpool University.

By these adjustments, the services of pathology in the provinces were divided into regions of considerable size, each containing a medical school. The nature of the affiliation varied at the different universities, being closest at Manchester, Liverpool and Bristol, and less intimate at Cambridge and Newcastle. In all cases, the Honorary Regional Advisers in Pathology acted as friends and advisers of all pathologists in the Region and assisted them in all matters of professional difficulty. So far as circumstances allowed, each Region came to have a self-contained and co-ordinated service of hospital pathology, which was departmentally independent of the public health service set up by the Medical Research Council, but worked in close co-operation with it.

LESSONS LEARNT FROM THE WORKING OF THE SCHEME

The difficult problem of laboratory supplies was adequately solved by central issue to designated laboratories from the Supply Division of the Emergency Medical Service. The consumable stores, such as reagents and culture media, were provided through the London County Council service both to the London sectors and to the Regions. Apparatus was ordered in advance and issued by the Supply Division. The help of both the London County Council service and the Supply Division was freely extended, to such non-designated laboratories as had difficulty in obtaining supplies and were prepared to pay for them. It is a remarkable tribute to those responsible for supplying all these laboratories that there was never any shortage of materials and, still more remarkable, no serious criticisms from any pathologists.

The survey of hospital laboratories in England and Wales, and the subsequent organisation of the service into a loosely co-ordinated whole, disclosed certain facts bearing upon the future medical services of the country. These may be briefly enumerated:

(1) *The pre-war inadequacy of clinical laboratory services* over large areas and in very many general hospitals. The belief was widespread that a hospital could undertake the treatment of acutely ill patients without one of the principal means of diagnosing their conditions and, though the war has seen a great advance, this belief is not yet entirely dissipated.

(2) *The cost of laboratory services.* This was very considerable and led many voluntary institutions to impose intolerable conditions of service both on pathologists and technicians, as well as to regard a laboratory as a financial asset instead of an essential charge. The cost of laboratory investigations, from data supplied mainly by the London County Council before the war, was expected to be in the neighbourhood of 3s. a 'specimen'. The estimated cost in the fifth year of the war was found to be approximately 9d. a 'unit'. The average number of units per specimen may be taken as four.

(3) *Technician laboratories*. These still exist, and were very numerous. The practice, both in voluntary and local authority hospitals, of asking a member of the clinical staff, with no special training in, or knowledge of, pathology, to supervise the laboratory work, is inexcusable. Some technician laboratories were not even managed by trained technicians, but apportioned as a part-time duty to such officers as dispensers, radiographers, clerks and even hall porters. The war produced a great improvement, but much remains to be done, particularly in mental institutions.

(4) *The isolation of laboratory staffs*. This was a very bad feature of pre-war pathology and has been considerably improved by a co-ordination of laboratories in large areas and the linking of area laboratories to university centres. It will be difficult to surmount all the disadvantages of local services, unless the areas assigned to hospital groups are sufficiently large and sufficiently co-ordinated to allow a free interchange of staff and technical assistance between a large series of laboratories. It will be necessary, further, to co-ordinate the groups so as to ensure that every laboratory in the country is attached to a university school. This connection proved of the greatest importance during the war.

(5) *Postal Service*. This was to a very large extent abolished during the war. The necessity of bringing the pathologists and the clinician into close personal contact had become widely recognised, and the laboratory test became less and less regarded as a penny-in-the-slot method of diagnosis.

(6) *The effects of a clinical laboratory service upon general medical practice*. The diffusion of laboratory services played a very important part in the general improvement of medical practice which followed the distribution of specialists from university centres to outlying districts. The establishment of a laboratory in a county hospital was often effected against considerable local opposition; any subsequent suggestion to remove it or curtail its activities came to be even more strenuously resisted. The improvement of medical practice within and outside these hospitals was in many cases revolutionary. The laboratory services were made readily available to all general practitioners, and it has been possible in some institutions to give patients direct access to the laboratory without passing through the out-patient department, thus bringing the practitioners into direct contact with the pathologist.

(7) *Laboratories in local authority and voluntary hospitals*. The principle adopted in every town lacking laboratory facilities was to house the laboratory in that institution, whether under voluntary or local authority management, which was agreed to be most convenient to the service. Rival claims could usually be met by calling the laboratory after the name of the town and not of the hospital in which it was situated, as an indication that it was equally at the disposal of all institutions or practitioners in the town who wished to make use of it.

It happened more frequently than not that the voluntary hospitals had some sort of laboratory which could be extended and made use of, and that the local authority had little or no interest in general hospital practice, but was prepared to co-operate in local public health needs.

(8) *Relation with the Public Health Laboratory Service.* An important matter to which the war has drawn particular attention is the relation between the Hospital Laboratory and the Public Health Laboratory Services. This cannot be too close and, indeed, there is no sharp dividing line. Except in the large centres, there is much routine public health bacteriology which can properly be undertaken in the hospital laboratory, but the more complicated investigations and all 'field work' should be left to the specialist bacteriologist. Much bad bacteriology has come from hospital laboratories and equally bad clinical pathology from public health departments. The proper integration of the two services will need very careful adjustment throughout the country.

(9) *The growing demand for Laboratory Services.* There was remarkably little delay on the part of clinicians in making use of the newly opened laboratories, and one of the most striking features of the new service was the rapid increase, year by year, in the number of investigations carried out. This increase has been maintained, and the close of hostilities found most pathologists and technicians grossly overworked. With the return to civil life of doctors from the Services, more accustomed to the use of laboratory facilities in diagnosis and during treatment of the patient, it was apparent that in the future there will be an even greater demand for all types of laboratory workers, and that a large number of new laboratories will have to be established to provide a reasonably accessible service to all general practitioners.

CHAPTER 11
THE CIVILIAN BLOOD TRANSFUSION SERVICE

Based on contributions by
JANET M. VAUGHAN
O.B.E., D.M., F.R.C.P.
Principal, Somerville College, Oxford

and

SIR PHILIP N. PANTON
M.B., B.Ch.
Consultant Adviser on Pathology to the Ministry of Health

PRE-WAR ORGANISATIONS

UNTIL the outbreak of the war no adequate blood transfusion service can be said to have existed, although in London and in certain large provincial towns 'blood banks', which were purely local voluntary organisations, had served the needs of the large hospitals and the surrounding areas. These blood banks maintained lists of voluntary donors who were called upon to supply fresh whole blood for individual cases requiring such treatment. Experiment in bottling and storing of whole blood was only beginning as was the separation of plasma and serum. Lessons had been learned from the experiences of the Spanish War, but had not been applied to any material extent in this country. Outside these few large centres, blood transfusion was almost unknown.

With the establishment of the Emergency Hospital Service, an organisation capable of supplying the large quantities of fresh or stored blood required to deal adequately with the expected influx of air raid casualties, was obviously necessary. There were informal discussions a few months before the outbreak of the war, and a scheme for the London area was worked out by a group of pathologists and others interested in transfusion practice and submitted in a memorandum to the Medical Research Council. This scheme was approved in principle and brought to the notice of the Ministry of Health, who officially adopted it.

THE LONDON BLOOD TRANSFUSION SCHEME

INITIAL ORGANISATION

The Medical Research Council undertook, on behalf of the Ministry of Health, the organisation of four depots for the collection, storage and supply of blood for transfusion purposes. After surveying several areas, two sites north and two south of the River Thames were chosen at Luton, Slough, Sutton and Maidstone. These centres were primarily intended to augment the existing arrangements in the London area and to enable hospitals to cope with all calls that might be made upon them, but they were also required to conduct research into the problems of providing and preserving large quantities of blood. The decision to prosecute active research was, as events proved, amply justified.

By July 1939, skeleton staffs, medical, technical and clinical had been appointed to take up their duties; the necessary alterations in depot premises and the supply of essential services were well forward, and basic equipment was ready for despatch to the depots and to the Sector hospitals. Donor panels had been established and were growing steadily. By the end of August such equipment as large refrigerators for blood storage and autoclaves had been installed. On September 1, telegrams were received from the Medical Research Council instructing depots to begin 'bleeding' and at the outbreak of the war on September 3, stocks of blood were available for issue and were being sent to the London hospitals. A plan which had been worked out entirely on paper was put into action with surprisingly few difficulties and continued to develop along the lines originally suggested throughout the war, eventually merging with the cessation of hostilities into the National Blood Transfusion Service.

ADMINISTRATION

As already stated, the four London depots were under the administrative control of the Medical Research Council. At first Professor Topley and subsequently Dr. A. N. Drury assisted by Dr. Chalmers for a time, were responsible for depot policy. Depot directors were, however, allowed considerable elasticity in developing the services under their charge, and depots developed along different lines, for they had different problems to meet and no precedents to follow. Though this independence increased the difficulties of the central administrative staff, it contributed to a rapid development of work of both academic and practical importance on blood transfusion in its widest terms. Technical developments, methods of staffing, of record keeping and of liaison with the hospitals and medical practitioners, tried and proved successful by one depot, were readily applied to others. The work of co-ordination was greatly facilitated by replacing the Depot Committee by the Blood Transfusion Research Committee set up in 1940 under the chairmanship of Dr. A. N. Drury.

STAFFING THE DEPOTS

All depots worked with a nucleus of trained and paid staff but this was supplemented to a varying degree by voluntary workers, whose help was invaluable. Voluntary workers were trained as technicians, nurses and drivers, and many gave full-time service, and by the end of the war were highly skilled.

In addition to the depot director each depot had four or five other medical officers, who bled donors, gave transfusions on request and engaged in research, and research assistants with B.Sc. degrees were often attached to the depots for special work. In some cases a State registered nurse was in charge of the V.A.D. nurses, in others the whole nursing staff employed belonged to Voluntary Aid or St. John detachments. The number employed varied according to whether they worked full-time or part-time, but on the average each depot employed the equivalent of ten to twelve full-time nurses. They were used primarily on the 'bleeding' teams, but they also cleaned and sterilised transfusion apparatus, and some did laboratory work such as blood grouping. In some depots they were also trained to give transfusions under supervision and were used in resuscitation teams. All depots were able to supply blood, blood products and equipment at any time in response to a telephone call.

RECORDS

All depots kept standardised records of the donors on their panels by means of cards on which were recorded the donor's name, address, occupation, blood group (ABO and subsequently in a large number of cases, Rh), the date of 'bleeding' and the result of the Wassermann test. In many cases also the titre of the donor's serum and therefore its value for the purpose of supplying test sera was also noted. In one depot throughout the war a record was kept of the fate of every bottle of blood taken; i.e. whether it was given as a transfusion and, if so, with what result, or whether it was turned into plasma or serum. Similar records of blood products were kept. This follow-up was initiated in the first instance to check the reaction-rate with both stored blood and blood products, but subsequently proved of value in a follow-up of transfused cases in order to determine the incidence of homologous serum jaundice.[19]

DONORS

Donors were recruited from every section of the population. From a practical point of view the easiest to handle were those who were already gathered together in large groups in one place, such as factory hands, army units or office staffs, but the housewife in the country village and small town was often a most faithful and regular donor. Many of them gave regularly every three months throughout the war, feeling it was the one personal contribution they could make to the war effort. The London depots never found it necessary to refuse a call for help for lack of blood. In times of crisis such as severe raids or the invasion of the

Continent, the enthusiasm of donors became almost an embarrassment, but in quiet times their recruitment was a considerable problem.

Recruitment of donors was encouraged in various ways. On a national scale there were broadcast appeals, sponsored by the Ministry of Health, and a wide distribution of posters at different times. A film covering the history and development of blood transfusion was also prepared and made available, in full for special audiences and in abbreviated form for general display. A pamphlet covering much the same ground, but giving a more detailed account of the use of blood and blood products in the field was also prepared.

Locally, use was made of special meetings addressed by members of the depot staff, propaganda articles in the local press, personal contacts with different organisations, loud-speaker vans and leaflets. Great help was given by organisations such as the Red Cross, the St. John Ambulance Brigade, Rotary Clubs, Women's Institutes and the Women's Voluntary Services. In many places a local organiser was found who was responsible for producing a given number of donors on any given date.

Bleeding of donors was undertaken both in the depot itself and by mobile teams sent out into the surrounding small towns and villages, where they set up temporary 'bleeding' centres in town hall, factory rest rooms, church hall or village public-house. Such teams consisted of one or more medical officers, nurses, secretarial help, and sometimes technicians capable of doing blood grouping on the spot.

No serious results of blood donation occurred in any donor in the London area. Special investigations were carried out into the incidence and cause of fainting during 1942 and 1943 by all the depot medical officers. (Brown and McCormack[3]; Greenbury[8]; Report to Medical Research Council, 1944[16].) In a study of 5,897 unselected donors, the incidence of fainting while still in the 'bleeding' centre, was 4·93 per cent.; only 13 per cent. of these donors who were described as fainting actually lost consciousness while in the depot. In an investigation of the symptoms occurring in 4,212 donors after they had left the depot, under 1 per cent. of both sexes reported having lost consciousness, and only 14 per cent. felt any ill effects after leaving the depot. Ten per cent. in fact said they felt unusually fit after bleeding. Methedrine was shown to be effective in treating the more prolonged falls of bloodpressure.

THE RECIPIENTS

As records accumulated, it became apparent that few reactions either mild or severe occurred in casualties after transfusion as long as uninfected blood was used. Mild reactions were far more common in sick patients and normal controls. An attempt was made to ensure that all severe reactions were fully reported to a special sub-committee of the Blood Transfusion Research Committee for further study. Exact figures for such severe reactions could not be given without being misleading, since it is known that not all cases were reported and further it was often extremely difficult to determine whether the transfusion or some other condition was responsible for death. In most cases such reactions proved not to have been due to the transfusion itself. In a few instances, errors in grouping were responsible, rarely with fatal results. In maternity cases it was possible to prove during the later years of the service that the Rh factor was not infrequently responsible for a proportion of cases of severe anuria, followed sometimes by death and sometimes by complete recovery. One or two instances of fulminating toxaemia followed by death and due to the contamination of the blood by a coliform organism growing at a temperature as low as $+2°$ C. were reported at an early stage. It was thought this might be due to insufficient sterilisation of apparatus and considerable attention was then paid to the correct working of the autoclaves. Sterilisation except by autoclaves was given up. (Spooner and Turnbull)[18]

Except for jaundice no evidence was obtained of the transmission of disease by transfusion fluids. In 1942 the first cases to develop jaundice after serum transfusion were reported to the committee and subsequently published (Morgan and Williamson)[14]. In the following years much work was done by depot medical officers in collaboration with other workers in this field on the risks of transmission of jaundice by transfusion.[1] [11] [19] It was established by a follow-up of 2,040 patients transfused with pooled serum or plasma in one depot area, that 7·3 per cent. developed jaundice which could be attributed to the transfusion. In a group of 1,284 patients who received blood only, no undoubted case of homologous serum jaundice developed. Blood has, however, been implicated by other observers. In order to minimise the risk of jaundice, pools of plasma or serum were reduced to blood obtained from ten donors, while as far as possible the use of blood rather than its products was advised until some means of destroying the icterogenic agent was devised. Those responsible, however, were convinced that the life-saving effects of serum and plasma, especially in the case of air raid and battle casualties, far outweighed any danger or discomfort caused by an attack of jaundice, which was usually mild, though acute necrosis of the liver with death occurred in a few instances.

APPARATUS

It was recognised during the period of initial planning that the apparatus, both for taking blood and giving blood, must be extremely simple for the following reasons: firstly, it would have to be made available in very large quantities; secondly, it would have to be easy to clean and assemble, and thirdly, since it would have to be used by relatively unskilled personnel, it was essential to make its method of use obvious and easy. The apparatus suggested proved extremely satisfactory, the only significant alteration made being in the type of filter used. The fact that a standard pattern was available for the whole country proved of great benefit in the stresses and strains of war-time practice. In the later stages of the war the value of the bone marrow route for administering fluid in certain cases was demonstrated and a standard needle for sternal puncture was issued (Fig. 6), and a modified transfusion needle was frequently employed for tibial puncture in infants.

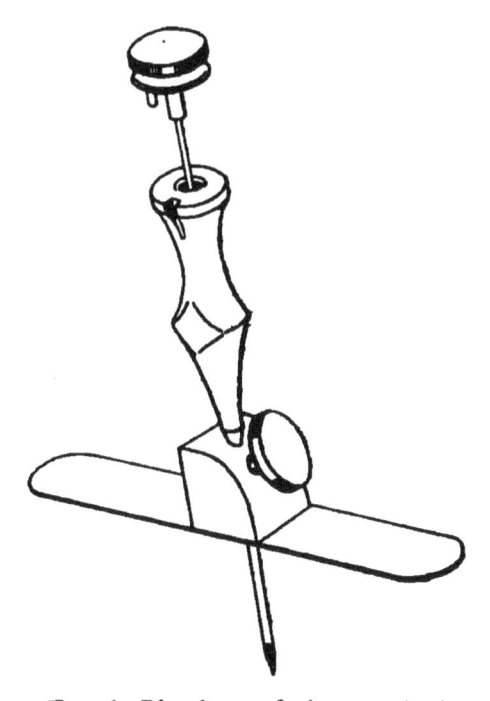

FIG. 6. Blood transfusion standard needle for sternal puncture

The apparatus used was described in appendices in both the first and second editions of the Medical Research Council War Memorandum No. 1 on the treatment of 'Wound Shock' (1940 and 1944).[13]

(1) The bottle used for taking, storing and giving blood or blood products was a modified pint milk bottle, slightly waisted to facilitate holding, fitted with an aluminium screw cap with a 4 mm. rubber liner inset and provided with a metal band and loop at the base for hanging the bottle in an inverted position.

(2) Apparatus for blood withdrawal was of two types, involving either :

   (i) Replacement of the cap by a rubber bung and glass tubing (see Fig. 7).

(ii) Perforation of the cap by two needles (see Fig. 8).

(i) *Replacement of the cap by a rubber bung and glass tubing*: The screw cap of the Medical Research Council bottle was removed and kept sterile. The bottle was then fitted with a sterile 'taking set', comprising a rubber bung pierced by two 3-in. glass tubes, one of which was lightly plugged with cotton wool, so acting as an air vent. To the other were attached a length of rubber tubing and a stainless steel needle which was protected by a small glass test-tube or short length of rubber

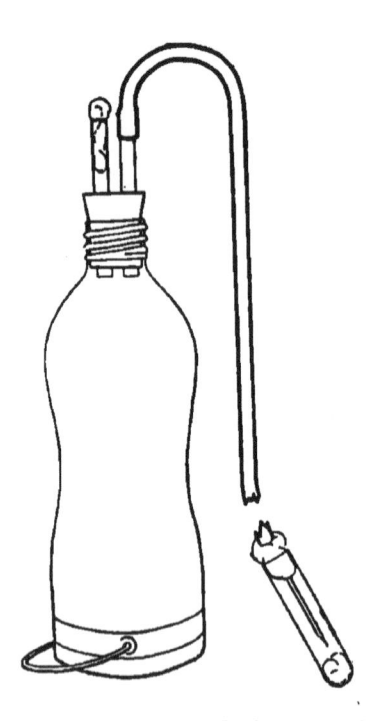

FIG. 7. Standard flask with rubber bung and glass tubing

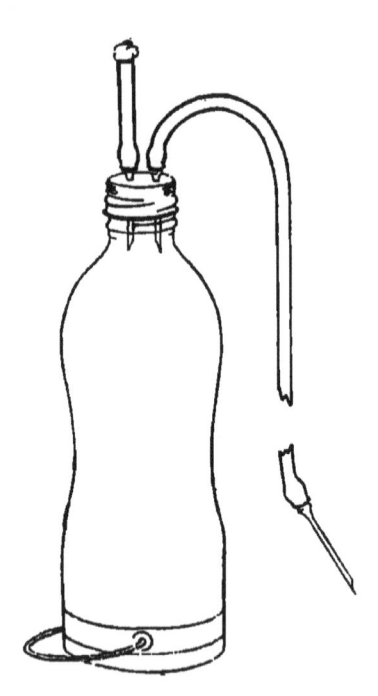

FIG. 8. Standard bung replaced by perforation cap

tubing plugged with cotton wool. (The glass tube only is shown in the diagram, for the sake of clarity.) A short length of glass tubing could be inserted near the needle, to serve as a window, so that the passage of blood down the tube might show the operator he had entered the vein. A sphygmomanometer cuff or tourniquet was applied to the upper arm of the donor, and the skin over the vein in the antecubital fossa cleaned, first by rubbing well with ether soap and water on a sterile swab, and then by two further swabbings with phenylmercuric acetate in 70 per cent. alcohol. The cuff was inflated to a pressure of 80 mm. Hg; the pressure was maintained at that level, and approximately 0·1 c.c. of a local anaesthetic was introduced intradermally over the vein. The needle of the taking set, after removal of the protecting tubing or glass, was then inserted in the vein, and held in position while the bottle filled. Gravity was sufficient to maintain a steady flow of blood. This could be facilitated by asking the donor to open and close his hand. It was essential to mix the blood and anti-coagulant by gentle rotation throughout the collection. Frothing was avoided by allowing the blood to flow down the side of the bottle rather than straight into the anti-coagulant. The blood having been withdrawn, and the rubber bung with its tubing removed, the bottle was again sealed by the screw cap after its neck had been flamed. Samples for a regroup and a Kahn test were obtained from the end of the rubber tubing after removal.

(ii) Perforation of the cap by two needles: In this method the aluminium cap of the blood bottle was perforated by machine with two holes 3 mm. in diameter. These were sealed after the bottles had been autoclaved, either by a viscose cap or a strip of adhesive tape. Immediately before blood withdrawal the perforations were exposed by removing the viscose cap or adhesive tape. Through one hole in the cap was pushed a taking (or administrating) needle, to which was attached a short length of rubber tubing carrying a second taking needle at the other end (protected by a short piece of tubing) for insertion into the vein. Both needles inserted into the cap were pushed through the rubber diaphragm. After removal of the blood as described with apparatus (i) the needles were withdrawn from the aluminium cap and the holes sealed with a fresh strip of adhesive tape.

The Administering Unit (Fig. 9). This consisted of a rubber bung pierced by two glass tubes, one of which was $9\frac{1}{2}$ in. long reaching almost to the bottom of the bottle, and was closed externally by a small cork. The other tube was $2\frac{1}{2}$ in. long; it was covered by a metal gauze filter or gas mantle filter (Fig. 10), and had attached to its outer end, in sequence, a length of rubber tubing, a drip feed, a further length of rubber tubing ending in a male metal adapter, a female adapter with a 'record' fitting, a short piece of rubber tubing and a narrow-bore stainless-steel needle protected by a small test-tube or piece of rubber tubing. A screw clip was attached to the rubber tubing just above the male adapter. A metal cannula attached to a short piece of rubber tubing and a female adapter could be used instead of the needle when it was necessary to cut down on a vein. If desired, the rubber tubing could be omitted and the cannula be attached directly to the male adapter.

The Wire Gauze Filter. The wire gauze filter consisted of a cylinder of close-meshed wire gauze, one end of which was open, the other partially closed by folding back the wire so as to leave a small hole for the passage of the $9\frac{1}{2}$-in. length of glass tubing. The gauze filter was fitted on to the $9\frac{1}{2}$-in. length of glass tubing, by pushing it up till the open end was pressed firmly against the rubber bung covering the open end of the $2\frac{1}{2}$-in. glass tube. A small ring of rubber tubing was then rolled up the $9\frac{1}{2}$-in. glass tubing until it came into contact with the other end of the filter (Fig. 9). This end, which was already partially occluded, was then firmly closed by pressure with artery forceps.

The Gas Mantle Filter. This type of filter consisted of an open cylindrical stocking of finely knitted cotton, as used in the manufacture of gas mantles. It was 3½ in. long, and was supplied by the makers threaded with a purse string at each end. The filter was supported inside the bottle by a ¼-in. piece of thick pressure tubing, which was pushed on to the long glass tube of the delivery set until it was about 2½ in. from the narrow end of the bung (Fig. 10). The stocking was slipped over the bung and the long tube; one end was fastened securely by tying its purse string beyond the pressure tubing, the other was fitted round the

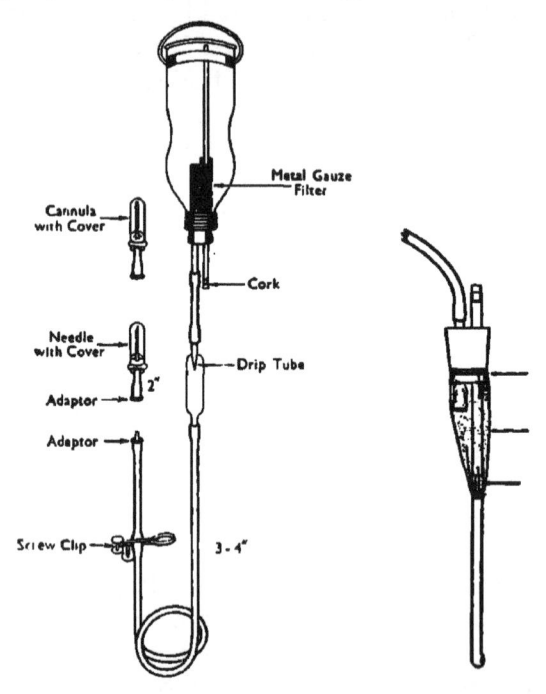

FIG. 9. Wire gauze filter   FIG. 10. Gas mantle filter

inner end of the bung (Fig. 10), where it could be fixed by fine copper wire (Fig. 10), or by grooving the neck of the bung so that the purse string could be tied tightly. In this way, the stocking was pulled into a stretched closed cone over the end of the delivery tube.

ANTI-COAGULANTS

After considerable experience with different anti-coagulant solutions the two following were generally used by the depot 'bleeding' teams as the most satisfactory:

(i) Trisodium citrate solution containing glucose;
(ii) Disodium hydrogen citrate solution containing glucose.

(i) Trisodium citrate solution containing glucose: This anti-coagulant consisted of 100 c.c. of 3 per cent. trisodium citrate in distilled water, to which was added 20 c.c. of 15 per cent. glucose in distilled water. The citrate and glucose were of a high grade of purity, and freshly distilled water was used for making up the solutions, which were filtered and autoclaved immediately. Glucose tends to caramelise during autoclaving in the presence of citrate; it was, therefore, necessary to sterilise the citrate and glucose solutions separately, and to mix after sterilisation; 120 c.c. of anti-coagulant solution was used for 420 c.c. of blood, making a total volume of 540 c.c. (approximately one pint).

(ii) Disodium hydrogen citrate solution containing glucose: Red cell preservation is most satisfactory when small amounts of disodium citrate are used, but clotting is then likely to occur unless brisk shaking is maintained throughout the period of blood collection. Solution (*a*) below is the better preservative. Solution (*b*) was used when it was impossible to ensure constant shaking throughout the collection :

(*a*) This solution consisted of 1·66 per cent. disodium citrate and 2·5 per cent. glucose; it was prepared by taking 2 g. disodium hydrogen citrate and 3 g. glucose, and making up to 120 c.c. with distilled water.

(*b*) This solution consisted of 2·08 per cent. disodium citrate and 2·5 per cent. glucose; it was prepared by taking 2·5 g. disodium hydrogen citrate and 3 g. glucose, and making up to 120 c.c. with distilled water.

Both mixtures were autoclaved with the production of a negligible amount of caramel, the amount varying with the quality of the glucose and the duration and temperature of autoclaving.

BLOOD GROUP DETERMINATION

When the depots were set up it was appreciated that the success of the service would largely depend upon the soundness of the blood grouping technique. At first supplies of suitable high titre grouping serum were made available by Dr. George L. Taylor of the Galton Serum Unit, administered by the Medical Research Council. Gradually, however, the depots became self-supporting in this respect. Each week as a routine the sera of large numbers of donors were tested to determine their titre and in this way a panel of high-titre donors was built up. At the same time valuable experience was gained in the technique of routine group determinations on a large scale. At one depot the error in group determinations during the first year was of the order of 8 per cent., but fell rapidly to less than 1 per cent., as the necessity of using high quality high titre sera and trained personnel was increasingly appreciated. The errors in later years were almost always secretarial, rather than technical. As the result of experience certain members of the Blood Transfusion

Research Committee prepared for the Medical Research Council a Report on Blood Groups, published as War Memorandum No. 9, in 1943.[12]

In addition to routine ABO determinations, Rh determinations also became in 1943 a routine depot procedure. Rh negative blood was kept in stock for maternity cases and patients needing repeated transfusion; transfusion reactions were investigated to determine if Rh incompatibility were possibly a responsible factor, and suspected cases of erythroblastosis foetalis were also studied. In some cases routine tests were made on all expectant mothers attending certain ante-natal clinics. Individuals shown in the course of testing to be Rh negative were issued with special group cards. This proved an important means of educating both the public and the general practitioner in the importance of Rh tests in maternity cases.

RESEARCH UNDERTAKEN BY THE DEPOTS

Apart from work mentioned elsewhere, a considerable body of research was carried out by depot staffs. This work was usually presented in the form of a report to the Blood Transfusion Research Committee and if of sufficient importance, was subsequently published in the scientific press. Many advances in the technique of preparing liquid serum and plasma were due to work done by Maizels in collaboration with the staff of the Medical Research Council Drying Plant at Cambridge. Fundamental studies were made particularly by Mollison and his colleagues on the Rh factor and its relation to erythroblastosis foetalis and on red cell survival. The latter has led to increased understanding of the haemolytic anaemias and to improvement in blood preservatives. Observations were made on the uses of serum and plasma in conditions other than 'shock', on the importance of massive and repeated transfusions after haemorrhage, on the anaemia and hypoproteinaemia associated with trauma, on blood volume changes following bleeding and transfusion, on the titre of ABO agglutinins in normal serum and their possible effect on transfusion reactions. Close liaison was maintained with workers in allied fields at the Lister Institute, the Wellcome Laboratories, the National Institute for Medical Research and the Galton Serum Unit, particularly those concerned with the preparation of blood products. The availability of large quantities of normal blood samples and the contacts maintained with widely scattered hospitals by a blood depot clearly offer unique opportunities to workers engaged in many different fields.

DEVELOPMENT OF THE DEPOTS

Contrary to expectation, there were no air raid casualties during the early months of the war. The depots were able to use this period to consolidate their organisation and improve their technique. Research was begun on improving the anti-coagulant solution used for the preservation of whole blood—the advantages of the addition of glucose to the citrate solution were thus shown (Dubash et al., 1940).[4] Controlled observations on the relative value of fresh and stored blood, made by medical officers especially appointed to carry out this work, demonstrated that in haemorrhage stored blood of good quality was of equal value to fresh blood (Brewer et al., 1940).[2]

At this time Group O blood was used almost entirely for transfusion, since it was thought that under emergency conditions it would be impossible to group all recipients. This led to repeated bleeding of a small section of the population, a far from satisfactory situation. A beginning was however made early in 1940 in the preparation of serum and plasma and in their clinical trial. This greatly simplified bleeding procedure as it meant that donors of all groups could be called up, the A, B and AB blood being used for the preparation of plasma or serum. At first serum and plasma were prepared according to their blood group and given after cross matching as in a blood transfusion, but it was soon appreciated that the pooling of all groups reduced the titre of ABO agglutinins to insignificant levels and therefore made the plasma and serum a universal donor product.

The depot organisation was first called upon to supply transfusion fluids in bulk at the time of Dunkirk. The availability of large quantities of blood and limited amounts of plasma or serum together with the necessary apparatus then proved its worth. During the first six months of the war the hospitals learnt to rely on the depots for prompt help in need and constant reliable service during quiet times and in many instances the sector transfusion organisation was to a large extent taken over by the depots. In others both continued to work together in a satisfactory manner for some time, though increasing shortage of personnel gradually led to a still further use of the centralised and therefore rather more economical depot service.

After Dunkirk, when plasma and serum had clearly proved their worth, intensive work was done on the best methods of collecting serum and plasma and on their final preparation in both liquid and dried forms. This work was done by the depot staffs, later with the co-operation of certain regional transfusion officers, and the staff of the Medical Research Council Serum Drying Unit at Cambridge. All new products received clinical trial by depot medical officers, thanks to the willing collaboration of the staffs of certain hospitals, especially those of the Middlesex County Council, before being issued for general use. In the course of these clinical trials, both medical officers and nurses developed valuable technical skill and much of interest was learnt about reactions after transfusion.

When severe air raids began in the winter of 1940, the depots found themselves able to meet all the demands made upon them, and most valuable experience was gained by many of their medical officers in treating traumatic conditions requiring transfusion. It was then first appreciated that many cases required very large doses if life was to be saved. The healthy individual suddenly subjected to trauma reacted to transfusion in a very different way from the medical case. At this time it was shown that the original calculation that 10 per cent. of casualties would require transfusion, on which the depot organisation had been built up, was correct. On the average each casualty received $2\frac{1}{2}$ bottles of fluid, and roughly 2 bottles of blood were used for every bottle of plasma. However, in two sectors supplied only with dried serum and no blood, satisfactory results were reported. When constant heavy bombardment ceased in the spring of 1941 it might have been expected that the demand for blood and blood products would decrease. Far from this, it continued to rise. Both surgeons and physicians had learnt to appreciate the value of transfusion as a therapeutic aid. The supply of standardised equipment ready sterilised and of a simple type had greatly reduced the difficulties of giving a transfusion, and further, the necessary technique had been learnt during the blitz period by a large number of medical men. Throughout the war there was a steady increase of the practice of transfusion all over the country. In many cases no doubt the pendulum swung too far and unnecessary transfusions were given, but on the whole the educative value of the war transfusion service was great.

In addition to bleeding in order to maintain blood stocks, the depots throughout 1941 and 1942 undertook an increasingly heavy programme in order to maintain adequate supplies of dried products. By 1943 it was considered that adequate stocks of dried material were available in the London depots and the surplus could be given to the Armed Forces, the Colonial civilian services and the Merchant Navy. In times of stress also the depots proved able to supply whole blood to the Forces and to regions whose organisation had been temporarily impaired by enemy action. Up to the end of 1943, Group O blood had been used extensively for transfusion as whole blood, while the other groups were pooled for preparing serum and plasma. It now became depot policy to encourage the use of group-to-group transfusion, for two reasons. Firstly, it was recognised that if very large demands were made for whole blood, as were made indeed by the Army in 1944, there would not be sufficient universal donor blood. Secondly, it was increasingly recognised that the most satisfactory results were obtained from group-to-group transfusion. When the Continent was invaded, the capacity of a depot organisation suddenly to increase its bleeding to meet a greatly increased demand was clearly demonstrated. One depot which had been bleeding 800 to 1,000 donors a week raised the figure to over 3,000. Even at this time of emergency, group-to-group transfusions were given at the majority of hospitals.

During the last year of the war plasma was also supplied to the Lister Institute for the preparation, at first on an experimental scale, of other blood products, especially thrombin, fibrinogen and fibrin foams. The value of these, particularly to the cerebral and plastic surgeons, became increasingly apparent, and production soon passed beyond the experimental stage.

Figures showing the gradual expansion of the depot work from 1939 to 1945 appear in Table I. In every case a large proportion of the material was used for civilian sick, particularly for maternity cases, so demonstrating the essential importance as a therapeutic aid of adequate supplies of blood products under all circumstances. The depots which were designed to meet a war emergency had proved themselves by 1940 to be, with the Regional transfusion laboratories, an essential part of the medical service of the country. The two were merged in 1946 to form the National Blood Transfusion Service under the Ministry of Health. This service will continue to supply blood, serum, plasma and apparatus for transfusion; it will also provide the Lister Institute and other centres with raw material needed for the preparation of essential blood products. This liaison of a practical service in the field with active centres of research, which proved so successful during the war, should yield an even richer harvest under conditions of peace.

THE REGIONAL BLOOD TRANSFUSION SERVICE

Up to the latter half of 1940, no central provision for a comprehensive transfusion service had been considered outside the London area. The provincial arrangements were, as in London before the war, local, voluntary and in many areas non-existent. Blood panels were organised by voluntary bodies such as the British Red Cross and St. John Ambulance Association, or by private individuals, as was the very large and efficient panel service at Birmingham, by medical schools, as in Liverpool and Manchester, or by municipal authorities in some large towns. There was little or no co-ordination between the local services and no standardisation of apparatus. It was therefore decided to establish a regional blood transfusion service under the E.M.S., and in July 1940, a draft scheme was drawn up by Dr. P. N. Panton (afterwards Sir Philip Panton) and Dr. A. N. Drury of the Medical Research Council, which after certain modifications, was approved by the Ministry of Health and sanctioned by the Treasury.

Blood transfusion centres, very much on the lines of the London blood banks, were set up in each Civil Defence Region, except in Region 7 which was covered by the Army blood transfusion service at Bristol. These additional centres were formed at Newcastle, Leeds, Birmingham, Nottingham, Cambridge, Oxford, Cardiff, Manchester and Liverpool, so that with the exception of the Nottingham bank, all were closely associated with a university department of pathology. This association was found to be so valuable that after the war it was decided to move the Nottingham bank to Sheffield.

These centres were thus situated at the headquarters of each Civil Defence Region with the following exceptions:

In Region 10 with its population of about seven millions, there were already two highly efficient blood transfusion organisations connected with the Universities of Liverpool and Manchester, which normally supplied the needs of large populations in considerable areas. This Region was therefore divided into two parts, with the Directors of the Liverpool and Manchester organisations respectively in honorary charge. The Liverpool area under Professor T. B. Davie, Professor of Pathology, Liverpool University, comprised the counties of Cumberland and Westmorland and the northern and western area of Lancashire, the adjoining portions of Cheshire and the four northern counties of Wales in Region 8, which were much more accessible from Liverpool than from South Wales and in peace-time had looked to Liverpool for their supplies. The Manchester area was under Dr. J. F. Wilkinson, the Director of the Medical Research Department of Manchester University; it included the densely populated south-east portion of Lancashire, the greater part of Cheshire and the small part of Derbyshire west of the Pennines. Each honorary director was provided with a whole-time assistant transfusion officer.

In Region 6, the transfusion centre was at Oxford under the direction of Dr. Robb-Smith, Director of Pathology, Radcliffe Infirmary, in an honorary capacity.

In Region 12, the portions not already covered by the London Scheme were provided for by extending this scheme to the rest of the counties of Kent and Sussex. For this purpose sub-depots were opened at Canterbury and Chichester under the charge of whole-time assistant transfusion officers.

At headquarters, Lt. Colonel L. W. Proger, R.A.M.C., who had been in charge of the blood transfusion services of the B.E.F. in France, was appointed to the staff of the Director-General of the Emergency Medical Services to assist Dr. P. N. Panton in dealing with the blood transfusion scheme. A central plant for drying plasma had been originally proposed to provide a national pool, but as the Medical Research Council were already producing large quantities of dried plasma and the R.A.M.C. also had very largely increased their output as a reserve for the supply of Forces overseas, a national plant was not considered to be necessary.

A senior whole-time transfusion officer was appointed to each of the other centres and, with only two changes, carried on throughout the war.

The duties of these officers were to organise transfusion services throughout their Regions. The service was to include:

1. A Regional laboratory for processing and storing plasma and serum, to be fed from blood-taking centres chiefly located in the main hospitals.
2. The supply of equipment for all large casualty hospitals for taking as well as giving blood.
3. The training of medical personnel at each of the selected hospitals in the technique of taking and giving blood.
4. The transport of blood in special blood vans to and from hospitals.
5. The recruitment of blood donors and the grouping of bloods.
6. The maintenance of close liaison with the transfusion officers of the Army to avoid overlapping.

As in the London depots, an adequate staff of assistant medical officers, scientific workers, nurses and technicians was appointed and the necessary transport provided. This transport maintained an almost daily link between all the hospitals in England and Wales and, as it was the only organisation on this scale available to the Ministry, came to be of great value for other purposes than those of the transfusion service. The preliminary and rapid distribution of penicillin, for example, could not have been effected in any other way.

PROGRESS OF THE SCHEME

As in London, at the start of the service the transfusion officers were instructed to make all possible use of existing organisations and of voluntary effort and all active panels were soon incorporated in the Regional organisations or very closely affiliated with them. The voluntary bodies, of which the British Red Cross and St. John Ambulance Association were the most important, provided much of the personnel both at the depots and at the centres connected with them. Other voluntary help was freely given. Many members of hospital staffs and general practitioners helped at the bleeding depots either on a voluntary or a paid sessional basis. Large donor panels were enrolled at each Regional depot and at all centres of population within the Region; blood was always available for routine hospital use for every air raid emergency and for supplementing the Service organisations, including those of the United States. The Air Force and the Navy were largely supplied from the civilian depots, and the Army blood transfusion service was considerably supplemented. From D-day onwards regular supplies of blood were driven or flown to Bristol from Leeds and other supplies came from Nottingham, Cardiff and the London banks. In addition to the E.M.S. hospitals, all civilian patients were provided for and a special service, including the provision of Rh negative blood, was arranged for maternity homes. The transfusion officers not only supplied, blood but gave transfusions when required, and frequently advised on the treatment of shock cases. The service became an indispensable part of ordinary medical practice, and the demand for blood and blood products rose out of all proportion to the special circumstances of a state of war.

Citrated whole blood, serum, plasma and suspensions of concentrated red cells were prepared at each depot the grouping, including Rh grouping, was carried out there, in most depots the Wasserman or Kahn tests also. Cleaning, assembling and sterilising apparatus occupied a considerable staff, much of which was unpaid.

In 1942, the weekly output of the drying plant in Cambridge, which had been greatly enlarged, reached a peak of some 2,000—2,500 bottles, a number sufficient to supply the Regions as well as to supplement the Services' needs; a very considerable additional supply was also sent from Canada. The Cambridge plant was fed with serum and plasma from the London and Regional banks, as well as from the Navy, Army and, to a lesser extent, the Air Force bleeding teams. By the end of the war sufficient stocks of dried product had been accumulated to justify an early closing down of the Cambridge plant and to consider replacing it with a much smaller one, possibly in the London area.

Throughout the war the donor response never failed; indeed, the numbers enrolled in most Regions were excessive and the chief complaint of the volunteers was that they were not called upon often enough. This response was largely due to the appeal of the Services and the civilian air raid victims, but the need for blood was constantly kept before the public by the judicious use of posters and newspaper articles, as well as by the radio and the screen. The necessary publicity, no doubt, over-emphasised the place of blood transfusion in medical practice but will still be essential when the circumstances of war are no longer present. Voluntary blood donation is now popular and there is every indication that, if constantly kept before the public, it will continue in the time of peace.

The war-time blood transfusion service never failed to provide what was asked of it; there were no large-scale calamities, and the number of complaints from donors, recipients or doctors was negligible; the service was enthusiastically supported at the beginning, and the end of the war found it still more popular and above criticism in the public mind. But for those engaged in the service there was constant anxiety, there were individual calamities, many minor reactions and, while such known disasters as the transference of syphilis were successfully avoided, the later stages of the war disclosed a danger hitherto unsuspected. The danger of the transmission of the virus of infective jaundice was not recognised until relatively late in the war, chiefly because of the long latent period between the transfusion and the onset of the disease.

WORK OF THE REGIONAL TRANSFUSION CENTRES

It will be seen that the work of the Regional centres was carried out on much the same lines as that of the London depots with which they were in many respects integrated; a fuller account of the work of these centres would therefore entail much unnecessary repetition.

As in the London depots much independent and correlated research work was carried out in the provincial Regions with the object of improving the methods of preparing blood products and their storage, the prevention of contamination, the avoidance of transfusion reactions in the recipients and the transmission of infectious diseases. The methods found valuable were reported to the M.R.C. Research Committee, who circulated all useful information in M.R.C. memoranda to the other Regions and to the London depots. Where applicable, these were also circulated by the Ministry of Health to the E.M.S. hospitals for the information of the hospital transfusion officers. The results of many of these researches were also published from time to time in the medical press. For example:

1. (a) The first attempt at drying plasma in this country was made in the Liverpool Transfusion Centre. This method was published in an article which also described the methods of withdrawing, storing and delivering plasma used at this centre.[5].

(b) An investigation was carried out into the reactions to the administration of blood, fresh or stored. These reactions were divided in three grades [17] and tended to establish that the incidence of reactions with preserved blood was probably no greater than with fresh blood.[5] The authors also found that Grade 3 reactions were increased by the age of the blood and further analysed the results of transfusion in a great variety of clinical conditions.

(c) An analysis of the incidence of fainting among 3,241 donors was also made. The percentage fainting proved to be 6·848 in both sexes of all ages and suggested that fainting was much commoner in donors under 30 than among the older groups and that males fainted more frequently in the younger groups and less frequently in the older ones.[20]

2. In the Manchester Centre much valuable work on the drying of plasma was also carried out.[21] [22]

Note: These and all other methods of drying plasma were soon superseded by freeze drying in vacuo. The technique had been known for many years but was only developed to a high standard of efficiency during the war, and this became the procedure of choice for preserving a variety of biological materials both in the laboratory and on a commercial scale. The story of the development of the technique for preserving proteins by drying was related in detail by Greaves.[7]

3. The Regional transfusion centre at Cambridge carried out research into 'Defribrination'[9]; 'The Separation of Serum in Bulk'[9]; 'Plasma utilisation in Serum Processing'[15] and the 'Transfusion of Filtered Liquid Serum'.[10] This laboratory—unlike most of the other Regional centres, which stored filtered liquid plasma and very little serum—after October 1940, stored filtered liquid serum only, for the reasons given in the last-named article above and which can be summarised as follows:

(i) As about 80 per cent. of all citrated blood is eventually processed and stored as plasma, there is no reason why this percentage of blood collected should not be processed immediately after collection, avoiding the interval during which bacterial growth by contamination can occur.

(ii) If blood is processed at once citration and filtration of plasma is unnecessary. It is simpler to collect clotted blood and filter the serum. It is also more economical and the product has a much higher protein content. When dried 400 c.c. of serum yield about 28 g. of protein, compared with about 18 g. from the same volume of citrated plasma, as no anti-coagulent has been added.

(iii) No filter is required in the giving set in transfusing serum.

(iv) In a sample of 838 transfusions of which records were kept and communicated to the centres, the reaction rate was 4 per cent.; 5 patients showed rigor and a rise of temperature; 18 rise of temperature without rigor and 5 slight rigor without rise of temperature.

Liquid serum separated from the clot within forty-eight hours of collection and sterilised by Seitz-filtration was therefore deemed a non-toxic safe material for transfusion.

APPARATUS

The apparatus used in the Regional centres was the standardised type as used in the London depots, which has been fully described by Dr. Janet Vaughan, with certain small modifications introduced by the directors in some of the centres to meet variations in technique.

Table I summarises the blood donations in London and the Provinces during the war period, while Tables II and III give some indication of filtrations done in the Provincial Depots, at Cambridge and at the Lister Institute, and the drying of plasma at Cambridge in each of the war years.

TABLE I
Blood Donors and Donations, 1939–1945

	Approximate number of active donors on panels at end of year						Number of blood donations					
	1940	1941	1942	1943	1944	1945	Sept. 1939 to Nov. 1941	1942	1943	1944	1945	1939–1945
Area served by the 4 London Blood Supply Depots.	160,000	200,000	266,000	279,000	373,000	208,000	186,493	107,000	141,032	214,566	142,502	791,593
The remainder of England and Wales, excepting the South-Western Region (Region 7) which was covered by the Army Blood Transfusion Service. (a)	Not known	563,000	616,000	675,000	632,000	245,000	Late 1940 to Nov. 3, 1941 215,252 (b)	281,163	321,981	454,684	293,932	1,567,012
Totals		763,000	882,000	954,000	1,005,000	453,000	401,745	388,163	463,013	669,250	436,434	2,358,605

(a) These figures include civilian organisations in the Southern Region (Region 6). The large number of donors in this Region who were bled by mobile teams from the Army Blood Transfusion Service in 1942–45 are excluded.
(b) From the opening of the Regional Transfusion Centres which occurred during the period July to September 1940.

Table II

Bottles of 400 c.c. of Plasma or Serum Filtered

PROVINCES*

September 1939 to November 1941	1942 (a)	1943 (b)	1944 (c)	1945 (d)	Total
64,866	86,050	68,781	30,036	13,614	198,481

(a) 50,251 bottles filtered, to Services.
(b) 63,112 bottles filtered, to Cambridge.
    3,099 Winchester quarts unfiltered, to Cambridge.
    1,661 bottles filtered, to Services.
    9,148 litres unfiltered, to Services.
    15,594 bottles dried products, to Services.
(c) 54,644 bottles filtered, to Cambridge.
    16,088 Winchester quarts unfiltered, to Cambridge.
    49,954 bottles whole-blood, to Services.
    9,119 Winchester quarts unfiltered, to Services.
    3,582 bottles dried products, to Services.
(d) 22,575 bottles filtered, to Cambridge.
    8,231 Winchester quarts unfiltered, to Cambridge.
    40,801 bottles whole-blood, to Services.
    3,850 litres, unfiltered, to Services.
    1,975 bottles dried products, to Services.

* There are no corresponding figures for the London depots as serum and plasma from these were sent in bulk to the Cambridge Unit for filtration. The output of the Cambridge Plant is shown in Table III.

Table III

Work of the Cambridge Filtration and Drying Plant and of the Lister Institute

	1940	1941	1942 (a)	1943 (a)	1944 (a)	1945 (a)	1940–5
Filtration: Cambridge	638 (a) 10,825 (b)	9,857 (a) 7,995 (b)	12,694	33,750	51,110	31,761	139,810 (a) 18,820 (b)
Lister Institute	—	—	—	5,599	31,720	13,913	51,232 (a)
Drying: Cambridge	9,400 (b)	4,600 (a) 9,457 (b)	9,160	69,246	101,602	49,096	233,704 (a) 18,857 (b)
Totals (bottles)	20,863	31,909	21,854	108,595	184,432	94,770	462,423

(a) = transfusion bottles each containing 400 c.c.
(b) = "medical flats" each containing 200 c.c.

Raw material was supplied to the Cambridge Unit chiefly from the London and Provincial Blood Transfusion Services, but also from the Army, and Navy, while the Lister Institute received its material solely from the London Depots.

GENERAL COMMENTARY

In the practice of blood transfusion the war has taught us three main lessons:

(1) Until such time as a safe and equally effective substitute can be discovered, blood transfusion has come to stay and the practice of it has increased prodigiously and will increase still further.

(2) The demand can be met, provided the appropriate organisation is available.

(3) Blood and the blood products are highly dangerous materials, but the dangers can for the most part be avoided under constant supervision by highly skilled personnel. False grouping, the transmission of infectious diseases other than jaundice, the use of the proper kinds and amounts of transfused fluid, the serious danger of infected material, can only be successfully dealt with if the utmost care is taken. The prevention of jaundice is still under investigation and this unsolved problem serves as a reminder that blood transfusion is not in its final phase but is still in urgent need of further research.

Transfusion is a procedure directed to the treatment of disorders of the circulation. There is little in medicine on which the study of the circulation does not impinge and it is for this reason that the advances stimulated by war in this field have had profound repercussions in many fields of civilian medical practice, and are likely to have more.

REFERENCES

[1] BRADLEY, W. H., LOUTIT, J. F., and MAUNSELL, K. (1944). *Brit. med. J.*, 2, 268.
[2] BREWER, H. F., MAIZELS, M., OLIVER, J. O., and VAUGHAN, J. (1940). Ibid., 2, 48.
[3] BROWN, H., and McCORMACK, P. (1942). Ibid., 1, 1.
[4] DUBASH, J., CLEGG, O., and VAUGHAN, J. (1940). Ibid., 2, 482.
[5] EDWARDS, F. R., and DAVIE, T. B. (1940). Ibid., 2, 73.
[6] —— KAY, J., and DAVIE, T. B. (1940). Ibid., 1, 377.
[7] GREAVES, R. I. N. (1946). Medical Research Council publication on the *Preservation of Proteins by Drying*. Special Report Series No. 258, H.M.S.O. London.
[8] GREENBURY, C. L. (1942). *Brit. med. J.*, 1, 253.
[9] HARRISON, G. A. and PICKEN, L. E. R. (1941a, b). *Lancet*, 1, 405. Ibid., 1, 536.
[10] —— —— and Ackroyd, S. (1943). Ibid., 1, 268.
[11] LOUTIT, J. F., and MAUNSELL, K. (1945). *Brit. med. J.*, 2, 759.
[12] MEDICAL RESEARCH COUNCIL (1943). *War Memorandum No. 9; Determination of Blood Groups*. H.M.S.O. London.
[13] MEDICAL RESEARCH COUNCIL (1944). *War Memorandum No. 1; 2nd ed. Wound Shock*. H.M.S.O., London.
[14] MORGAN, H. V., and WILLIAMSON, D. A. J. (1943). *Brit. med. J.*, 1, 750.
[15] PICKEN, L. E. R. (1941). *Lancet*, 2, 190.
[16] REPORT TO MEDICAL RESEARCH COUNCIL (1944). *Brit. med. J.*, 1, 279.
[17] RIDDELL, V. H. (1939). *Blood Transfusion*. Oxford Univ. Press, London.
[18] SPOONER, E. T. C., and TURNBULL, L. H. (1942). *Bull. War Med.*, 2, 345.
[19] SPURLING, N., SHONE, J., and VAUGHAN, J. M. (1946). *Brit. med. J.*, 2, 409.
[20] WILLIAMS, G. E. O. (1942). Ibid., 1, 783.
[21] WILKINSON, J. F., AYLWARD, F. X., and MAINWARING, B. R. S. (1940a, b and c). *Lancet*, 1, 685. Ibid., 2, 385. *Brit. med. J.*, 2, 583.
[22] —— BULLOCK, K., and COWAN, W. (1942). *Lancet*, 1, 281.

CHAPTER 12
RADIOLOGY

by
A. E. BARCLAY
O.B.E., M.D., F.R.C.P.
Consultant Adviser in Radiology

RADIOLOGY IN THE WAR OF 1914-18

It was natural that the experience gained in the last war should be taken as the basis of planning for the Emergency Medical Services. During the War of 1914-18 radiology was virtually in its infancy and had not yet become an essential pre-requisite of practically all treatment and operative procedure. Although the application of radiology had been considerable in that war, its use had been confined almost entirely to the examination of fractures and the localisation of foreign bodies, as radiography had not as yet been universally recognised as essential for the proper treatment of many disabilities. In fact, there had been little demand for anything more than the examination of casualties and even then only if circumstances made it relatively easy; in rush periods of offensives, X-ray examinations were usually omitted.

ADVANCES DURING THE INTER-WAR PERIOD

When war came in 1939, radiology was on a wholly different plane from that of twenty-five years before. Now recognised as an essential component of medical service, it found its allotted place in the scheme for an Emergency Medical Service planned during the threatening months of 1938-9.

SUPPLY OF APPARATUS

The Emergency Hospital Scheme proposed to use a considerable proportion of the beds in all existing hospitals which had adequate equipment and staff to deal with the X-ray work, but further accommodation was to be provided in mental hospitals, public assistance institutions and sanatoria, to many of which hutted accommodation was to be added, and also in a few *ad hoc* hutted hospitals. There were no X-ray facilities in most of these emergency hospitals and, even in those where X-ray plant existed, provision for X-ray service was on a scale that was inadequate for the expected volume of work. In most of these hospitals, therefore, either extension of existing facilities or new departments were required, and in most cases the latter alternative had been adopted. Contractors were provided with standard plans of these hutted extensions and in them the detail of the X-ray department was laid down. It was to be placed at one end of the operating theatre hut and consisted of a good X-ray room, a dark room and a store. Unfortunately, these plans were not submitted to the consultant advisers and it was not till well on in the autumn of 1939, when the buildings were far advanced, that they saw these plans. It was then too late to alter the layout, in which the only access to the X-ray department was through the operating theatre, to which very naturally surgeons made strenuous objections. Radiologists also objected to the fact that the department was not centrally sited to save the transport of cases. Nothing could be done about the siting, but access was provided by an outside path for which, in some cases only, authority was obtained for providing a covered way (see Fig. 3, page 38).

In the department itself there were many mistakes and deficiencies. For instance, the store room had to be made into the radiologist's room, leaving no store room; there was no hatch or light trap for the darkroom; the black-out blinds were deemed adequate for the X-ray room and even for the dark-room, and no furniture of any kind had been ordered. There were many other similar if minor mistakes. The X-ray rooms were all to be lined with lead, which was entirely useless and unnecessary, but the orders had gone forward and could not be corrected. The many and various alterations required to make these departments usable cost between £250–£300 in each case. The fundamental error of siting these X-ray departments so far away from the centre and without satisfactory access inevitably caused increase of transport and made difficult the essential collaboration of radiologist and clinician.

These X-ray departments were expected to deal only with casualty work for which mobile units and simple X-ray couches would meet the needs, and in the summer of 1939 a number of these sets, together with complete outfits of all accessories, including dark-room equipment, had been ordered. The departments gradually came into use as they were completed in 1940.

In the general scheme London was to be divided into ten Sectors, each based on one or more of the teaching hospitals, and on the outbreak of war the bulk of the work of the London hospitals was to be evacuated to the Sector hospitals in the country. This would need complete reorganisation of the X-ray services and Sector Radiologists were therefore appointed to work in conjunction with the Consultant Adviser in Radiology to deal with the problems in these sectors. For E.M.S. purposes the rest of the country was divided into Regions and for some of these Regional Radiologists were also appointed.

When war came, the E.M.S. scheme was put into action. These were busy days, particularly for the London Sector Radiologists who were faced with the organisation of an X-ray service in emergency hospitals in which there were often neither mains supply of current nor suitable accommodation. Their work for the most part was accomplished by transferring such personnel and apparatus as could be spared from the parent teaching and other hospitals, and by improvising departments in such accommodation as was available. Naturally, apparatus was very scarce and the Sector Radiologists begged and borrowed from any source they could find. Within a fortnight of the outbreak of war they had succeeded in providing at least a skeleton X-ray service in all the main Sector hospitals which had come into being. This was no mean achievement even though, in the event, their facilities were not called into use for months. In the provinces, however, the scheme for evacuating main hospitals to the country was not complete on the outbreak of war, nor was it ever carried into effect. These hospitals carried on as usual but with reduced numbers, a proportion of beds being allocated for E.M.S. work; and the special E.M.S. hospitals of various types, as already described, came into being as rapidly as the supply of material and labour permitted, priority being accorded to those most urgently required.

In all these emergency hospitals there was difficulty in obtaining a satisfactory electric supply. In most of them heavy cables had to be laid, often for considerable distances, in order to draw current direct from the mains. This problem, however, was most difficult in the mental hospitals used for E.M.S. purposes as they were often far distant from a 'grid' supply. These institutions usually developed their own electricity and it was always direct current. This raised a difficult problem for X-ray work for it had to be converted to alternating current and this inevitably entailed loss of efficiency, usually reducing the output of X-ray apparatus by about 30 per cent. Moreover, in many of these institutions the generating plant was underpowered and could not take an additional load. In spite of running special cables from the power house direct to the X-ray department, this inefficiency could not be much reduced and sometimes this handicap had to be accepted as there was no 'grid' current available within miles.

TYPES OF APPARATUS SUPPLIED

A brief description of the types of apparatus employed and how it was provided seems to have its place at this point. X-ray apparatus may be classified under four main types: (*a*) the portable set, (*b*) the mobile set, (*c*) 2-valve fixed set and (*d*) 4-valve fixed set.

(*a*) The portable set could be dismantled and easily transported either by hand or on a trolley; it was shockproof and was employed mostly at the bedside, but its output was small (5 or 10 ma.) and only suitable for the radiography of limbs.

(*b*) The mobile unit, more usually styled the ward trolley unit, was considerably heavier; it moved on castors and was transportable rather than mobile. It was much used in X-ray departments as a fixed unit, but was mobile on smooth surfaces and could be taken to the wards and used as a bedside unit if necessary. Most of these sets were moved about a good deal and many were damaged by the shaking they received when wheeled over rough surfaces. The set was self-rectified, i.e. without valves, the X-ray tube utilising one half of the electric cycle and suppressing the other; it was shockproof and simple to operate, and the X-ray tube stand was an integral part of the unit. The capacity was considerable (30 ma. 90 kv.) and its output was capable of dealing with the thick parts of the body, though with relatively long exposures. Chest work, for instance, could be done but the exposure required was too long to give the fine detail that is necessary for this class of work. The set was accompanied by a simple couch, fitted with a Potter Bucky diaphragm. In practice these sets did admirable work and dealt with the bulk of the fractures and other relatively simple cases. Provision was made for locating foreign bodies, but none for upright screening and it was not intended that the apparatus should be used for that purpose. In a number of hospitals, however, home made screening stands were fitted by enthusiastic resident medical officers; this led to ill-conceived surgery based on valueless or misleading X-ray examinations, and this use of the apparatus had to be prohibited.

(c) The 2-valve fixed set, which also utilised only half the cycle, the other half being suppressed by the valve, was coupled to a fixed couch, at the end of which was a screening stand. This combination apparatus was more powerful than the mobile sets and could deal with all kinds of work provided that there was time to make the necessary adjustments, particularly from screening with the tube below the couch to examination of the patient in the erect posture. A number of these sets was ordered in 1940 when it was realised that E.M.S. hospitals must deal with gastro-intestinal and other 'heavy' cases, but delivery was much delayed largely by the blitz. When the sets came into use, however, it was evident that they were too slow in operation to cope with the unexpectedly large volume of 'heavy' work that then had to be dealt with in the larger E.M.S. hospitals.

(d) The unexpectedly large demand for all types of X-ray work in E.M.S. hospitals rendered it essential to provide many of them with a full-scale apparatus capable of dealing with all classes of work. For this purpose a unit was selected that comprised a 4-valve generator and a motor-driven combined couch and screening stand. This made a compact unit that could be easily housed in the rather limited space that was usually available.

Most of the above apparatus was obtained from manufacturers in this country, but on account of the labour shortage, by 1943 a considerable number of the 4-valve sets were obtained from the U.S.A. under lend/lease. In addition to these main sources of supply, the American Red Cross generously presented units either direct to the hospitals or through the Ministry of Health.

The following table gives the total apparatus provided during the war, showing the year of supply:

X-Ray Apparatus Supplied

Date	Portable units	Mobile units	Fixed Units 2-valve	Fixed Units 4-valve	Fixed Units Unrectified	Dental units	Skin therapy units	Deep therapy units	Total
1939	—	50	—	—	1	—	—	—	51
1940	61	117	29	18	3	11	14	—	253
1941	43	44	13	15	1	—	4	—	120
1942	6	5	6	12	—	—	—	—	29
1943	3	4	5	4	—	—	—	—	16
1944	20	1	1	6	—	7	—	—	35
1945	3	1	1	3	—	5	1	1	15
1946	—	—	—	9	—	—	—	4	13
	136	222	55	67	5	23	19	5	532

Of the above, 20 portable units, 42 mobile units, 16 fixed units, 1 dental unit, 19 skin therapy units and 5 deep therapy units (94 by gift and 9 by purchase or lend/lease) were supplied from America. The remaining 429 were purchased in Britain except for 2 portable units, a gift from the Silver Thimble Fund, and 13 mobile units lent by the British Red Cross Society.

DIFFICULTIES TO BE OVERCOME

All through the autumn and winter of 1939-40 very few of the E.M.S. beds were occupied either in the metropolitan area or in the provinces, thus giving time for organisation and equipment. It was not till the spring of 1940 that a small proportion of the beds was filled by convoys from the military hospitals overseas, evacuated in view of the coming offensive. Although the number of patients was not large in proportion to the hospital facilities available, they at once showed the weakness of an organisation built up to deal only with casualties, for the bulk of the cases were of classes that required X-ray examinations of ordinary civilian type, with an extraordinarily high proportion of gastro-intestinal cases with which mobile units could not deal. The number of gastro-intestinal cases was far greater than could be dealt with as intended, by transfer to properly equipped ordinary civilian hospitals, and it was therefore necessary to instal more adequate apparatus in some of the larger E.M.S. hospitals. X-ray apparatus of the 2-valve type was chosen and a simple design of combination unit was evolved by the Sector Radiologists, but it was about eighteen months before these sets came into use.

In the meantime Dunkirk had been evacuated and, with the consequent occupation of many of the E.M.S. beds, it was realised that the casualty work, far from being the major charge on the X-ray department, even after this tragedy, was of minor importance as compared with the cases of ordinary civilian type that were sent for X-ray examination. It was only for short periods during blitzes and after offensives that the casualty work sometimes brought long hours of duty before all cases had been dealt with. Hence, a further effort was made to equip as many as possible of the major E.M.S. hospitals with apparatus that could deal with 'heavy' X-ray cases, but this was not possible on a large scale and had to await the delivery of the 2-valve sets already on order. When eventually this apparatus was delivered, it was found that although competent to deal with small numbers of these 'heavy' cases, it was altogether too slow in adaptation to meet the needs of a busy department in which the bulk of the work was of the ordinary civilian types. It was decided, therefore, to use these sets in the less busy E.M.S. hospitals and to replace them with 4-valve sets and tilting couches in as many as possible of the important and busy hospitals. By degrees all hospitals were adequately equipped for the work with which they had to deal.

It might appear from this account that the problems of apparatus supply were comparatively simple. This was far from being the case, and work was often carried on under very great difficulties until, gradually, suitable apparatus could be installed. For instance, in one outlying hospital which was allocated for head injuries, the electric supply was direct current produced in the hospital. It was quite impossible at the time to provide apparatus for the important and highly specialised work in this hospital. Yet work was successfully carried on by a very ingenious and resourceful radiologist who adapted his own portable apparatus, using many make-shift devices, and employed it with satisfactory results, overloading it unmercifully and always at the risk of complete breakdown, until the position was relieved by the provision of suitable apparatus. To obtain satisfactory ventriculograms with such apparatus and with the handicap of direct current was a very fine achievement—an achievement that was paralleled in other hospitals under equally difficult circumstances.

The shortage of X-ray tubes and valves, virtually all of which came from America, was serious, and in the early years of the war held up not only the delivery of apparatus but sometimes the work in departments. But on the whole the requirements of the X-ray service for apparatus were met, and during the last two years of the war there was no serious difficulty.

At no time was there any shortage of X-ray films. In 1942, a great advance was made by the introduction of a new type of X-ray film which was so much more sensitive that it reduced the exposures by half. This advance was of considerable importance in that it so increased the efficiency of the portable and mobile sets that they were able to cope with many of the difficult cases that otherwise would have had to be transferred to hospitals where more powerful apparatus was available.

Throughout the war the closest co-operation in all matters existed between the E.M.S. and the Army authorities, and particularly in regard to the supply of X-ray apparatus; in order to avoid conflicting interests the Army confined itself to certain firms while the Ministry dealt with others.

STAFFING OF X-RAY DEPARTMENTS

The problem of staffing all these new X-ray departments was one of considerable difficulty. It was a first principle that all new X-ray departments should be controlled by a radiologist, but the number of radiologists available even at the beginning of the war was limited, and some of them would certainly go to the Forces. It has already been stressed that the work to be undertaken in the new E.M.S. hospitals was expected to be simple and not to take much of the radiologist's time. Hence, one radiologist might undertake the supervision of several of these E.M.S. hospitals in addition to his normal commitments. In the event, this arrangement threw a very heavy strain on most of the radiologists, particularly when it became obvious that the E.M.S. hospitals must deal with many cases of ordinary civilian types for which, in the circumstances, they had not the time that is essential for radiology on a consultant basis. Surgeons also became equally busy, and, as the close co-operation that is essential for satisfactory work was usually absent, a written report had often to take the place of consultation.

TRAINING OF RADIOLOGISTS

Early in 1941, representations were made that the number of radiologists in H.M. Forces and in the E.M.S. was likely to be seriously short of what was required for efficient service, and it was suggested that the Ministry of Health should enrol radiological house officers at hospitals where training for degrees or diplomas in radio-diagnosis could be given. The proposal was accepted and a selection board comprised of a number of consulting radiologists and a representative of the E.M.S. interviewed each applicant. Only those young practitioners who had held at least one hospital appointment, and intended to make radiology their career, were considered eligible.

Between 1941 and 1945 out of about 250 applications, 70 practitioners in four groups, were selected and posted for duty in London and the provinces, usually to hospitals at which there was a medical school. The only obligation they were asked to meet was to give one year's service, after special qualification, in the E.M.S. at an appropriate salary. Those in the final group were medically examined by the War Office before acceptance, as it was intended they should be recruited as soon as they had taken a diploma in radiology. By this time the course of training had been extended to eighteen months. Of the 70 selected, 61 qualified as radiologists, usually at the first attempt, but an extension of six months was permitted to those who were at first unsuccessful. Five of the unsuccessful candidates resigned for private reasons, within a month or two of entering on their training; two resigned on account of ill health and two failed twice in the examination.

RADIOGRAPHERS

On the technical side it would have been impossible to cope with the work had it not been for the fact that radiography was made a reserved occupation early in 1940. The Society of Radiographers was responsible for training and examining large classes of students, and, although there was sometimes an acute shortage of radiographers, no department was ever brought to a standstill for lack of staff. Radiographers, however, frequently had to work long hours to cope with the work, particularly during blitz periods. Moreover, there was a continuous increase in the volume of X-ray work, which in the aggregate over the whole country, more than doubled in the war years.

PROTECTION OF X-RAY WORKERS

A feature that calls for a passing note is the fact that in the early years an increasing number of radiographers were being sent off sick because of diminished white blood-cell counts which were attributed to X-ray dosage. Radiographers suspected that theirs was a dangerous calling and became health conscious. Steps were taken, therefore, to test all X-ray tubes, a small number of which were found to have faulty protection. The suspicion that many of these workers were suffering from the effects of X-ray dosage led the National Physical Laboratory to establish, at the instance of the Ministry of Health, a test of the radiations to which the workers were exposed. This took the form of a film to be worn by the worker for a certain period, after which it was to be returned to the N.P.L. for assessment of the dosage received. The returns from the N.P.L. showed a most satisfactory degree of protection and only in a few instances was the dosage received by radiographers more than a small fraction of the safety tolerance dose. Since this service came into operation less and less has been heard of blood changes among radiographers, and during the last three years of the war not a single case was reported. Another factor that probably had considerable bearing on this problem was the systematic inspection of all dark-rooms in which radiographers must perforce spend much of their time. In many instances dark-rooms were too small and the ventilation very inefficient. Steps, therefore, were taken to remedy bad conditions by installing fans and getting the radiologist in charge to organise the work in such a way that none of the staff spent overlong hours in dark-room work.

In the War of 1914–18 many radiologists and surgeons received severe X-ray burns in the search for and location of foreign bodies and also in setting fractures under X-ray guidance. In this war, as already stated, the foreign body was a minor consideration and in any case protective devices had been so perfected that there was no longer much risk attached to screening. But the attraction of setting fractures under X-ray guidance is a constant one to surgeons, particularly in America where the number of accidents arising from this cause is still considerable. In this procedure it is inevitable that the hands of the surgeon should be exposed to the direct beam of X-rays and it is only with knowledge and meticulous care that danger can be avoided. In the early days of the war 2 cases of severe X-ray burns resulting from setting fractures under X-ray guidance were reported. The Ministry therefore sent out directives that this procedure must never be undertaken except in the presence and under the guidance of a radiologist. No further accidents are known to have occurred.

PREPARATION FOR D-DAY

The approach of D-day demanded much preparation in the localised region of disembarkation which could not be disclosed until the last moment. Radiographers were included in the extra staff that was sent to reinforce the resources of the local hospitals. Additional apparatus of mobile and portable types had been accumulated and placed at the disposal of the radiologists in the area who were to be responsible for providing the necessary X-ray service. The number of casualties, however, was not as great as had been expected and nowhere was the reinforced organisation stretched beyond capacity. The efficiency and smooth working of all the arrangements, in which the X-ray service took its vital share, were truly remarkable and drew unstinted praise from all who had the privilege to observe the scene.

The work in the E.M.S. during the war was virtually a duplication of that carried on in the civilian hospitals, and there were no striking advances either in technique or procedure other than the introduction of more sensitive films referred to above.

UNFORESEEN FEATURES

There were four major surprises. (1) There was no call for the accurate location of foreign bodies which was the chief pre-occupation of the radiological service in the War of 1914–18. This was due to the revolution in surgical procedure in which the drainage and irrigation of wounds has been completely replaced by excision of all dead tissues, in which the presence of a foreign body was an incident, whereas in the last war its removal was a prime objective of the surgeon. (2) It had not been realised how essential X-ray procedure had become in investigating abdominal conditions. It was proved that these examinations were no longer a luxury but a vital pre-requisite of all medical and surgical treatment, so much so that even during the most intense rushes of casualty work the demand for these examinations continued without pause. (3) Proportionately the number of gastro-intestinal cases admitted to hospital was considerably larger than in civilian practice, so much so that in ordinary convoys as many as 25 per cent. would require opaque meal examination. (4) The number of patients in whom active ulceration of the stomach and duodenum was reported was much higher than that found in civilian practice.

GENERAL COMMENTARY

In spite of the excessive work thrown on the radiologists, and the barely adequate technical assistance, coupled with the improvised character of many of the X-ray departments and the persistent increase in the volume of work, the standard of work maintained throughout was on a surprisingly high level. The greatest deficiency was the impossibility of maintaining collaboration between radiologists and surgeons. Each was working beyond capacity and adequate time for consultation could not be found. Written reports from a radiologist are all right up to a point, but in a large proportion of cases personal consultation is essential if full value is to be obtained from the work done in the X-ray department.

CHAPTER 13
PHYSICAL MEDICINE

by

SIR ROBERT STANTON WOODS

M.D., F.R.C.P.

Consultant Adviser in Physical Medicine

INTRODUCTION

PHYSICAL medicine is that branch of medical art which employs physical agents in diagnosis and treatment. These agents comprise heat, electricity, massage, passive movements and active movements, including gymnastics, games and productive occupation. As the boundaries of physical medicine are not determined by either nosological or anatomical considerations, the approach to a record of its activities over a given period must differ from that of almost any other special branch of medicine. It would be possible to select certain diseases or disease groups into whose diagnosis and treatment physical medicine enters and survey this aspect of the effect of war. This specialty, however, is applicable in such a wide range of conditions, occurring in practically every tissue or region of the body, that it may be said to extend throughout the whole field of medicine and surgery.

The vast scope of physical medicine was, until comparatively recently, appreciated only by the few specialists in this subject and its full practice was limited to a few centres. The extent of its applicability to the relief of human suffering and disability was purely potential.

The history of physical medicine during the war years is one of ever increasing appreciation of its importance by the medical profession as a whole and by the health and hospital authorities throughout the country.

No new discovery has resulted from the impact of war conditions but there has been a complete re-orientation of physical medicine itself and such a widening of its facilities, organisation and scope as to present almost a revolution in the treatment of disease.

This chapter contains, therefore, an account of the growing recognition of this specialty as it occurred during the war—a recognition attributable mainly to the effect of the war itself but also partly to the mere passage of the years—and a record of its most immediate concrete result, the great development of facilities for physical medicine in the Emergency Medical Services.

PRE-WAR SITUATION

Massage Department. Twenty years ago the hospital department which is now called the 'Department of Physical Medicine' was almost universally known as the 'Massage Department', and even as late as 1939, it was only in the most progressive communities that this would not have been a fairly accurate description. Except in a few hospitals in which the department was controlled by a specially appointed member of the staff, the sprains and rheumatics were rubbed and baked and electrified week by week, month by month—nay, year by year. In some hospitals there was not even a massage department. On the other hand, at certain progressive hospitals where, during the inter-war decades, new buildings had been erected to house physical medicine, two notable advances had been made—a gymnasium had become an essential provision and unified medical supervision had been established.

PHYSICAL MEDICINE IN THE EMERGENCY MEDICAL SERVICES

Until April 1939, the consideration of physical medicine had been almost entirely lacking in the organisation of the Emergency Hospital Scheme, but in May 1939, on the advice of the Physical Medicine Group Committee of the British Medical Association, a Consultant Adviser in Physical Medicine was appointed.

At first there was some lack of appreciation of the scope of physical medicine, and some considerable time elapsed before this special field was adequately recognised and established. After 1940, however, difficulties gradually disappeared and, with the passage of time and the influx of casualties, real progress was made in all the Regions.

A general survey made during 1945 provided a most interesting comparison with conditions as they had existed in 1940. Modern rehabilitation did not exist in 1940; in 1945 it appeared to be firmly established. (See Comparative Survey later in this chapter.)

The Regional Hospital Officers were co-operative to a high degree and to them, therefore, with their wide sphere of influence, must be accorded a considerable share of the credit for the advances made. Over a somewhat smaller clinical field, the orthopaedic surgeon took full advantage of the facilities at hand; here and there a progressive medical officer of health provided the needed push; and occasionally the influence of the lay house governor or secretary was obvious.

ORGANISATION

The war-time physical medicine service was organised under four main sections: (1) Accommodation; (2) Medical Personnel; (3) Technical Personnel; and (4) Equipment.

ACCOMMODATION

As already stated, up till 1939, except in the larger hospitals in the chief cities, space facilities were either of the most meagre description or non-existent. At the outbreak of hostilities, by the force of circumstances, the official attitude was that 'no bed space must be sacrificed to physical medicine', and for some months after, the only accommodation available was such as had always been used for the purpose, with the addition in a few instances, of disused sheds and whatever physiotherapy could be administered in bed. Even at most of the nineteen orthopaedic centres selected late in 1939, physiotherapy was being carried out partly on bed-patients and partly by adapting discarded indoor space. This not only hampered treatment through lack of room, but gave rise to many technical difficulties from unsuitable electrical supply and wiring, inefficient water supply, etc.

In December 1939, the first hurdle was successfully negotiated with the Ministry's decision that each of the nineteen orthopaedic centres was to be equipped with a department of physiotherapy. The first of these was established at Park Prewett Emergency Hospital, where a first-floor ward was converted for massage, thermotherapy and electrotherapy. Later, at a few other orthopaedic centres permission was given to use part of a ward-hut for physiotherapy but at non-orthopaedic hospitals patients were still to be treated in bed.

In spite of the increasing recognition of the importance of physical medicine, at this early stage no special arrangements had been approved in any type of hospital for allocating physiotherapists to the hospital staff, while the suggestion of such special facilities as gymnasia for general reconditioning was still less acceptable. Active reconditioning by means of group exercises and games had also perforce to be limited to those rooms or wards which were not at the moment in demand for any other purpose. In March 1940, a decided step forward was taken when sanction was given for the erection of a special building for physiotherapy. One was actually built, but even this was inadequate as it had to be shared with X-rays.

It had, however, been obvious for some time that physical medicine would have to be accommodated in standard huts, specially designed and constructed for this purpose. The drawing up of a plan for a standard physiotherapy hut was, consequently, one of the earliest tasks of organisation.

STANDARD PHYSIOTHERAPY HUT

In 1939 the two most important types of hospital were (*a*) the hospital which housed an orthopaedic centre and (*b*) the Class I general hospital. One of the most difficult decisions in connexion with the whole organisation concerned the minimum amount of floor space for a department of physiotherapy which would at the same time be large enough for efficiency. It seemed most practical to base the new hut, as far as possible, on the E.M.S. standard hut already in production for general purposes, and to conform to the fixed width (24 ft.) and fixed height of the latter, making the necessary adjustments in the length only. The length required was considered under two headings: (1) the type of hospital—was it a general hospital or one housing an orthopaedic centre? (2) The size of the hospital reckoned in number of beds.

(1) *Type of Hospital.* The opinions of orthopaedic surgeons were widely sought as to the percentage of their in-patients which would, at some period, call for physiotherapy. These opinions varied between 'none whatever' and '100 per cent.' of cases! The size of department selected for an orthopaedic centre was, therefore, on the assumption that 60 per cent. of patients would need this form of treatment—i.e. mid-way between the two extremes of view, with an added 10 per cent. for safety. An assessment of the corresponding size which would be in demand at a general hospital was arrived at by means of statistics of the percentages of in-patients in the main hospitals in London which, before the war, had had physical treatment. This estimate again varied between wide extremes of 11 per cent. and 75 per cent. (the latter a truly remarkable figure); after due consideration 30 per cent. was judged to be a fair average. These two percentages, 60 per cent. and 30 per cent., which ultimately proved to be approximately accurate, provided a basis for the estimation of the average number of patients in the two types of hospital which would require treatment by physical methods.

(2) *Size of Hospital.* A more complicated problem was provided by the question of the length of a 24 ft. wide hut which would be required by a given number of patients. This involved such matters as the width of the treatment plinth and the proper spacing of neighbouring plinths; the average length of time occupied by each patient who might be having one, two or even three different kinds of treatment at any one visit; the allocation of technicians on the reckoning that an individual physiotherapist can supervise one, two or three patients simultaneously, according to the kind of treatment; the number of hours in a working day; the use to be made of the central part of the hut (economy of floor space being strictly enforced); cupboard space, water and current supply, lighting and heating, offices and waiting-room. After prolonged calculation, two simple formulae emerged, relating the length of the department in feet to the bed-states of an orthopaedic centre and a general hospital respectively.

In April 1940, therefore, a standard specification was drawn up for a hut to accommodate physiotherapy, the size to vary in accordance with the type and bed-state of the hospital. Since no provision for a gymnasium was allowed, exercises, whether undertaken individually or in groups, had to be carried out in the space allotted to passive physiotherapy. The specification was presented to the Ministry and later adopted with modifications but there was little immediate result, owing to the demands from many departments of Government on the limited supply of labour and materials.

In June 1940, Circular 2066 containing the following direction was issued:

> In Class I hospitals with 300 beds and over, a 'special' room with six to twelve power points and a basin with running water was to be used; this room, however, if a ward, was to revert to its former function in times of stress. At orthopaedic centres there was to be a special physiotherapy department—if necessary in an *ad hoc* hut. At hutted hospitals half a ward hut was to be set aside unless there was a more suitable space in the building.

The building of standard physiotherapy huts was, therefore, strictly confined at first to the nineteen orthopaedic centres. Indeed, in August 1940, a sudden ban upon all building in the E.M.S. having descended, those orthopaedic centres at which such special provision had not already been started, as well as the remaining 122 hospitals of 300 beds and over, were compelled to carry out all physical treatment for ambulatory patients in a corner of a ward or other comparable site.

GYMNASIA

Later on in the year the Ministry took up the question of the demand for gymnasia, the essential character of physical re-education having received more general recognition. In December 1940, therefore, the Consultant Adviser in Physical Medicine was authorised to put forward proposals and a long-prepared plan for a second type of hut was presented. This hut allowed 63 ft. for a gymnasium, 24 ft. for 'offices' and space for passive physiotherapy which was to vary, as in the earlier hut, with the type and bedstate of the hospital concerned. The plan was officially agreed to in January 1941, though not put extensively into effect till later in that year.

FRACTURE CLINICS (See Chapter 5)

Early in the course of the war it became obvious that the nineteen orthopaedic centres would not be sufficient to accommodate more than a small percentage of all fractures. Three further types of fracture department, therefore, came gradually into being.

The first of these, the Fracture A Clinics, were housed in non-vulnerable general hospitals and admitted long-stay fractures. They were staffed by general surgeons who had had extensive fracture experience, whereas at orthopaedic centres fractures were treated by purely orthopaedic surgeons.

Fracture B Clinics, situated in hospitals mainly in more vulnerable areas, were for the admission of cases of fracture whose stay should not extend beyond seven days.

In common with the rest of the E.M.S., Fracture A and B Clinics dealt with both Service and civilian in-patients. As, however, the length of stay of civilians in hospital has always been much shorter than that accorded to Service patients, certain smaller hospitals and clinics were later selected to function as Fracture C Clinics, where the subsequent out-patient treatment of civilian industrial fracture cases was undertaken.

RESUMPTION OF BUILDING

In March 1941, building was resumed in the E.M.S., and the provision of special physical medicine huts at orthopaedic centres was continued. At this stage, also, special hutted accommodation began to appear at Fracture A Clinics. Owing to the short stay of patients in Fracture B Clinics, no special physical medicine facilities were provided but this apparent lack was compensated by the facilities at the Fracture C Clinics.

Later still, at neurosis centres and even at some purely general hospitals there was a gradual but extensive provision and adaptation of space facilities for this specialised work.

REHABILITATION

The term 'rehabilitation' caused at first considerable confusion of thought to those not acquainted with physical methods of treatment; they looked upon it as an entirely new form of therapy. Accordingly, in January 1942, an attempt was made to clarify the situation by the issue of E.M.S. 'Supplement 28—Preparing the Sick and Injured for Return to Work'—and, some months later, by Supplement 28a. Both these memoranda were intended for the guidance of medical superintendents and hospital staffs in the use of such measures as would rehabilitate their patients and return them as soon as possible to the ever-shortening roll of available man and woman-power.

Although the importance of activity and self-help in convalescence had been stressed in limited medical circles before the war, the greatly increased war-time opportunities of gaining experience, especially in the surgery of injury, caused the importance of this factor of self-help to be more and more widely appreciated. This led to increased demands for indoor space.

From April 1942, a third type of physical medicine hut, one shared equally between a gymnasium and an occupational therapy department, was being constructed at some orthopaedic centres and Fracture A Clinics, thus bringing the space accommodation for physical medicine at certain hospitals up to a relatively high level. In addition, more of the first two types of hut were being erected and even at Red Cross auxiliary hospitals, building for gymnastic purposes was sanctioned.

Towards the end of the war, the erection of special physical medicine huts was discontinued. Fortunately, about this time the E.M.S.

Standard 24 prefabricated and sectioned hut began to make its appearance and was found to fill the gap very adequately. Designed for general purposes, it was admirable in every way, except that its height of only 7 ft. 11 in. at the eaves made it unsuitable for ball games.

One further allocation of space may be mentioned. During the period of intensive bombing, many large hospitals in populous centres were compelled to close their top-floor wards and some of these vacated wards were very efficiently adapted for use as physiotherapy departments but were not suitable as gymnasia because the noise of this activity disturbed patients in the wards below.

Up to the early part of 1943, rehabilitation facilities were provided exclusively for Service and civil defence patients, air raid casualties and certain specified evacuees. After that date, civilian industrial fractures were added to this list. It therefore became necessary to survey the facilities throughout England and Wales and to this end the Ministry issued a questionnaire. This involved a great deal of work in Regional offices, necessitating as it did a personal visit by responsible officers to each hospital before the questionnaire could be adequately filled in. Besides asking for information of existing physical medicine facilities, this questionnaire also requested suggestions for practical improvements in the provision for all sections of rehabilitation. The survey occupied all the spring and summer months of that year and when finished proved that there was a good deal of keenness to carry out the scheme often under great handicap, a certain amount of apathy in places where extension was possible and in many cases, utter inadequacy mainly owing to lack of staff and space. Further consideration and experience have tended to show that such rehabilitation is not suited to outpatient conditions.

SUMMARY

During the war years, the space allotted in hospitals and clinics to physiotherapy and remedial gymnastics throughout England and Wales underwent very considerable enlargement. Whereas in 1939 space facilities for this service, in accordance with modern requirements, were almost non-existent, except at the teaching hospitals in London and the large provincial centres, in 1945 serious inadequacy in this respect had been very largely overcome.

MEDICAL PERSONNEL AND SPECIALIST ADVICE

An unbiassed observer must be impressed with the increased efficiency of physical medicine departments where the work is under the unified medical control of an expert. Before the war, this condition hardly existed outside London. Experts were therefore not available for the staffing of such departments in the Emergency Medical Service, especially as these departments rapidly increased in number as soon as the authorities were convinced of their importance. Nine were accordingly selected for London but only two in the other Regions. Just before the war began, five of the nine, although not yet officially employed, surveyed their Sectors, checking equipment lists and reporting on the condition of available apparatus, on the accommodation and on technical personnel.

Unfortunately, before the war and in its early stages, it was impossible to establish the principle of unified medical control of each physical medicine department. When in October 1940, it was finally agreed to be desirable, many of those who might have been selected for an intensive training in this work had been absorbed into other essential duties.

In February 1942, 'D.G.L./80—Medical Officers i/c Physical Medicine Departments' was issued. This contained instructions that staffs should seek the advice of a medical officer in touch both with the clinical requirements of patients and with the methods of treatment available. If a suitable medical officer was available, he was to be made responsible for the work of the physical medicine department. If a medical officer wished to undertake these duties but lacked experience he was to be transferred for one or two months to a hospital where he could gain experience and instruction.

In July 1942, therefore, in order to satisfy this requirement as far as possible, several of the best physical medicine departments in the Service were selected to provide intensive training of medical men for this work on a part-time basis. This course was to extend over at least one month and, if possible, over two or three. It was soon found that no medical men could be spared from their war-time posts to undergo so long a training and by the following year the scheme had to be replaced by another which was considered more practical in application, though it was otherwise less satisfactory.

This latter scheme provided short 'week-end courses' occupying many Fridays, Saturdays and Sundays from October 1943, at Ashridge, Botley's Park, Harlow Wood, Horton (Epsom), Morriston, Orpington, Pinder Fields, Whitchurch and Winwick Emergency Hospitals, and much credit is due to the staffs of these hospitals for undertaking the additional work involved in the supervision of the courses. About 250 hospitals in England and Wales took advantage of this opportunity by seconding a member of the medical or surgical staff. Naturally, only the barest outline of the organisation of a modern rehabilitation department could be taught in thirty-six hours. But even this afforded some help to those who had few, if any, ideas on the subject and the results gradually became apparent.

The proper clinical function of the medical man in charge of a physical medicine department is two-fold. Not only does his experience of the use of physical agents and of the more active forms of this therapy enable him to exercise expert day-to-day supervision of their application by technicians, but he is also in a position to form a necessary liaison between the rehabilitation department and the physicians and surgeons who have been responsible for the primary treatment of the patients and who continue to be responsible until the final results are attained.

TECHNICAL PERSONNEL

As was only to be expected, the provision of technical personnel was also inadequate.

During 1938 and 1939, the Chartered Society of Massage and Medical Gymnastics (now the Chartered Society of Physiotherapy) expended much time, money and effort in compiling from among its 11,000 members a register of 3,000 who agreed, in the case of war, to serve in hospitals in the Emergency Medical Service. This register was divided into mobile and immobile sections and by September 1939, had increased to 5,000.

These technicians were not included on the establishment of hospitals under the Emergency Hospital Scheme and it was therefore difficult to persuade hospital authorities to employ them. At the outbreak of war their private practices in the evacuated areas almost ceased and there was in consequence widespread unemployment—even serious hardship—over a large part of the country. Indeed, some masseuses worked in hospitals without remuneration, while many qualified physiotherapists entered the forms of national service, having been officially encouraged to do so.

The picture was completely altered when in June 1940, E.M.S. Instruction Gen. 330 was issued, not only authorising but urging hospitals to engage masseuses and recognising the Chartered Society rates of salary as the authorised standard. This instruction was responsible for the immediate solution of the unsatisfactory situation in the organisation of physical medicine in the Emergency Hospital Scheme. It coincided with, or just anticipated, the first real rush of Army casualties from abroad and was therefore opportune.

After this, the demand for trained technicians in the E.M.S. hospitals rapidly increased.

As late as the middle of 1940, unemployment had been almost the rule; in January 1942, there were only 114 trained physiotherapists not engaged in individual or hospital practice and yet, in the search for man-power, prospective trainees were being discouraged. By February 1943, the available supply had been completely absorbed.

Since physiotherapy was not among the 'reserved' occupations, control of the movements of these workers was lacking; until 1943 resignations from and appointments to hospital departments occurred without any reference to a central body. In September 1943, the

Ministry of Labour and National Service issued a 'Control of Engagements' Order which banned private practice, unless it allowed some time for work in hospitals, and ruled that physiotherapists could not transfer to other occupations. At the same time the Chartered Society of Physiotherapy became the recognised Employment Agency under the Ministry of Labour and National Service. From that date some semblance of order appeared in the physiotherapy service.

During 1943, 1944 and 1945, however, the supply situation became steadily more difficult, during the year ending May 1945, out of 1,104 vacancies in hospitals in the E.M.S. only 442 could be filled. The chief reason for the increased demand was the great expansion of physiotherapy in the emergency hospitals. Military hospitals, too, were making more and more use of physiotherapy and several hundred female physiotherapists had been sent to the Middle East, to Italy, to France and to India; by the end of May 1945, the Army was employing 414—all with at least two years' seniority. Physiotherapists employed in Royal Naval hospitals did not exceed 50 in number, while Royal Air Force hospital departments were staffed partly by members who had joined the W.A.A.F. with sergeant's rank, and partly by civilian members who had 'officer' status—an arrangement which did not promote harmony.

The supply of trained personnel, already seriously diminished by transfer to other occupations, was further rendered inadequate by a falling off in the number of physiotherapists undergoing training. This was cumulative in its effects and was still operative after the war.

TRAINING IN PHYSIOTHERAPY

In the early months of the war the London schools of physiotherapy were closed owing partly to the withdrawal of trainees by their parents from vulnerable areas and partly to the evacuation of the sick population, but in January 1940, schools began to re-open at the new base hospitals outside the London area.

In the early years of the war, the Ministry of Labour and National Service would not recognise this training as 'essential'. Even by February 1942, the cases of candidates were merely being considered individually, and it was not until later in that year that a policy was formulated, according to which girls were allowed to take up this career but only if they could qualify before attaining their twentieth birthday—a very early age for serious responsibility. The reason given for this restriction was that otherwise they might make use of the training to evade call-up for munitions or for the women's services. To comply with these conditions, it became necessary to accept candidates for training at the age of $17\frac{1}{2}$ and some schools reported that the nature of the training required a higher degree of physical stamina than was shown by these youthful trainees.

From the pre-war number of about 500 newly-qualified yearly, the numbers consequently fell, whereas, as already stated, the demand rose steeply. After many representations, however, first one and then another concession was made. In August 1943, the qualifying age was raised to 21 and in the autumn of 1944, a further relaxation raised it to 22. But even though age relaxation resulted in a considerable flow of applicants for training, obviously it would bring no relief for some years.

A further and equally potent factor in bringing about this relative dearth of physiotherapists was that whereas, under pre-war conditions, the number of these young women who qualified yearly was sufficient, the greatly increased demand resulting from war casualties could not possibly be satisfied. Moreover, the educational facilities in the training schools could not accommodate a considerable increase in the numbers of pupils without seriously interfering with efficiency. There was, therefore, an urgent need to increase the number of schools and, as a consequence, to increase the number of teachers. Such extended educational facilities could not be effective for at least $4\frac{1}{2}$ years—a 3-years' course for qualification as a physiotherapist, followed by practice in physiotherapy before even starting on the $1\frac{1}{2}$ years' training in actual teaching.

The number of physiotherapists undergoing training would have fallen even further had it not been for the hospitality which was extended to evacuated schools by many hospitals in areas less vulnerable to bombing.

This problem of the scarcity of physiotherapists, unlike other problems in physical medicine, was never solved during the war, but in 1946 a scheme was initiated by the Ministry of Health for training teachers with the view of meeting the rapidly growing post-war demand for trained technicians in the hospitals.

MASSEURS

The number of masseurs employed in the E.M.S. was very small. This was due to several reasons but mainly to the call-up of men into the Fighting Services, though partly to the fact that men and women were paid at equal (and, therefore for men, inadequate) rates. For the latter reason male technicians almost always preferred to engage in private practice. There were a few blind physiotherapists in hospital departments, but except in massage, they cannot work without special apparatus.

REFRESHER COURSES

Early in the war it was realised that, if their work was not to suffer, refresher courses for serving physiotherapists were essential. In 1941, the proposal to finance such courses was rejected and the suggestion remained in·abeyance until 1943. After the latter date many such courses were held at several of the largest and best equipped orthopaedic and Fracture A centres. These fulfilled a very important instructional function, especially in the experience they offered of organising physical medicine departments and of the working of social security services.

EQUIPMENT

This specialty makes use of a wide range of physical agents and a modern department would be to some extent defective if any of them were lacking. In the summer of 1939, because of the uncertainty of economic conditions in the previous years, manufacturers had almost no stocks and it was in consequence necessary to confine new manufacture to as few types as possible, giving first consideration to those which would probably be in greatest demand for war casualties, especially in the treatment of soft tissue wounds and fractures. The provision of the minimum estimated quantity of purely basic equipment, including only sources of heat of different kinds, faradic coils and direct current apparatus, was therefore proposed to the Ministry early in September 1939. As expense at that time was still a consideration, this estimate was cut down by two-thirds by the Treasury, and orders were placed in November 1939. As delivery was not expected for some months and the presumably unavoidable delay caused some anxiety and inconvenience, the purchase of ordinary commercial gas lamps as sources of heat was considered, in order to bridge the gap between low peace-time stocks and augmented war-time demands, but subsequently, some standard radiant heat lamps were procured to meet the most urgent needs.

For some time hardly any additions were made to the types of equipment originally provided owing to a large extent to an increasing shortage of labour and materials and to the relatively low priority afforded to physical medicine equipment. Certain more elaborate types of apparatus which were considered 'standard' for a modern department could not at first be sanctioned; later, orders were given for a limited supply.

During the summer of 1940, the addition of portable ultra-violet lamps for local treatment was recommended and approved, but the suggestion that apparatus for general irradiation should also be supplied to a few of the largest centres was not approved. In 1942, however, the demand was revived and the purchase of ten carbon arc lamps was allowed; these were installed in some of the principal centres in the latter half of 1943. One of the problems which complicated the selection of both the portable radiant heat and the portable ultra-violet units was the large variety on the market and although requests were made by the Ministry of Health that, in war-time and in the interests of economy, only one 'standard' model should be allowed, the manufacture of unapproved types did not diminish; a large proportion of these units were mechanically unsound.

In December 1942, the supply of a further heat source, namely, paraffin wax was allowed for certain special centres—particularly for burns. After the first two or three war years, the ever-increasing length of time required for delivery of each new order gave evidence of the lack of skilled workmen and of the difficulty of obtaining substitute materials.

ULTRA SHORT-WAVE THERAPY

An item of equipment for the supply of which sanction was refused early in the war was the ultra short-wave apparatus. This refusal gave rise to a certain amount of criticism from those who regarded it as of considerable value as a therapeutic agent, especially for the treatment of localised, deep-seated, septic conditions. Not only was its use objected to, however, on account of 'interference' with radio communications, caused by high frequency apparatus, both medical and industrial, but the surgical advisers of the Ministry of Health were not convinced that the extensive use of this form of therapy was essential in the E.M.S.

In July 1940, the Wireless Telegraphy Board decided to ban the use of private high frequency apparatus and only to allow it to hospitals by special permit, provided that the plant was efficiently screened. In August 1940, all private plants were confiscated. This action roused considerable protests from medical men who used this form of treatment in practice.

The Physical Medicine Advisory Committee pressed for the provision of this apparatus, at any rate in certain orthopaedic centres. Sanction was obtained to instal suitably screened apparatus at Horton, Orpington and Winwick Emergency Hospitals, to which patients suffering from disabilities in which this form of therapy had been found especially beneficial, such as osteomyelitis, etc., could be transferred. In July 1942, the ban on this apparatus for use by private individuals was lifted and it was allowed by special permit if properly screened.

In February 1944, the Physical Medicine Advisory Committee again pressed for a very considerable extension of supplies to E.M.S. hospitals and recommended that a hundred machines be ordered for this purpose, it being pointed out that Ministry of Labour centres and 'partially' E.M.S. hospitals could obtain this equipment, while sanction for their provision for '100 per cent.' E.M.S. hospitals was still being withheld. Eventually, in January 1945, sanction was accorded to the supply of 25 additional sets, but owing to the diminishing responsibilities of the emergency hospitals after VE day, this number was reduced to 10, none of which had been delivered before VJ day. There is no evidence that the ultimate recovery of any patient was prejudiced by failure to use this method of treatment, in fact, when penicillin became more generally available, it is doubtful whether any more extensive supplies would have been justified.

ELECTRO-DIAGNOSIS

For some time the lack of an efficient apparatus for electro-diagnosis was a real handicap and it was not until late in 1940 that a specification for a muscle-nerve testing unit to remedy this defect was approved, and supply began in April 1941. The principles underlying this apparatus had for long been well known, being simply those of the presence or absence of the so-called 'reaction of degeneration', and no clinically practicable alternative method was available before the war ended. The importance of the 'time intensity' factor in both diagnosis and treatment in cases of peripheral nerve injuries had been realised for many years but it was not until 1945 that an apparatus was produced which allowed of the principle of so-called 'chronaxie' being put into practical clinical use in diagnosis and treatment. Nevertheless, the apparatus based on the 'reaction of degeneration' was very efficient.

Another recent diagnostic innovation was the electromyograph, which makes use of the significance of fibrillation in muscle fibres. The supply of this apparatus in certain centres for peripheral nerve injuries was recommended, but on the grounds of shortage of labour and materials it was disallowed.

GYMNASTIC AND GAMES EQUIPMENT

In the early stages of the war the standard gymnastic equipment supplied was very meagre, being such as could be housed in a strictly limited space. The gradual appearance of a gymnasium for general body reconditioning has already been mentioned and this entailed a corresponding extension of equipment.

The earliest allocation, in August 1941, allowed wall-bars, medicine balls, step-with-risers, ropes-and-pulleys, etc., etc., for the use of orthopaedic and Fracture A hospitals.

From May 1943, onwards, further types of apparatus were supplied and by 1944 the range of these was adequate for all practical purposes, a major principle being one of conservatism in respect of varieties.

Equipment for indoor and outdoor games included footballs, skittles, darts, deck quoits, netball, deck tennis, etc.

SWIMMING BATHS

Hydrotherapy, in its commonly accepted sense, is discussed in the clinical section which records the history of spa treatment as it was applied to war casualties or was affected by war conditions.

With the increasing appreciation of the part to be played by active exercise in rehabilitation, a swimming bath is now considered as almost essential by the expert. Very few hospitals are provided with this equipment and it is probable that its provision will be reserved for the residential rehabilitation centre of the future.

COMMITTEES

The Ministry of Health had the benefit of the advice of the following committees, of which the Consultant Adviser in Physical Medicine was a member:

The Committee of Consultant Advisers to the Ministry of Health.

The Physical Medicine Advisory Committee. After two abortive attempts in 1939 and 1940 to form an advisory committee for physical medicine, this committee first met in July 1940, and continued to meet at headquarters until the end of the war, though its personnel underwent many changes. As the scope of physical medicine widened, the number of purely physical medicine members was reduced; a representative of orthopaedic surgery and one of spa practice were asked to join; the attendance of the medical officer in charge of equipment in the E.M.S. was found to be indispensable, and a representative of the Department of Health for Scotland was also usually present as an observer at the meetings. The Ministry's Adviser in Occupational Therapy and the Secretary of the Chartered Society of Physiotherapy were invited to attend whenever any matter of particular interest to them was upon the agenda; and in 1944, the newly-appointed Director of Physical Training in the E.M.S. became a regular member.

Rehabilitation Committee. In November 1940, the preliminary meeting of a committee to consider certain general aspects of rehabilitation was held at the Ministry of Health. The Director-General, E.M.S., was chairman and certain individuals were enrolled as permanent members, while from time to time others were asked to attend if it was considered that their advice might be helpful. This committee met on nine occasions until January 1943, when it lapsed. Its deliberations and advice covered a wide field.

Orthopaedic Consultants' Committee. From June 1940, until February 1946, the Orthopaedic Consultants to the E.M.S. and the Army met in committee once a month. In December 1942, the Navy and the Air Force were invited each to send a representative, and in January 1943, the Consultant Adviser in Physical Medicine was elected a member.

COMPARATIVE SURVEY

The Provincial Regions. In the following statistical survey of 67 selected hospitals, the four large mental institutions which were taken over by the E.M.S. are not included as these had reverted to their pre-war functions. Had these been included, the picture would have been even more encouraging.

Almost without exception, the Regional Hospital Officers selected hospitals whose progress was characteristic of their Regions. The choice was therefore not confined to the best, as it included some of the least progressive in order to produce a fair average sample.

The space facilities under consideration were confined to three categories, namely, those for physiotherapy (massage, thermotherapy, electrotherapy and actinotherapy); those for active rehabilitation, viz., gymnasia and adapted outdoor space; and those for occupational therapy.

Conditions existing at these hospitals before September 1939.

(1) At 24 of the 67 institutions no physical medicine facilities whatever had existed before September 1939. (Four of these were new hospitals.)

(2) At 34 some space had been allotted to passive physiotherapy—often very small.

(3) Gymnasia had been in existence at 9 out of the 67 institutions.

(4) Two hospitals possessed a department of occupational therapy.

Conditions existing in 1945. Of the 67 institutions, at only one was there no space whatever for physical medicine; at 58 there was ample accommodation for physiotherapy and active rehabilitation (gymnasia) and at all but 20 of these there was also provision for occupational therapy. Three hospital centres had reached the present acme of rehabilitation, namely, the establishment of a 'residential rehabilitation annexe'.

The progress recorded in this brief summary of the results of a nine months' survey is conclusive evidence in itself of the revolution which took place during the war years. If the results recorded are taken as characteristic of the whole of England and Wales between 1939 and 1945 the percentage of hospitals with physiotherapy (massage, etc.) departments had risen from 65 per cent. to 98·5 per cent.; the corresponding percentages for gymnasia are 13·5 per cent. and 86·5 per cent.; for occupational therapy, 2·9 per cent. and just over 70 per cent.

Such remarkable increase of space facilities in general is in itself a matter for congratulation, providing as it does for the treatment of very many more patients than formerly. This, however, is not the sole or even the main reason for hopefulness. As indicated elsewhere, it furnishes incontrovertible evidence of a much greater awareness on the part of the medical profession of the function of this specialty, and the mere existence of a department in a hospital is of considerable educational value in itself.

A further indication emerges from an analysis of the relative parts played by passive physiotherapy and physical activity in after-treatment. Before September 1939 (excluding the main hospitals in London and in the large provincial towns), the physical methods employed in rehabilitation were confined to massage, electrotherapy, thermotherapy and actinotherapy, and even for these the provision of space was in general relatively meagre. In 1945, accommodation for physiotherapy had not quite doubled; for active rehabilitation, the provision had multiplied six times; for occupational therapy, twenty-three times.

The London Region. The end of the war prevented a final survey of the hospitals in the Sectors similar to that of the other Regions. The organisation of the Emergency Hospital Scheme in and around London differed fundamentally from that which was found suitable for the rest of England and Wales, and to no branch of medicine did this apply more than to physical medicine. The great majority of beds in this Region before 1939 were concentrated in a comparatively small area, the whole of which became at once highly vulnerable to bombing. In-patients were therefore, as far as possible, evacuated either to the periphery or even further afield and this applied to the whole extent of the Region and not, as in the rest of England and Wales, merely to a comparatively few hospitals in each large city. Physical medicine for in-patients, therefore, almost ceased at the teaching hospitals and to a great extent at the large municipal institutions within the area. In the case of out-patients also there was for a long time practically no demand here for physiotherapy. At the periphery of London, on the other hand, a great reorganisation of the large general hospitals and adaptation and extension of special hospitals took place, as well as the creation of entirely new ones. In the peripheral sectoral areas, therefore, space for physical medicine underwent wide expansion comparable with conditions outside the Sectors. Some of these peripheral hospitals reverted to specific or even non-medical functions, but others continued as general hospitals and to that extent the increased space for physical medicine was preserved. Some of the most distant of these could be converted into residential rehabilitation annexes of the central hospitals. So far as the centrally situated hospitals are concerned, those at which there are schools of physiotherapy are adequately equipped; others are by comparison defective. In densely populated and especially in highly industrial areas, although there will always be a demand for physiotherapy for out-patients, it is probable that physical medicine facilities for in-patients will, in the nearer or more distant future, be situated at residential rehabilitation annexes rather than at the 'acute' centrally placed institutions.

SUMMARY

As a direct result of war conditions, the Emergency Medical Services have revolutionised not only the organisation, administration and provision of facilities but even the clinical picture of physical medicine in hospitals throughout England and Wales. Much remains to be done, indeed, it can be said that hardly more than a start has been made. The results, however, of these changes have been so encouraging that it is possible to look forward with confidence to continuing progress and the consolidation of many of the gains that have already been made.

Plates XXXVI to XLI illustrate some types of remedial exercise and occupational therapy.

LESSONS FOR THE FUTURE

EXTENSION OF OUTLOOK AND SCOPE

The most important change in the physical medicine picture in the hospitals was in the general outlook, concept and scope of the specialty.

Largely owing to the additional opportunities for gaining experience, afforded by the great increase of clinical material, which necessitated the increased provision of facilities in the E.M.S. hospitals, there occurred a revolution in outlook on the part of the profession generally. It is true that in addition to passive measures of physiotherapy, active exercise of the injured part had long entered into the remedial scheme. Until quite recently, however, at most hospitals, after-treatment was limited to the affected limb or region of the body. Physical medicine in the treatment of localised disabilities did not as a rule directly concern itself with the body as a whole. There were, of course, notable exceptions to this rule, but the provision of gymnasia in the E.M.S. hospitals gave opportunities for the widespread introduction of general exercises and games into the physical medicine programme and was thus largely instrumental in altering the conception of rehabilitation from that of purely local remedial measures to one which included the whole body. A further educational advance consisted in considering re-establishment of morale as part of the rehabilitation aim, with the obvious corollary that a greater emphasis was accorded to the part which the patient's own efforts could play in his recovery. Hitherto, so far as this branch of therapy was concerned, the convalescent was happy to be entirely passive and to enjoy his massage, his heat and so forth. He was now called upon to contribute active assistance. This is not a universally popular rôle with the individual patient, but there is little doubt that it is sound psychology, the psychology of self-help, and it gives the patient a yard-stick for the assessment of his own progress, with a consequent fillip to his morale.

The building of gymnasia at hospitals could not of itself have effected much. At certain progressive centres an up-to-date department, including a gymnasium, was all that was necessary, but these were exceptional and at the majority of hospitals further educational stimulus was called for.

This enlarged concept of the function of physical medicine is beginning to spread beyond the field of traumatic surgery. The results attained in accident cases by active exercise for general reconditioning are leading to the employment of this form of therapy in connection with general surgery. It is therefore not uncommon for patients within the first week after even major abdominal operations to start a course of general reconditioning, with supervised activity of all four limbs accompanied by a régime of breathing exercises. It is probable that something is gained if this procedure can be initiated even before operation. Clinical observation has, of course, its own pitfalls but it is worth recording that experienced personnel, such as ward-sisters, are at times enthusiastic about the effect of this comparatively recent innovation upon the physical and psychological state of patients. Even that conservative body, the hospital physicians, are here and there introducing a similar régime as soon as such procedure is both safe and advisable.

For the sake of emphasis, it may be repeated that this enlistment of general bodily activity as a factor in the planning of convalescence after injury or illness from any cause, has a two-fold rationale. Its aim is not solely one of physical betterment; perhaps indeed, this is not its chief object. Of at least equal importance is the uplift to the morale which it brings about. The steady progress in physical activity, which can be registered from day to day, has been found to have a profound influence upon the recovery of self-confidence which had temporarily degenerated.

OCCUPATIONAL THERAPY

Passive physiotherapy and active reconditioning by gymnastics and games, especially during the early stages of convalescence, cannot be undertaken for longer than a strictly limited part of the convalescent day, and yet in many patients it is obviously necessary to engage the attention with other thoughts than those of life's worries. Partly with the aim of diversion, therefore, convalescence-planning is making more and more use of productive occupation.

Occupational therapy, until 1939 almost confined to mental hospitals, received very wide extension in the Emergency Medical Services. Different experts placed widely varying emphasis upon the relative importance of the diversional and physically remedial features of this form of treatment but most were agreed upon the desirability of its inclusion in rehabilitation, at any rate for in-patients.

TRAINING IN THE PHYSIOTHERAPY SCHOOLS

For some years before the war, a number of the hospitals at which students were trained for the Diploma of the Chartered Society of Physiotherapy had introduced into the curriculum an intensive course in general physical re-education as part of routine rehabilitation. This applied not only to cases of limb trauma but even to those of general illnesses whenever such after-treatment was suitable. In the physiotherapy schools therefore it is not uncommon now to find on the teaching staff a woman holding the Diploma of one or other of the recognised Physical Education Colleges. This training is very much in advance of generally accepted medical practice, but it is in accordance with the views of the more progressive traumatic surgeons and even of a few general surgeons and physicians. The wide dissemination of these trained technicians in hospitals throughout the country is not without its influence on the introduction of general physical exercise as part of rehabilitation.

ARMY PHYSICAL TRAINING COACHES

This influence was accentuated when, in February 1940, the Army authorities began to second N.C.O.s of the Army Physical Training Corps to work in the Emergency Medical Services and B.R.C.S. Auxiliary Hospitals, after a short preliminary training in remedial gymnastics. Originally intended to help in the reconditioning of Service patients only, these instructors were later permitted to include a percentage of civilians in their remedial classes. Their work soon became a prominent and indispensable feature of rehabilitation in the Emergency Medical Services and when the war ended there were about 250 physical training instructors thus engaged. The usefulness of these N.C.O.s was much heightened by the appointment in 1944 of a Director of Physical Training (formerly Inspector of Physical Training in the Army) to supervise their technique and their discipline.

In order that the incorporation in civilian hospital technique of the principle of general body activity in rehabilitation should not lapse from lack of personnel, in October 1945, a first course for ex-Service physical training instructors was established at Pinder Fields Emergency Hospital, Wakefield. This was intended to give additional remedial instruction; elementary instruction in anatomy, physiology and relevant medical and surgical conditions; and generally to re-orient the trainees into conditions governing civilian hospitals where these differ from those in Service institutions. It is most encouraging that all the trainees from the first course, which ended in August 1946, have been placed in civilian hospitals.

DIPLOMA IN PHYSICAL MEDICINE

One further result of the growing recognition of the importance of physical medicine should be recorded. For several years before the outbreak of war, the establishment of a diploma had been under discussion but the negotiations threatened to be long drawn out. That these suddenly came to a head in 1943 and 1944 is certainly not unrelated to the influence of war conditions.

In 1943 the Royal Colleges instituted a diploma in physical medicine and the first examination was held in July, 1944. Whether this step was a premature one, taken before conditions were suitable, remained to be seen. No individual was in a position to comply with all the regulations for entry to the examination and certain of these had to be modified for all the candidates. On the other hand, the opportunities offered in rehabilitation departments of certain E.M.S. hospitals enabled candidates to acquire qualifying experience which would not have been otherwise available. Further, the inherent nature of physical medicine itself and its recent growth and development rendered necessary a lack of definiteness in the syllabus although, in this respect, there was much less to criticise than at first sight appeared inevitable.

The early examinations at least made clear the intention of the Royal Colleges that the standard demanded should be a high one; and this was clearly desirable for a specialist diploma. The maintenance of a high standard was also to the advantage of the men serving in the Forces, as it avoided the risk of their returning to find less experienced persons holding the diploma and, possibly in consequence, occupying key positions. Up to July 1946, there were nine successful candidates out of twenty-two entrants.

RESIDENTIAL REHABILITATION

From what has been written above, it is possible to estimate the profound effect which the war has had upon the planning of the convalescent period for in-patients. Hitherto, this phase of illness had been neglected. Patients had gone almost haphazard from the ward either to their own homes or to convalescent homes. In the former they had probably drifted towards full health (or in the opposite direction) without skilled advice as to the correct stage at which to take up life's burdens once more and, in the majority, without any supervision in the spending of the interim period. Even in the latter the only planning consisted in a period of rest. There was no organisation at convalescent homes for active reconditioning, no guidance in the use of leisure, no systematic help with the problems to which the patient was soon to return. Sooner or later this will almost certainly be altered and the phase between either the lessened activity of an illness, or a quite early stage in the history of an injury, and the final return to a full working life will be the subject of intensive supervision, guidance and treatment. Reconditioning will start long before the bed-fast stage is ended; it will continue during the remainder of the in-patient period and after discharge from the hospital ward, and become progressively more strenuous up to the time of resumption of work.

OUT-PATIENTS

The convalescence of out-patients cannot be undertaken on the same lines. During 1943, a campaign of education, almost one of propaganda, was carried out in the E.M.S. with the aim of instituting a comparable scheme for former in-patients and out-patients. They were to attend a rehabilitation centre; they would spend about six hours daily at this centre; their régime of treatment would consist of physiotherapy, general and local reconditioning exercise and occupational therapy, and an essential part of the scheme would be an organised social service with, of course, a substantial midday meal.

In densely populated districts, a scheme of this nature for out-patients is feasible for certain limited classes of disability. Ambulatory fractures and other injuries, certain chronic joint affections, expectant mothers (for part of a day)—to mention a few groups—would benefit. A review, however, of the disabilities for which the great majority of patients attend an out-patients department forces the conclusion that the basic causes of these disabilities are not 'medical'. The debility, the 'rheumatism', the indigestion, in the vast majority are no more amenable to so-called rehabilitation than they ever have been to the bottle of medicine. Indeed, the only features of modern rehabilitation which would be applicable to a large percentage of hospital out-patients are those which are directly concerned with the betterment of the material and psychological background of the living conditions generally.

CHAPTER 14
THE PROVISION OF MEDICAL PERSONNEL

ADMINISTRATIVE AND CLINICAL ESTABLISHMENTS

THE organisation created by the Ministry of Health to administer the Emergency Medical Services at Headquarters and in the Regions has been described in Chapter 2. Appointments to administrative posts were made partly from the permanent medical staff of the Ministries of Health and Pensions, and partly by the recruitment of suitably qualified officers from other sources. Specialists were, as stated in Chapter 1, appointed on the advice of the Committee of Reference of the Royal Colleges, whilst the ordinary staffs of hospitals were supplemented by practitioners recommended by the Regional and Sector Hospital Officers, Group Officers and Local and Central Medical War Committees. The latter committee was, in 1941, made responsible for fixing the main medical establishments (i.e. the 'A', 'B2' and 'B1' posts, defined later) of all civil hospitals whether in the E.M.S. or not.

The governing authorities of each hospital were responsible for the provision of their own establishment within the limits laid down by the Central Medical War Committee, but as time went on they had to rely on the E.M.S. to supply suitable officers for vacancies which they were unable to fill. This procedure was necessary, particularly in *ad hoc* E.M.S. hospitals, hospitals which had been largely expanded by taking over additional accommodation and hutted extensions, and in special hospitals. House appointments, however, were filled by the hospital authorities from newly qualified practitioners before their recruitment to the Armed Forces, women practitioners and those ineligible on medical or other grounds for recruitment to the Forces. Thus the civil hospitals were staffed by:

(*a*) Practitioners not liable for military service or, if liable, not yet required for such service, who were normally appointed to the honorary and whole-time staffs of the hospitals and, while carrying on their normal civil duty, also treated E.M.S. patients, military or civil, who attended or were admitted to their hospitals;

(*b*) Whole-time and part-time practitioners enrolled in the E.M.S. chiefly to staff new *ad hoc* E.M.S. hospitals, largely expanded and upgraded pre-existing hospitals and the E.M.S. wings of mental hospitals.

As mentioned in Chapter 3, the arrangements for mobilising practitioners enrolled in the E.M.S. were put into force at the beginning of the war, and after some preliminary difficulties had been dealt with, proceeded smoothly and rapidly; the medical establishment of the Civil Defence Services, the organisation of which was proceeding at the outbreak of the war, continued throughout the winter of 1939-40 and was more or less complete before the invasion of France and the air attacks on Britain began in May 1940.

CONSCRIPTION OF PRACTITIONERS

From the outbreak of hostilities until the German invasion of France the problem of staffing the E.M.S. hospitals, although it presented considerable difficulties because of the general shortage of medical personnel, had more or less kept pace with the gradually increasing demands which were being made on these hospitals.

In April 1940, however, the Ministry of Labour and National Service announced that the National Service (Armed Forces) Act, 1939, would apply to medical practitioners, who might be called up for service in H.M. Forces in their professional capacity. This liability extended to all practitioners, whole-time and part-time, subject to the age limit of 41, but certain exceptions were made, such as persons holding whole-time teaching appointments, etc.[1]

EFFECT ON E.M.S. HOSPITALS

As the result of this decision many useful junior members of the medical staffs of E.M.S. hospitals were called up, but certain 'key' men were permitted to be retained as the result of strong representations made by the hospital authorities, endorsed by the Ministry of Health. The effect was chiefly felt in the new *ad hoc* hospitals and in large base hospitals which had been established in mental hospitals, upgraded public assistance institutions, etc., because in this type of hospital no suitable pre-existing medical staff was, as a rule, available. These vacancies had to be filled, and in addition large numbers of practitioners were required for the organisation set up to deal with the expected invasion of this country by the enemy. For this latter purpose the Ministry of Health issued an E.M.S. Instruction laying down the procedure for calling up practitioners to supplement the staffs of hospitals. County and county borough medical officers of health, in consultation with Local Medical War Committees, were required to compile lists of general practitioners in their areas who could be called upon, in the event of urgent need, to work in hospitals for short periods on sessional fees in addition to carrying on their general practices. Practitioners already allocated for duties in the Civil Defence Services, or employed part-time by the War Office for medical attendance at camp reception stations, etc., were not to be included in these lists.[2]

As time went on, the difficulties of providing adequate medical staff of all grades for the E.M.S. hospitals progressively increased as the strength of the Fighting Forces expanded.

The arrangements made by the Central Medical War Committee with the Services, under which no newly qualified men would be called up until they had done six months as house surgeons or physicians or in practice, ensured that the teaching hospitals still had an adequate supply of the best material. The old-established non-teaching voluntary and local authority hospitals also had little difficulty in filling vacancies, but a number of newly qualified men, who failed to obtain house appointments in large well-known hospitals, seemed to fight shy of taking appointments in the newly constituted or expanded E.M.S. hospitals and preferred to take posts as assistants or locum tenens in general practice until they were called up for the Services.

Some of these large hospitals with military wings had barely sufficient staffs to deal with the convoys from overseas and had to call on local practitioners to work part-time on sessional fees. In other cases some of the members of the junior house staffs of the large teaching hospitals in towns had to be temporarily transferred to these new base hospitals in rural areas. But even when these expedients had been applied, many of these hospitals had to include considerable numbers of fully equipped beds in their lists of reserve beds owing to the shortage of medical and nursing staffs.

With a view to meeting the increasing shortage, discussions took place on the question of bringing in doctors from Canada and the United States. It soon became evident that the Canadian authorities would require all their available doctors to meet the needs of their own civil population and their Fighting Forces overseas, but it was considered that the question of importing doctors from the United States might be taken up, it being known that many were anxious to place their services at our disposal if the obstacles in the way could be removed. Indeed, a number of American doctors had already come to this country at their own expense as volunteers.

THE 'ROBINSON' COMMITTEE*

In December 1940, as the result of these discussions and the increasing shortage of medical personnel, the Rt. Hon. Malcolm Macdonald, M.P., Minister of Health, appointed a committee, with Sir Arthur Robinson, G.C.B., G.B.E., as chairman, as a matter of urgency to consider, in relation to the needs of the civilian population and of H.M. Forces, the recruitment of doctors to the Services, and to report what steps should be taken to secure a proper allocation of medical man-power between the civilian and military Services.

---

* See Army Medical Services, Volume I, Chapter 9.

This committee met daily and heard evidence by representatives of the Central Medical War Committee, the Ministry of Health, the Fighting Services, the Ministry of Labour, the General Medical Council, etc. They found that the number of medical practitioners in active practice in peace-time in Great Britain and Northern Ireland was in round figures 45,300, of which 1,400 held regular commissions in H.M. Forces and that since the outbreak of war until December 1940, 7,500 additional practitioners had been embodied in the Services. This left 36,400 in civil practice, but of these 16,700 were over 50 years of age, including about 5,000 over 70 and therefore, either unfit for practice or unlikely to be able to bear the strain of additional work.

In the Emergency Medical Services in England and Wales 1,653 doctors were employed whole-time and 552 part-time. There was also a reserve pool, which was not heavily drawn upon, of 4,615 doctors who undertook to serve as and when required on a sessional basis. It was estimated, however, that there might be available for practice about 36,000 practitioners, i.e. 0·82 per thousand of the civilian population that remained after recruitment of some 3,000,000 to the Fighting and other Services. In H.M. Forces the ratio of medical officers to total personnel per thousand was stated to be 4·1 in the Royal Navy, 2·8 in the Army and 2·9 in the Royal Air Force. The additional requirements of the Services up to the end of March 1941, were stated to be 1,757 and the average annual intake into the profession was found to be about 2,100. This was not a net increase as allowances had to be made for withdrawals, deaths, etc.

The distribution of medical personnel in the hospitals was found to be in the London area, with 90,550 beds, one whole-time medical officer for 56·3 beds; and in the rest of England and Wales, with 338,337 beds, one medical officer for 170·3 beds. The Committee's report,[3] January 1, 1941, contained the following recommendations:

(i) That the medical establishments of hospitals should be examined and revised forthwith.

(ii) That the use of civil practitioners in proximity to concentrations of troops might be further extended.

(iii) That where three Fighting Services were represented in the same area, the principle of area service should be adopted.

(iv) That the possibility of the release of Service medical officers for civilian work in the winter should be carefully examined.

(v) That the question of the employment of alien doctors should be re-examined and extended as far as possible.

(vi) That the employment of final year students as house surgeons and physicians should be set on foot at once.

(vii) That the employment of practitioners from the Dominions should be further explored.

(viii) That the possibility of recruitment of practitioners from the United States of America should be considered.

(ix) That an effective organisation for the settlement of questions of priority should be established.

ACTION TAKEN BY THE MINISTRY OF HEALTH

The Ministry of Health at once took action on the recommendations which concerned them:

(i) *The Establishments of Hospitals*. This recommendation was communicated to all large hospitals and it was agreed that the Central Medical War Committee would review the establishments of all hospitals with special reference to A, B2 and B1 posts.

In March 1941, after consultation with the Central Medical War Committee the Ministry laid down the following as an 'ideal' establishment per thousand occupied beds in E.M.S. hospitals:

Medical Officers on salaries of £500 per annum part-time and £800 per annum whole-time or on the higher rate of sessional fees	13
Medical Officers at £550 per annum whole-time or on the lower rate of sessional fees	8
Junior Medical Officers at £350 per annum whole-time	3·5
House Surgeons and House Physicians	10·5

This 'ideal' establishment was circulated to all hospitals[4] and they were required to submit their present establishments to the Central Medical War Committee who then laid down a sanctioned establishment for each hospital which was not to be exceeded.

(v) *Employment of Alien Practitioners*. Hospitals were urged to employ alien practitioners and certain restrictions on their employment laid down by the Security Departments were modified for the purpose.[5] This resulted in the number of practitioners with only alien degrees employed in the E.M.S. being raised to 301 by June 1941, which permitted the release of 126 British practitioners for service with the Armed Forces. The extent to which aliens were employed will be found in the section dealing with the work of the Central Medical War Committee at the end of this chapter.

(vi) *Employment of Final Year Students*. Many teaching hospitals were found to have already given effect to the principle laid down in this recommendation which from this time was adopted to the fullest extent commensurate with efficiency.

(vii) *Employment of Dominion Doctors*. No action was taken on this recommendation for the reasons already mentioned.

(viii) *Employment of American Doctors in the E.M.S.* The Ministry of Health had already taken action on this recommendation. After several conferences on the subject steps were taken to legalise the employment of American doctors in the civil hospitals in the United Kingdom by obtaining their temporary registration by the General Medical Council, and the British Embassy in the United States was instructed to find out whether the United States was willing to co-operate and permit American doctors to volunteer for such service. No difficulty whatever was made by the United States Government, and the Embassy was instructed to get in touch with the American Medical Association to ascertain their views and enlist their co-operation to obtain suitable volunteers. This co-operation was willingly given, but the American Medical Association expressed the view that they could not undertake to become a clearing house for the engagement of suitable volunteers.

The Embassy was then informed that present requirements would be met if twenty surgeons of about ten years' experience and thirty practitioners of five years' experience could be selected from among those volunteering for service. The former would be paid as specialists at the rate of £800 per annum, plus free board and lodging and the latter £550 per annum plus the same allowances.

About this time, however, the military authorities expressed a desire to employ a large number of American doctors if they were available, and the demand in the E.M.S. continued to increase; it was therefore agreed in December 1940, to endeavour to obtain one thousand doctors, nine hundred for the Services and one hundred for the E.M.S. It was also arranged at the request of the American Red Cross that the recruiting of these doctors should be done through them in liaison with the British Red Cross in this country.

The first American doctors under this scheme began to arrive in June 1941, but a few had come over earlier in the year at their own expense. Dr. Howard R. Ives was the first to be employed in the E.M.S., and was posted to Hill End Hospital, St. Albans. Shortly after this twelve more, including two women, arrived, and by September 30, fifty-five altogether had been accepted, of whom forty-two had sailed and thirteen were ready to sail. By October 31, fifty-seven had sailed. Of the total recruited for the E.M.S., ten were women.

The United States having come into the war in December 1941, all recruitment of American doctors for the British Army and the E.M.S. was stopped in January 1942. Of those who had already come over, any who chose and were suitable were transferred to the U.S. Army and some returned to America; but at December 23, 1942, there were still thirteen male and seven female U.S.A. doctors in the E.M.S.

The American Hospital in Britain. (See Appendix I). In the meantime an orthopaedic unit called 'The American Hospital in Britain, Ltd.' with the approval of the United States Government and the Government of the United Kingdom was established under Dr. Philip D. Wilson, the well-known orthopaedic surgeon, for service in Britain in civilian hospitals. This unit, which consisted of five orthopaedic surgeons, one plastic surgeon, one neurosurgeon, three operating nurses and one medical recorder, arrived in England by sea in September 1940.

The Harvard Field Unit. (See Appendix II). In addition to Dr. Wilson's unit, an epidemiological unit organised by Harvard University, with the agreement of the Ministry of Health, arrived in England in 1941, under the direction of Professor John Gordon. The object of this unit was to assist in dealing with outbreaks of infectious diseases which it was expected would occur owing to the dislocation of the health services by war conditions. This unit brought with it a prefabricated hospital and full equipment, which was established by agreement on a site on the outskirts of Salisbury, where there was a demand for hospital accommodation for infectious diseases, the D.D.M.S. Southern Command having found difficulty in obtaining beds for such cases among the troops in the Command.

The medical officers of health of scheme-making authorities were requested to assist the objects of the unit in any way they could. The hospital gradually filled up and was nearly full, when after the arrival of the U.S. Forces in this country, the unit was taken over by the U.S. Army.

(ix) *A Priority Organisation.* Action on this recommendation was deferred in the hope that the steps recorded above would make it possible to supply Service needs without recourse to standing priority machinery, but eventually the Rt. Hon. Ernest Brown, M.P., who had succeeded Mr. MacDonald as Minister of Health, announced in the House of Commons on June 19, 1941, that it had been decided to set up a committee to be known as the Medical Personnel (Priority) Committee.[6]

THE MEDICAL PERSONNEL (PRIORITY) COMMITTEE*

Terms of Reference. 'To investigate in the light of recommendations made in January 1941, by the Committee of Inquiry on Medical Personnel' (the 'Robinson' Committee), 'what further steps can usefully be taken to secure the utmost economy in the employment of medical personnel in H.M. Forces, the Civil Defence Services, the Emergency Hospital Scheme and all other medical services, including general practice, and having regard to any recommendations made as a result of such investigations to report from time to time what should be the allocation between the above-mentioned services of the available medical personnel'.[7]

Interim Report. Mr. Geoffrey Shakespeare, M.P. (afterwards Sir Geoffrey Shakespeare, Bart.), Parliamentary Secretary for the Dominions, was appointed chairman and the members included representatives of the Royal Colleges and the Medical Departments of the Services. The committee first met on July 3, 1941, and after 25 sittings and several visits to selected areas, submitted an Interim Report to the Minister of Health on August 6, 1941.[7]

---

* See also Army Medical Services, Volume I, Chapter 9.

The committee found that as a result of the recommendations of the 'Robinson' Committee each Service had reviewed its establishment and requirements and had effected considerable economies. Further economies had been secured during the committee's inquiries and, in the view of the Services, demands had been reduced to a minimum if the efficiency of the medical services was to be maintained and further expansion programmes met. These minimum demands at that time were Royal Navy 100, Army 1,200 and Royal Air Force 300, a total of 1,600.

The committee stated that they were not yet in a position to give an opinion upon the medical personnel requirements of the E.M.S., and the other hospital and health services, but expressed the view that the withdrawal of a further 1,600 practitioners would impose a severe strain on the existing resources. Their general recommendations were as follows:

(1) That in each Region, a committee composed of senior medical Officers representing the various Services, civil and military, should be set up, and that a neutral person, preferably the Regional Commissioner, should be the chairman. These committees should meet regularly and be charged with ensuring the maximum co-operation to meet civilian and Service needs and review at once, and from time to time, the position in the Regions as regards medical personnel in order to effect economies in medical manpower and eliminate overlapping and under-employment.

(2) That the Central Medical War Committee should in the meantime continue to provide medical officers for the Services at the present rate.

(3) That in order to facilitate the work of the Central Medical War Committee in obtaining the numbers of medical officers, some of whom would have to come from the hospital staffs, the Ministry of Health should obtain complete particulars as to the bed accommodation and staffing of all civilian hospitals in Great Britain.

(4) That, in the case of medical practitioners, the Minister of Labour should consider the advisability of raising the age limit for compulsory military service from 41 years to 46.

This suggestion of enlarging the field of recruitment by extending the age limit five years beyond that for the general population indicated the committee's sense of the urgency of the problem. According to the Central Medical War Committee's Register there were about eleven thousand male practitioners under 41 years of age unevenly distributed throughout the country, from whom it would be difficult to obtain the number required by the Services without seriously depleting certain areas. The possibility of compulsory transfer of practitioners into areas where there was more urgent need for their services had been considered, but, while it was thought possible to effect transfers from one salaried post to another, the difficulties in transferring doctors from one general practice to another were regarded as insuperable.

(5) That, as Service requirements must be met in part by further decreasing hospital staffs, powers should be taken to move whole-time

medical staffs in A, B2 and B1 posts from one hospital to another so as to ensure greater mobility to meet any periods of strain.

(6) That the medical officers of the Anti-Aircraft and Balloon Barrage Commands of the Army and Air Force should be pooled.

The Ministry of Health immediately took steps to obtain the information required as regards civilian hospitals and their staffs referred to in recommendation (3) above. 'A' posts were defined as whole-time resident posts which could be filled by practitioners not having previous hospital experience. 'B' posts were those for which previous experience was required and, although whole-time, were not necessarily resident appointments. They are more exactly defined in the section of this chapter which deals with the work of the Central Medical War Committee.

After presenting their first Interim Report the committee continued exhaustive enquiries into all the sources of supply of medical man-power in every branch of the profession. They periodically framed further resolutions in the form of recommendations to the Minister of Health, which resulted in:

(a) The rapid calling up for the Services of all 'A' practitioners found fit after six months' hospital experience, and the cessation of granting of extensions;

(b) The mental hospitals being required to release 100 medical men of military age for the Services by January 1942;

(c) The reduction of whole-time personnel of military age holding A and B posts by 15 per cent. in hospitals in the London area and 10 per cent. in the provinces;

(d) The replacement of male by female practitioners to the fullest extent possible in hospital posts;

(e) Action to release as many young medical men as possible from pathological and research work for special or general duty in the Fighting Services;

(f) Action to obtain the release from the public health services of the local authorities of more medical officers of both sexes for service with the Armed Forces.

At the same time a detailed scrutiny of the demands of the Services resulted in further economies in medical man-power. The Royal Air Force accepted cuts of 37 per cent. on their original demands for the previous six months, the Army reduced their demands by 40 per cent. and the Navy reduced theirs for the last three months of the year by 50 per cent. By these methods the deficit in the requirements of the Services was met by the end of June 1942.

As regards the E.M.S., in addition to the percentage cuts in hospital staffs, recommendations to increase their mobility in emergencies were made, so that the staffs of hospitals in areas being attacked from the air could be supplemented from hospitals in areas not under attack.

These recommendations were accepted and put into force by the Ministry of Health and were included, together with the action taken, in the second Interim Report of the Committee submitted on February 11, 1942.[7]

The general conclusions of the committee as a result of their investigations were:

(*a*) That the Combatant Services were now fully alive to the limited resources available to meet their needs;

(*b*) That the co-operation of the Services had resulted in a substantial reduction in their demands;

(*c*) That their recommendations for the saving in medical man-power in the civilian hospitals would help to solve the problem, but that continued vigilance in the economical use of the available resources was essential;

(*d*) That no more recruits from alien sources other than those already obtained could be expected.

FURTHER TRANSACTIONS OF THE MEDICAL PERSONNEL (PRIORITY) COMMITTEE

Between July 1942, and the end of hostilities the committee held eighteen further meetings and from time to time made recommendations to the Ministry of Health with the view of endeavouring to meet the continually increasing shortage of medical personnel.

The following is a summary of the most important of these which were accepted and put into force:

(1) *March* 1942.—That the clinical portion of the medical curriculum be reduced from three years to thirty months; on this subject the General Medical Council addressed the Universities and the licensing bodies who, by May 1943, had all accepted the proposal.

(2) *May* 1942.—That the holders of A and B2 posts in hospitals be recruited to the Forces after six months' tenure and only exceptionally be permitted to take higher posts in hospitals.

(3) *May* 1942.—That part-time officers be required to undertake a greater share in hospital work in order to release more whole-time officers.

(4) *July* 1942.—That post-graduate teaching entailing the whole-time attendance of practitioners for a considerable period be abandoned for the duration of the war.

(5) *September* 1942.—That all newly qualified practitioners who had not secured a hospital appointment within three months should be forthwith recruited to the Forces.

(6) *September* 1942.—That the holders of A posts in hospital be released for recruitment after three months instead of six, the release in each hospital to be up to 50 per cent. of the A posts. This direction was afterwards applied to B posts also.

(7) *December* 1942.—That the age for recruitment for male practitioners be raised from 46 to 51 and for women from 31 to 41, and that powers be taken to transfer civil practitioners to paid hospital appointments. The recommendation to increase the age of recruitment for male and female practitioners was not accepted, but it was agreed that powers of direction into salaried posts should be obtained.

(8) *December* 1942.—That the further demands of the Services were such that any attempt to meet these demands would have serious consequences which should be brought to the notice of the Minister of Health. The committee pointed out that the situation permitted only one of two alternatives: (*a*) a drastic reduction of the basis and scope of general practice and of the public health organisation. Some public health services would have to be closed down, and the burden placed on general practitioners would be such that members of the public would often find themselves unable to secure the services of a doctor in cases of urgent need; (*b*) that the Services should be required to content themselves with a recruitment rate of not more than 200–225 practitioners a month.

The allocation of doctors between the Forces and the civil population was considered by the War Cabinet, who decided to ask the Lord Privy Seal, Lord Cranborne, to investigate the medical organisation of the three combatant Services and of the E.M.S. (see Army Medical Services, Volume I, Chapter 9).

The result was that whereas the committee had been faced with the problem of finding about 5,000 practitioners for the Services in 1943, these demands were by various expedients reduced to 3,600 or 300 a month. The committee, however, reported to the Cabinet that they could not provide more than 220 practitioners a month and then only by a further call-up of general practitioners and a further cut in the whole-time staffs of hospitals. To go beyond this figure, such essential services as public health, maternity and child welfare, the school medical service, etc., would have to be further cut down.

Eventually, in July 1943, the committee were instructed to make arrangements to provide 2,016 practitioners for the year 1943.

(9) *January* 1943.—That the restrictions on the holders of A and B posts to higher posts in the hospitals be removed so that the hospitals may be free to propose these promotions, subject to their obtaining the approval of the Central Medical War Committee in each case.

(10) *September* 1943.—That the direction of women practitioners to salaried posts should be applied to unmarried women up to the age of 46.

(11) *February* 1944.—That the Service departments should be asked to recruit more women doctors and that steps should be taken to raise the recruitment age to 40.

(12) *October* 1944.—That the arrangements in force for the recruitment of doctors might for the present be allowed to continue.

(13) *February* 1945.—The committee reviewed the shortage of medical man-power in various civil hospital services and recommended that in such services as the laboratory services, radiotherapy for cancer, radiological service, miners' medical service, tuberculosis service, although all of great importance, no increases should at present be permitted, but that no recruits from these services could be expected for the Forces.

(14) *October* 1945.—That the recruitment of newly qualified practitioners should continue on the present basis as a means of ensuring the maximum release of doctors from the Forces under the Government release scheme.

(15) *October* 1945.—That short-term commissions of at least one year should be offered to surgeons and physicians over the age of 40 of recognised consultant status in civil employment, in order to facilitate the return of officers of similar status in the early release groups in the Forces, whose release would otherwise have to be deferred, as it was essential that the professional standard of medical officers in the Forces of specialist status must be maintained.

(16) *January* 1946.—In order to provide the maximum recruitment of young practitioners to the Forces and at the same time to avoid dislocation in the civil health services, the committee recommended that medical officers other than specialists should now be recruited for a short-term employment of two years.

These recommendations made by the M.P.P.C. from time to time indicate the difficulties that arose in an endeavour to meet the essential requirements of the Services, and at the same time to safeguard the interests of the civil population by limiting the depletion of the numbers of private practitioners and maintaining the hospital staffs at a standard and level sufficiently high to deal adequately with civilian and Service patients.

Recommendation (8) above is an important example of the policy followed to attain these ends. In the light of experience it can be said that these objects were in the main attained, but only by the cordial co-operation of both the civil and military authorities. The civil practitioners had to undertake long hours of work, many having to carry on single-handed a practice previously served by two or three partners, and many retired practitioners had to return to harness in practice and in hospitals.

The Services made every possible endeavour to limit their demands to the barest minimum. Certain civil practitioners, however, on translation to military spheres of action, ventilated their opinions in the press, and created the impression that they had little or nothing to do and would be better employed assisting their overworked colleagues in civil practice. They did not appreciate at first that their chief duty in the Services, when not in action, was not to attend on sick men, but to prevent them being sick during the periods of strenuous military training and to prepare both themselves and their men to meet the heavy strain of military action against the enemy.

The M.P.P.C., to assist them in their duties, naturally took steps to obtain all relevant information about the distribution of the numbers of the various grades of the medical profession available for civil and military duties.

The figures given in Table I below show the distribution of the profession in 1940, 1943 and 1945, periods which have been taken as samples. These figures include temporarily registered practitioners but not officers with regular commissions in the Services. At the beginning of the war the latter amounted to 1,440 officers:

TABLE I

Occupational Distribution of the Medical Profession

(England and Wales)

	March 1940 Services	March 1940 Totals	January 1943 Services	January 1943 Totals	February 1945 Services	February 1945 Totals
1. Consultants or specialists	383	3,979	730	3,841	724	3,693
2. General practitioner	2,360	18,877	4,157	18,682	3,995	18,332
3. W.T. voluntary hospital	845	1,995	2,632	4,498	3,998	6,105
4. W.T.L.A. general hospital	126	850	1,078	2,418	1,685	3,385
5. W.T.L.A. special hospital	92	934	505	1,432	608	1,468
6. W.T.P.H. service	116	1,931	310	2,253	377	2,172
7. W.T. government services	60	500	123	602	145	775
8. W.T. teacher	21	259	55	313	66	359
9. W.T. research	58	322	90	388	102	396
10. W.T. non-government post	54	285	63	472	65	581
11. Dentist	24	307	83	362	90	354
12. Retired	122	} 5,798	126	2,647	99	1,515
13. Totally ineffective	—		—	2,084	—	3,234
14. Unclassified	247	2,665	970	2,542	911	2,587
Totals	4,508	38,702	10,922	42,534	12,865	44,956

W.T. = Whole-time.   L.A. = Local Authority.   P.H. = Public Health.

Table II on the following page shows the gradual increase in the work which was being thrown on private practitioners owing to the increasing demands of the Services:

TABLE II

Ratio of General Practitioners to Civilian Population

(England and Wales)

Year	Estimated civilian population	Numbers of general practitioners	Ratio
1938	41,215,000	18,870	1–2184
1939	41,246,000	16,517	1–2497
1940	39,889,000	15,706	1–2540
1941	38,743,000	14,969	1–2588
1942	38,243,000	14,525	1–2632
1943	37,818,000	14,336	1–2638
1944	37,785,000	14,337	1–2635
1945	38,157,000	15,874	1–2404

NOTE: The population figures are the estimates of the population for the mid-year supplied by the Registrar General, while the numbers of practitioners in civil practice at the end of each year are taken from the figures supplied by the C.M.W.C to the M.P.P.C.

Table III below shows the numbers of medical men, women and specialists recruited to the Services during each year of the war:

TABLE III

Recruitment of Medical Personnel

(England and Wales)

	1939–40	1941	1942	1943	1944	1945
Men	4,880	2,355	2,827	1,820	989	908
Women	99	58	203	142	196	60
Specialists	395	177	411	139	46	80
Totals	5,374	2,590	3,441	2,101	1,231	1,048

Table IV on the following page, extracted from the Medical Register gives the annual increase of practitioners available, chiefly by the intake of newly qualified men and by the temporary registration of alien practitioners, together with the annual wastage through death and other causes:

TABLE IV

Number of Persons whose Names were registered in, added to, or removed from, the Medical Registers for each Year from 1939 to 1945 inclusive

| Year | Numbers added by registration ||||| Number restored | Number removed | Total numbers in register on December 31 in each year |
------	In England	In Scotland	In Ireland	Colonial	Foreign	Total				
1939	1,437	692	356	296	187	2,968	49	1,027	63,360
1940	1,323	673	315	57	16	2,384	37	1,102	64,679
1941	1,189	632	285	134	1,056	3,296	16	996	66,992
1942	1,663	593	381	206	713	3,556	7	1,127	69,428
1943	1,501	611	405	153	862	3,532	13	1,091	71,882
1944	1,196	619	307	320	529	2,971	11	1,218	73,646
1945	1,268	581	428	124	265	2,666	11	1,190	75,133
Totals	9,577	4,401	2,477	1,290	3,628	21,373	144	7,751	

Average net intake per annum 1966·5.

Table V below shows the number of medical men and women in the Services at the end of each year of the war and the sources from which they were obtained:

TABLE V

Numbers of Medical Personnel in H.M. Forces

(England and Wales)

Date	Total number on medical register	Specialists	General practitioners	Hospitals	Public health	Others	Totals
January 1942	41,671	639	3,704	2,855	210	1,381	8,789
January 1943	40,450	730	4,157	4,215	310	1,510	10,922
February 1944	41,428	739	4,173	5,631	381	1,504	12,428
February 1945	41,722	724	3,995	6,291	377	1,478	12,865
February 1946	42,213	281	1,771	5,735	258	935	8,980

The recommendations of the committee and the above tables indicate that every possible source of medical man-power was thoroughly investigated and depleted to such an extent that by 1943 it was recognised that any further reduction in their numbers might well cause a breakdown in the civil medical organisation.

In the E.M.S. hospitals, although many beds had to be transferred to the reserve for lack of medical and nursing personnel, the policy of mobility and elasticity and the concentration of essential effort in the form of special centres, enabled the depleted numbers fully to cope with the increased duties required of them. When it is recalled that the great majority of the 277,821 wounded of the Armed Forces and Auxiliary Services of the United Kingdom, and all the seriously injured civilian casualties (91,446, including Home Guard and Merchant Navy), as well as Service and civilian sick, were treated in E.M.S. hospitals, and that the E.M.S. casualty services dealt with 150,832 slightly injured civilian casualties, it will be recognised that this was no mean achievement on the part of the comparatively small army of medical men and women whose lot it was thus to serve on the Home Front. Theirs was indeed a gigantic task, which could only be carried out successfully, as it was, by the co-operation of all concerned in a great and sustained effort of devoted and untiring service. It was fortunate, however, that the number of overseas casualties admitted to hospitals in this country were far smaller than in the War of 1914–18 and that air raid casualties were far below the numbers considered probable.

Table VI below shows the establishment of the E.M.S. hospitals during each year of the war:

TABLE VI

Establishment of E.M.S. Hospitals

Date	Whole-time	Part-time
January 1 1939	1,661	—
January 1 1941	1,069	527
January 1 1942	1,345	482
January 1 1943	1,147	548
January 1 1944	1,088	462
January 1 1945	1,134	461
January 1 1946	865	412

NOTE: Excludes consultants and practitioners on sessional fees and medical officers in charge of first-aid posts.

THE CENTRAL MEDICAL WAR COMMITTEE

The following account of the work of the Central Medical War Committee in connexion with the recruitment and allocation of medical personnel and the employment of alien practitioners is based on contributions by the Secretary of the Committee.

THE PERIOD 1925–35

On March 4, 1925, a communication on the recruitment of medical practitioners in case of war was addressed to the British Medical Association by the Ministry of Health inviting the Association to co-operate with the Government by formulating proposals for the composition of a Central Medical War Committee for England and Wales, with separate committees for Scotland and Northern Ireland, and for the establishment of Local Medical War Committees. The functions of the proposed committees were described as follows: 'The main functions of the central committee will be to determine the quota of medical officers to be provided from time to time from the area of each Local Medical War Committee and to represent the profession in any negotiations with the Government departments concerned. The functions of the local committees will be to determine how the stipulated quota can be released for service with least injury to the civil population and to the personal claims of the practitioners affected'. The letter emphasised the importance of the establishment of the Central Committee and of the Scottish and Northern Irish Committees in advance of mobilisation, and that the instructions for the appointment of local committees should be ready for immediate use when required. The letter added that it was proposed to provide for the special needs of the consultant and teaching staffs of the London hospitals by inviting the Royal Colleges to appoint, as in the last war, a Committee of Reference (see 'Brock' Committee, Introduction).

On March 25, 1925, the Council of the Association resolved to cooperate with the Ministry in the way proposed, and drew up a memorandum which they sent to the Ministry on December 31. In this memorandum two main objects were kept in view: first, to provide a minimum of standing machinery with a maximum of efficiency in mobilisation; and secondly, to ensure sufficient elasticity to avoid any constitutional or social dislocation during adjustment to war conditions.

It was proposed, in the first place, that the Association should appoint a Central Emergency Committee with the following functions:

(1) To conduct any interim dealings with the War Office or the Ministry of Health pending emergency conditions;

(2) When such conditions arose, to function for all purposes until it was possible for a fully competent body to meet;

(3) To convene a fully competent body immediately on the receipt of intimation of necessity from the Ministry of Health; and

(4) On the intimation of necessity to send out instructions for the constitution of the necessary local bodies.

For Scotland and Northern Ireland similar committees were proposed, which would convene the fully competent bodies for these areas, acting on a request from the Central Emergency Committee for England and Wales. The personnel suggested for the Central Emergency Committee included three of the honorary officers of the Association (the Chairman of the Representative Body, the Chairman of Council and the Treasurer), the Chairman for the time being of the Naval and Military Committee and three members to be appointed annually by the Council, with a secretary and a deputy secretary.

Detailed suggestions were made for the composition of the Central Medical War Committee, which would replace the Central Emergency Committee when a national emergency occurred. The proposed personnel included the members of the Central Emergency Committee, additional members appointed by the British Medical Association, the Society of Medical Officers of Health, the Poor Law Medical Officers' Association, the Medical Women's Federation, the Royal College of Surgeons of England and the Royal College of Physicians of London, together with representatives (acting as liaison officers) of the similar committees for Scotland and Northern Ireland and the Committee of Reference.

Finally, the memorandum dealt with the local emergency plans. These were to be based on the local organisation of the Association. The executive committee of each division would function as an emergency committee for its area until such time as it was found necessary to constitute a Local Medical War Committee, which would not be a committee of the B.M.A., but would be elected by the whole of the local profession. On the declaration of war, the immediate functions of the Local Emergency Committee would be to make arrangements for the practices of local reservists and Territorial Army officers, to provide any assistance required by local military authorities and to summon a general meeting of the profession for the purpose of electing a Local Medical War Committee, representative of all types of practice in the area.

The plans described above were approved by the Ministry of Health, and in July 1926, the Council of the Association appointed Central Emergency Committees for England and Wales, for Scotland and for Northern Ireland. Thereafter these committees were re-appointed each year, but ten years passed before the Committee for England and Wales held its first meeting. In 1936 the personnel had been altered, and the committee was re-constituted as follows: the Chairman of the Representative Body of the Association, the Chairman of Council, the Treasurer, the Chairman of the Naval and Military Organisation, Public Health and Welsh Committees, a representative of the Royal College of Surgeons and a representative of the Royal College of Physicians, with a secretary and a deputy secretary.

THE PERIOD 1936–38

At its first meeting, in September 1936, the Central Emergency Committee reviewed the memorandum of 1925 and recommended that the Council should re-affirm its approval of the memorandum with certain amendments. These included a change in the composition of the committee, a provision that the Council should be free to vary the membership of the committee at its discretion and a recommendation that the membership of the Central Medical War Committee should be altered by including the Chairman of the Insurance Acts Committee of the B.M.A. and excluding representatives of the Poor Law Medical Officers' Association and the two Royal Colleges. The Council approved these changes in November 1936, and sent the revised memorandum to the Ministry of Health.

In 1936, the Secretary of the British Medical Association was appointed to represent the Association on a sub-committee of the Committee of Imperial Defence which was considering the question of co-ordination of medical services in time of war. In the same year the Association made a statistical survey to ascertain the exact distribution of the medical profession in its various sections throughout England and Wales and the distribution of hospital beds. The survey showed the numbers of practitioners in the areas of the various B.M.A. branches, classified according to sex, age (above or below 50) and type of practice.

In January 1937, the Central Emergency Committee held a meeting which was attended by representatives of the Ministry of Health, the Ministry of Pensions, the Air Raid Precautions Department of the Home Office and the Medical Departments of the three Defence

Services. The provision of medical personnel for the Services and for the treatment of air raid casualties in the event of war was discussed and it was considered that the arrangements for establishing war committees after the outbreak of hostilities were not wholly satisfactory. It was recommended that, subject to the approval of the Committee of Imperial Defence and the Ministry of Health, the British Medical Association should be authorised to prepare in advance, for the area of each home division, a register of practitioners who, immediately on the occurrence of a national emergency, would be willing to accept commissioned service with the Forces at home or abroad or to undertake the treatment of air raid casualties in their own localities or, on a short-term contract, in any part of the country. It was recommended also that the Central Emergency Committee should be empowered to co-opt representatives of the medical departments of the Royal Navy, the Army and the Royal Air Force, and of the Ministry of Pensions and the Home Office (see 'Goodwin' Committee Report, Chapter 1).

These recommendations were adopted and in October 1937, the Central Emergency Committee, which had been increased by the inclusion of a representative of the Medical Women's Federation in addition to the representatives of the departments mentioned above, discussed and approved plans for the establishment of registers of practitioners who would be available for national service during the period of voluntary recruitment immediately following mobilisation.

When the Central Emergency Committee next met, at the end of April 1938, the intentions of approximately 75 per cent. of the profession with regard to service were known and had been analysed. The analysis was sent to the Ministry of Health and the Committee of Imperial Defence. A central card register, containing all essential details, was prepared for ease of reference.

During the week of the Munich emergency in September 1938, the Central Emergency Committee invited all practitioners who had completed its war service questionnaire to reaffirm or amend their offers of service and to permit the disclosure of the information, originally given in confidence, to central and local authorities. At the same time the committee invited those who had not made a return to do so. The atmosphere of crisis produced an excellent and very prompt response, and by the end of September only 3,000 practitioners (less than seven per cent. of the 44,500 covered by the national register) had not informed the committee of their intentions of service. The emergency, however, had brought to light certain defects in the arrangements for the medical care of the civil population in time of war. It appeared that the work of providing the necessary medical personnel was likely to be hampered seriously by the fact that the Central Emergency Committee had no information about the Government's plans for the hospital treatment of air raid casualties and for evacuating the civil population from vulnerable areas. The responsibility for civilian medical services was shared by two Government departments, and there had been much confusion about the arrangements for the medical staffing of first-aid posts which were controlled, not by the Ministry of Health, but by the Home Office. Again, medical practitioners were being approached by local commanding officers of the Services and were being earmarked for Service duties without prior consultation with the Central Emergency Committee.

A deputation from the committee discussed these matters with the Minister for Co-ordination of Defence and urged the importance of central co-ordination of the civilian medical services and the medical services of the Armed Forces through the establishment of a single Government body to control all demands for medical personnel. The deputation recommended that the Central Emergency Committee, reconstituted to make it fully representative of all branches of the profession, should be given authority, in consultation with the appropriate Government organisations, to advise on the allocation of the available medical personnel to all the different services in time of emergency.

Early in November 1938 the Council of the British Medical Association reconstituted the Central Emergency Committee with an enlarged membership, which included the chairmen or other representatives of all the standing committees of the Association concerned with the various departments of medical practice, as well as four general practitioners appointed by the Association on a territorial basis, and representatives of the Society of Medical Officers of Health, the Medical Women's Federation, the Medical Committee of the House of Commons, and the Royal Colleges. Liaison officers of the Scottish and Northern Irish Committees were included and provision was made for the attendance of representatives of the Ministry of Health, the Home Office, the Ministry of Pensions and the Medical Departments of the three Services. The Council approved a recommendation that the Central Emergency Committee in its new form should continue in existence as the Central Medical War Committee in the event of a national emergency.

During the September crisis the Association asked its divisions throughout the country to set up Local Emergency Committees for the immediate purpose of preparing schemes to protect the practices of absentee practitioners in the event of war, a model scheme having been issued previously to the divisions for their guidance. It was proposed that these Local Emergency Committees should assume the functions of Local Medical War Committees in a national emergency. The central committee also issued to the local committees copies of the appropriate sections of the emergency register of medical practitioners, brought up to date in the light of the latest available information; and subsequent changes in the register were notified to the local committees at regular intervals.

THE YEAR 1939

In the early months of 1939, the Central Emergency Committee and its standing sub-committees held frequent meetings and considerable progress was made in the medical preparations for war. The Government accepted the principle that the committee, in consultation with the local committees, should be responsible for advising on the allocation of medical practitioners to the Services and to Government departments. Estimates were obtained from the Service departments of the numbers of practitioners they would require in the period immediately after mobilisation, and quotas were allocated to the Local Emergency Committees. The local committees began the provisional earmarking of practitioners for certain local duties, such as duties at first-aid posts (the control of which had been transferred to the Ministry of Health), casualty clearing stations and hospitals, and for recruiting medical boards.

Special arrangements were made in respect of consultants and specialists, except pathologists and bacteriologists, on the staffs of voluntary and municipal hospitals in the County of London or temporarily transferred to other hospitals outside this area. It was arranged that requests from the Services and from Government departments for consultants and specialists would be sent to the Central Emergency Committee, which would decide the proportion to be recruited from the London area and ask the Committee of Reference to make the necessary allocation from the pool at its disposal. At the request of the Committee of Reference, the Central Emergency Committee undertook the administrative and secretarial work involved in making a special register of London consultants and specialists, and appointed its secretary to serve on the Committee of Reference for liaison. The allocation of pathologists and bacteriologists was made on the recommendation of the Medical Research Council, this body having undertaken the planning of emergency pathological services.

Later in 1939, the Central Emergency Committee was consulted by the Ministry of Health regarding the staffing of civilian hospitals in time of emergency. Detailed proposals were later received from the Ministry and, after some revision, were approved by the committee in July. The membership of the committee was increased by adding representatives of the Medical Research Council, the Board of Education and the Board of Control.

When war was declared the national register contained particulars of 98 per cent. of the medical practitioners resident in Great Britain. There was no shortage of volunteers for immediate commissioned service in the Forces. Before the middle of September the considerable mobilisation demands of the War Office had been fully met, but the Local Emergency Committees were asked to scrutinise their registers and submit additional names of men who could be spared from their areas, in order that a central reserve list of volunteers might be established to meet future Service requirements. The local committees in evacuation areas were asked to submit also the names of practitioners who could be spared for, and were willing to undertake, civilian medical work elsewhere; and the committees in the crowded reception areas were invited to report any need of assistance. Many volunteers, including numbers of retired practitioners, offered their services for war work but the demand for civilian medical personnel was limited and many inquirers had to be informed that no opportunities of undertaking 'war work' were immediately available for them.

Among the practitioners with pre-war commitments, which had rendered them liable for duty with the Army on the outbreak of war, there were many specialists. The Central Emergency Committee scrutinised the qualifications of such practitioners and sent to the War Office lists of those who, if not already holding specialist posts, were recommended for appointment to such posts as vacancies occurred.

Many additional matters were considered in consultation with the appropriate departments, including the rank to be accorded to medical officers holding specialist posts within the authorised Service establishments, the rank given to officers with previous war service, the employment of women practitioners by the Service departments, and the pay of civilian medical practitioners employed by the Services and of the practitioners responsible for the organisation of first-aid posts and training the lay personnel attached to these posts.

MEDICAL CONSCRIPTION

It had been foreseen that, sooner or later, compulsory recruitment of medical practitioners for service with the Forces would be necessary. The voluntary system proved satisfactory during the first five months of the war but in February 1940, it began to show signs of breaking down. By the middle of that month approximately 2,500 volunteers had been provided by the Central Emergency Committee and some 2,000 practitioners with a liability for service had been mobilised. There was no longer a waiting list of candidates for immediate service in the Royal Army Medical Corps. In January those practitioners, numbering approximately 750, who had been registered in the Medical Register during 1938 and the first six months of 1939, and who had stated their intention of undertaking whole-time service at home or abroad were asked whether they were now free and willing to be recommended for commissions in the R.A.M.C., but only a small proportion replied that they were immediately available.

In February a circular letter was issued to all members of the profession in England and Wales except those serving with the Forces. This letter explained that heavy demands were being received from the Service departments, especially the War Office, and asked that those who were prepared to volunteer should inform their local committees. In addition, the central committee, which had now assumed its war-time title of 'Central Medical War Committee', wrote to the local committees, advising them of the quotas of practitioners which they were expected to supply for immediate military service and the steps to be taken to secure the requisite numbers of volunteers. At the same time, the local committees were invited to give their views on the suitability of the voluntary method of recruitment.

When the central committee met on February 21, some thirty Local Medical War Committees had replied, all criticising the voluntary system and advocating a measure of compulsion. The Committee therefore decided to represent to the Minister of Health and the Minister of Labour and National Service that medical practitioners within the age limits of current proclamations relating to general recruitment should be made liable for compulsory medical service with the Forces, the compulsion to be applied through the machinery of the Central Medical War Committee.

In April 1940, the Central Medical War Committee considered and approved an outline of the procedure proposed for applying conscription to the medical profession in England, Scotland and Wales. An explanatory letter issued to the English and Welsh local committees on April 9 was published in the *British Medical Journal* of April 13 for the information of all concerned. This letter stated that the Minister of Labour had excluded the medical profession from the Schedule of Reserved Occupations and had provided for the compulsory recruitment of medical practitioners as medical officers to the Forces. Male practitioners under the age of 41 were therefore liable to conscription. They would register with the Ministry of Labour in accordance with the programmes announced from time to time for male citizens generally of the age groups covered by the current proclamation.[8]

It was arranged that medical practitioners registering at the Employment Exchanges should fill up the Central Medical War Committee's war service questionnaire even if they had completed one already. The Ministry of Labour would send these forms to the committee, which would enter in the national register the up-to-date information thus provided and also convey it to the local committees. The central and local records of those who had registered would be marked with the letter R, and these practitioners would be designated R practitioners On receipt of a quota demand the local committees would select those volunteers and R practitioners who could most easily be spared and would recommend them to the central committee for recruitment.

The local committees were instructed to notify the selected R practitioners of the provisional decision to recruit them, and to allow them an opportunity to appeal against the decision and to appear before the committees for this purpose if they so desired. Other interested parties —principals, partners, insurance committees, hospitals and other employing bodies—were also to be given an opportunity of making representations. Should the local committee decide to recommend recruitment there would be a further right of appeal to the central committee. The only valid ground of appeal was the indispensability of the practitioner to the civil medical services of his area. Questions of physical unfitness were for the Service departments to determine. Appeals on the ground of excessive personal hardship would be heard by the Military Service (Hardship) Committees set up by the Ministry of Labour, and would be sent to that Ministry by the Central Medical War Committee, which would be informed of the results. Conscientious objectors would appear before the special tribunals established to consider their claims.

The Central Medical War Committee appointed a sub-committee, designated the Services Committee, to deal with the recruitment of individual practitioners and to consider the recommendations of the local committees on individual recruitment and appeals from the practitioners concerned. It was thought that the recruitment of recently qualified practitioners could best be arranged centrally, and for this purpose the Services committee was instructed to set up a Young Practitioners' Sub-committee. It was decided to regulate the employment of housemen in hospitals in order that the greatest possible number of recruits might be obtained from this source. Hospitals were asked to make a return to the Central Medical War Committee of their peacetime establishments of house posts and their proposed war-time establishments (which were expected, normally, to be smaller). The war-time establishments of hospitals in the provinces were scrutinised (and in some cases altered) by the Young Practitioners' Sub-committee after consultation with the Local Medical War Committees. The Committee of Reference examined and approved the establishments of hospitals in the London area.

The posts which the hospitals were asked to include in their returns were classified in three categories, designated A, B1 and B2. The A posts were the whole-time resident appointments normally occupied by practitioners without previous experience. The B posts were the whole-time appointments, usually but not necessarily resident, for which previous experience was required. B posts within the senior establishment were designated B1, while the intermediate category between the B1 and the A appointments was known as B2. Typical B1 posts in a voluntary hospital were those of registrar, resident medical or surgical officer and chief assistant. B1 posts in municipal hospitals were defined as those with a tenure of more than one year and carrying a salary not less than £350 a year with emoluments.

It was arranged that the recruitment of R practitioners holding B1 posts would be initiated by the Committee of Reference in London and by the Local Medical War Committees outside London. The recruitment of R practitioners in A and B2 posts was dealt with centrally by the Young Practitioners' Sub-committee, which was given the following terms of reference:

'To advise on the recruitment of young practitioners, including (1) practitioners qualifying on or after December 1, 1939, up to the completion of their tenure of hospital appointments within the authorised establishment or to their appointment to posts within the senior establishment of a voluntary or municipal hospital; (2) practitioners who qualified before December 1, 1939, and who now hold resident hospital posts other than those within the senior establishment.'

Having regard to the total number of posts in the approved hospital establishments and the number of practitioners normally qualifying each year, the Central Medical War Committee regulated the tenure of A and B2 posts in a way calculated to achieve a fair balance between the competing claims of the hospitals and the Services. An R practitioner who had qualified within six months was allowed to accept an A post for six months only, without renewal. His recruitment was then considered unless he had secured a B2 post. This he was allowed to hold for six months, normally without renewal, though applications for permission to renew a B2 post or to appoint the holder to another B2 post were considered on their merits. The tenure of B1 posts was not defined. If, before completing a B2 appointment, an R practitioner was selected for a B1 post, his recruitment was deferred and was left to the Local Medical War Committee or, in London, the Committee of Reference. Draft forms of advertisement, indicating the conditions imposed for A, B2 and B1 posts by the Central Medical War Committee, were supplied to the hospitals, and only advertisements which conformed with the committee's requirements were accepted by the medical journals. These measures of control made it possible to supply young practitioners to the Services at the rate of 1,000 to 1,200 a year.

AFTER DUNKIRK

After the arrangements for conscription had been worked out, the Local Medical War Committees were asked in May 1940, to provide fresh quotas of practitioners for service with the Forces. By the end of that month more than 4,000 practitioners had been recommended by the Central Medical War Committee for Service commissions. Then came the evacuation of the British Forces from France, resulting in a temporary suspension of the recruitment of medical officers for the

Army. The selection of practitioners to be recommended to the War Office was continued, those selected being informed that they were liable to be called upon at any time.

The halt in recruitment for the Army made it possible to adopt a more generous attitude to the claims of the hospitals for house officers. The regulations regarding the employment of these officers were reviewed in the light of experience and it was found that the limitation of A appointments to six months had resulted in a real deficiency of practitioners available for these posts. It was therefore decided to allow an R practitioner holding an A post to be retained in that post for a second period of six months or to be appointed for six months to another A post in the same hospital.

For the further assistance of hospitals in need of house officers, the central committee represented to the Government that powers should be exercised through the committee for the compulsory direction of medical practitioners to civil hospital posts and the public services. These powers were already possessed by the Minister of Labour under Defence Regulation 58A, and he decided to make use of them to direct medical practitioners to perform such services as he might specify. It was arranged that the compulsion would normally be applied only to practitioners within two years from qualification and would be exercised through senior officers of the Ministry of Health and the Department of Health for Scotland, appointed as National Service Officers and acting on the advice of the Central Medical War Committees for England and Wales and for Scotland. It was therefore possible to inform hospitals, in July 1940, that when they had failed to secure a candidate for an A, B2 or B1 appointment, they might ask the central committee to nominate a practitioner to be directed to the vacant post.

The evacuation of the civil population from certain towns on the East and South East coast after the fall of France created a difficult situation for the local doctors, who were temporarily deprived of their means of livelihood. After negotiations between the central committee and the Ministry of Health it was arranged that the Ministry would assume financial responsibility for the provision of the necessary medical services for the remaining population in these towns, the doctors required for this purpose being appointed whole-time medical officers of the Emergency Medical Service. The practitioners to be retained were selected by the local committees after consultation with the Regional Officers of the Ministry and the local medical officers of health.

In 1940, the plans for evacuating children from vulnerable areas included provision for their medical examination before they left. The necessary medical personnel for this purpose was provided through the Central and Local Medical War Committees. Some months before the evacuation, the central committee had written to all practitioners in the London County Council area who were over 35 years of age and had not been earmarked for service at first-aid posts or emergency hospitals, asking them if they were prepared to undertake this work; and the names of the volunteers had been given, with the consent of the local committees, to the Chief School Medical Officer of the London County Council. In the autumn of 1940, when provision was made for medical supervision and attendance at public air raid shelters and at rest centres, the practitioners required were nominated by the local committees.

During 1940, the Advisory Emergency Hospital Medical Service Committee reviewed the terms and conditions offered by the Ministry of Health to practitioners holding appointments of various kinds in the Service. As a result of representations to the Ministry, important modifications were made in the arrangements, some of which had given rise to considerable dissatisfaction. The Central Medical War Committee assisted the Ministry by making recommendations for the grading of practitioners employed in the Emergency Medical Services, particularly those engaged on a sessional basis; and continued the work of grading the practitioners (other than those within the province of the Committee of Reference) who, claiming specialist status, had offered themselves for service as specialists with the Forces. Those who, though entitled to be regarded as specialists, did not possess sufficient experience to justify the award of full specialist rank, were designated 'graded specialists'. Towards the end of 1940, the Central Medical War Committee appointed a special sub-committee, known as the Grading Committee, to advise on the grading of applicants for specialist commissions and of medical officers in the Emergency Medical Service.

THE PERIOD 1941–42

The machinery established in 1940 for the compulsory recruitment of medical officers for the Forces continued to work smoothly during the succeeding years, but it was necessary to adopt increasingly drastic measures in order to satisfy the continual demands of the Service departments. Recruitment for the R.A.M.C. had been resumed in September 1940, and in October the Local Medical War Committees had been asked to provide new quotas. A further quota demand was made in March 1941. By this time the services of a large number of alien practitioners had become available under the Medical Register (Temporary Registration) Order. The attention of the local committees was drawn to the possibility of some of the practitioners in B1 posts being replaced by aliens and the committees were asked to review the position of all such practitioners when they had held their appointments for one year. At the same time, the Ministry of Health called for further contributions to the Armed Forces from public health and hospital authorities, and suggested the employment of senior medical students, so far as was compatible with the law, as junior house officers in hospitals where adequate supervision of their work by members of the teaching staffs of the medical schools would still be available.

The C.W.M.C. regarded an independent priority organisation as an essential complement to its own machinery, and resolved to urge the immediate establishment of such an organisation in order to maintain the most efficient and economical allocation of the available medical personnel. In June 1941, the Minister of Health announced that, with the three Service Ministers and the Secretary of State for Scotland, he had appointed a Medical Personnel (Priority) Committee, with Mr. Geoffrey Shakespeare, M.P. (afterwards Sir Geoffrey Shakespeare, Bart.) as chairman, to secure the utmost economy in the employment of medical practitioners in H.M. Forces and in civil establishments,[6] (see page 394).

In 1941, the medical arrangements for the Home Guard received the attention of the Central Medical War Committee. In the previous year, the committee, in conjunction with the Council of the British Medical Association, had made an offer on behalf of the medical profession to provide, free of charge, first-aid treatment for members of the Home Guard wounded in action or injured when on duty. This offer had been gratefully accepted by the War Office, and the Local Medical War Committees had been asked to supply medical volunteers as required. Later, it became evident that a medical organisation within the Home Guard itself was desirable for such purposes as training medical orderlies and stretcher bearers and preparing plans for the collection and evacuation of battle casualties. Certain recommendations were made by the central committee to the War Office and were given effect in Army Council instructions. It was arranged that all nominations of medical practitioners for appointment as Home Guard medical officers would be made by the Local Medical War Committees or submitted to these committees for approval. A short course of training for Home Guard medical officers was arranged by the War Office at the instigation of the central committee.

Between January 1 and August 31, 1941, the central committee supplied approximately 1,900 medical officers to the Services, but the allocations approved by the Priority Committee for the remaining months of the year made it necessary to request fresh quotas from certain of the local committees in September. In assessing previous quotas consideration had been given to the classification of the territories of the local committees whether evacuation, reception or neutral areas, but it was now possible, with the aid of up-to-date population figures supplied by the Ministry of Food, to estimate the medical needs of the different areas more accurately. It was found that in England and Wales as a whole there was one general medical practitioner for every 2,588 civilians (as compared with 2,184 before the war) and it was decided to limit the September quota to those areas in which the ratio of general practitioners to the civil population was higher than the average for the country as a whole.

On December 5, 1941, the Central Medical War Committee, as a result of a recommendation of the Priority Committee, informed hospital authorities that the re-appointment of holders of A posts for a second period of six months could no longer be permitted, and that on January 5, 1942, the recruitment of R practitioners then holding extended A posts would begin, although in the interval it was permissible to appoint practitioners in their second six months' tenure of A posts to B2 posts within the authorised establishment. After January 5, only practitioners who had not yet completed six months in their first A posts might be selected for B2 appointments. In accordance with another recommendation of the Priority Committee, the Central Medical War Committee scrutinised approved hospital establishments of A, B2 and B1 posts with a view to securing a reduction of 15 per cent. in London and 10 per cent. in the Provinces.

Confronted by increasing difficulties in finding the medical personnel required by the Services, the central committee recommended that the age limit for conscription of medical practitioners should be raised to 51. This recommendation was not approved, but in March 1942, a Royal Proclamation extended the operation of the National Service Acts to men up to the age of 46 and the Minister of Labour made provision for the immediate compulsory recruitment of male medical practitioners up to this age. Early in May 1942, with a view to meeting outstanding Service requirements, the central committee asked the local committees to recommend for recruitment quotas of general practitioners calculated to reduce the numbers of such practitioners to 1 for 3,000 civilians in urban areas, 1 for 2,400 in rural areas and 1 for 2,700 in mixed areas. In the same month it was decided, again on the recommendation of the Priority Committee, to recruit all holders of A and B2 posts after six months' tenure of these posts. Hospitals were no longer permitted to appoint holders of A posts to B2 posts, or holders of B2 posts to B1 posts. At the same time the compulsory recruitment of women practitioners liable for service under the National Service Acts (mainly unmarried women below 31 years of age) was begun, but the promotion of such women from A to B2 posts and from B2 to B1 posts was allowed. On the recommendation of the Central Committee provision was made for the temporary 'freezing' of practitioners in B1 posts who were regarded as indispensable, the powers of the National Service Officers of the Ministry of Health being extended to permit of the compulsory direction of practitioners to remain in these posts.

It was decided that practitioners who had been graded as specialists could no longer be reserved for specialist employment, and such practitioners were recommended for general duty commissions on the understanding that they would be transferred to special work as opportunity occurred. The quest for new recruits was extended to medical schools and research establishments, and restrictions were imposed on the reservation, under arrangements previously approved by the central committee, of R practitioners as trainee pathologists and radiologists. But despite all the efforts made by the central committee, and the admirable co-operation given by the local committees in their increasingly difficult task, the number of practitioners available for recruitment in September 1942, fell considerably short of the Service requirements, which had been unexpectedly increased. As a temporary measure it was decided in that month to recruit R practitioners in A posts who had held their posts for three months or longer, with a proviso that no hospital should be required to give up more than 50 per cent. of the holders of its A posts; and to recruit also, at the end of three months after qualification, all male practitioners who had not then secured hospital employment. Because of the urgency of the situation, these practitioners were denied the right of appeal against their recruitment, except on the ground of conscience or of excessive personal hardship.

During September 1942, medical practitioners were recruited to the Services at the record rate of more than 100 a week. By December 31, 1942, the total number provided by the Central Medical War Committee since the beginning of the war (excluding those recommended for recruitment but rejected on medical or other grounds) had risen to 11,366, of whom 3,420 were provided in 1942. These figures included practitioners supplied through the central committee by the committee for Scotland, which had followed the same conscription procedure as had been used in England and Wales, and by the Committee for Northern Ireland, where recruitment had continued on a voluntary basis. They included also a relatively small number of practitioners supplied to the War Office for posting to the Indian Medical Service, arrangements having been made in 1942 for vacancies in the I.M.S. establishment to be filled by officers of the R.A.M.C. It was understood that 1,437 medical officers were serving in the Royal Navy, the Army and the Royal Air Force at the outbreak of war, and that there were 2,217 medical practitioners with a liability for service with the Forces on mobilisation. These figures, added to the number of practitioners supplied by the Central Medical War Committee up to the end of 1942, gave a grand total of 15,020.

In June 1941, a special sub-committee was appointed to consider modifications in the conditions of service of practitioners attached to first-aid posts, which had been proposed as a result of a recommendation of the Select Committee on National Expenditure. In September 1941, the central committee appointed an Aliens Committee to deal with problems arising in connection with the employment of alien practitioners; and in November 1942, it decided to set up a special committee to consider all questions relating to the post-war demobilisation of medical officers of the Services.

Although the central reserve of practitioners above military age who were available for civil employment had been very seriously depleted in 1940, the central committee continued during the next two years to give every assistance possible in providing candidates for vacancies of many kinds, including those in general practice, in the public health medical service, in industrial establishments and in the Merchant Navy. The Services committee advised on applications for exit permits from practitioners selected for overseas appointments. From time to time practitioners invalided out of the Services but fit for civil employment were helped to secure suitable work. The local committees continued to exercise their function of recommending candidates for local part-time appointments.

THE LATER WAR YEARS

During the remaining period of the war, the Central Medical War Committee continued to experience great difficulty in supplying the needs of the Services for medical officers. In 1943, various new expedients were considered with a view to increasing the number of recruits, and those found likely to produce useful results were adopted.

In May, recommendations made for the control of establishments of public health medical officers were accepted by the Ministry of Health, and local authorities were required to furnish the Minister with returns of the public health medical staff in their service, and to seek his consent to the filling of vacancies. Also, all whole-time public health medical officers of military age were notified that they must obtain the permission of the Minister before applying for other public health posts. These measures of control made it possible to secure the utmost economy in the staffing of the public health service.

Between the beginning of January and the middle of July 1943, the committee nominated 1,202 practitioners to the Service departments. The quota of recruits fixed for the remaining five and a half months of the year was 814, making a total of 2,016 for the whole year.

As it became evident that the number of practitioners available would fall below the total required, another expedient, which had been used in September 1942, was adopted with a view to satisfying the Service requirements. On the recommendation of the Medical Personnel (Priority) Committee, it was decided to accelerate the recruitment of young practitioners holding A and B2 posts in hospitals other than mental hospitals. Recruitment notices were sent to all male practitioners, liable for military service and not known to be medically unfit, who had held these posts for three months or would have done so on December 1. No hospital, however, was required to give up more than 50 per cent. of its A and B2 officers taken together. This procedure yielded 276 recruits and made it possible for the committee to complete the quota for 1943, although it had the effect of reducing the yield of young practitioners in 1944.

A procedure for initiating centrally the recruitment of general practitioners was applied to 43 areas where the local committees had failed to complete their quotas. When the number of fit R practitioners remaining in an area did not exceed the number required to satisfy the quota, all these practitioners received recruitment notices. When there were more R practitioners than could be demanded within the quota, the youngest were selected up to the number required. The local committees were given an opportunity, which they readily accepted, of making representations against the recruitment of these men, and of making alternative nominations when possible.

These investigations occupied much of the time of the Services committee during the first seven months of 1944, but the result was by no means commensurate with the labour involved. It became apparent that it was impracticable to insist on rigid adherence to the approved ratio of general practitioners to civilian resident population. Often there were local circumstances, connected with the geographical distribution of the remaining R practitioners in an area, which made it impossible for a local committee to provide its full share of recruits as assessed on a purely statistical basis. The report on this central recruitment experiment, presented to the Central Medical War Committee by the Services committee in January 1945, concluded with the following paragraph:

> 'The total number of practitioners considered is 251 and the number recommended for recruitment is 29, of whom 10 have been found medically unfit. Eleven have appealed successfully for deferment on hardship grounds. The number actually recruited is only 19. In view of the great amount of time and labour expended, this must be considered a very disappointing result. It is satisfactory, however, to be able to report that these investigations have convinced the committee that, in general, the local committees have been thorough and painstaking in their efforts to complete their quotas and that failure has usually been due to circumstances beyond their control. There is now no doubt that the supply of recruits from general practice has been exhausted.'

In 1942, the Services committee had absorbed the work of its Young Practitioners Sub-committee, but in the following year it remitted to the sub-committee the task of examining, at the request of the Medical Personnel (Priority) Committee, the staffing of the provincial medical schools in England and Wales. In November 1943, the sub-committee conducted an exhaustive investigation of the position of R practitioners on the teaching and research staffs of the provincial medical schools and associated hospitals, other than those holding B1 posts and those found medically unfit for military service. The observations of the Deans of the Schools had been obtained through the University Grants Committee, and the comments of that committee were available also. The Services committee adopted a recommendation of the sub-committee that the recruitment of practitioners holding whole-time posts as professors or readers should be deferred indefinitely, provided that they remained in these posts. As regards the other practitioners under review, it was decided in some cases to recruit at the end of the academic year, and in others to reconsider the question of recruitment at that time. The position of all these practitioners was re-examined by the sub-committee in June 1944, when it was found necessary to rescind some of the earlier decisions. In only four cases did the Services committee, on the recommendation of the sub-committee, resolve to proceed with recruitment immediately. The review of medical teachers was repeated in the two following years, but the number of recruits obtained from this source continued to be very small.

The number of recruits allocated by the Government to the Services for the first nine months of 1944 was 1,250. The committee estimated that the total yield of new recruits during the year would not exceed this number. Towards the end of the year the committee was informed that the figure of 1,250, although originally proposed for nine months, was to be regarded as the allocation for the whole of 1944. The number of practitioners actually recruited was within 20 of this quota.

During the first half of 1945 the committee received no instructions as to recruitment quotas but continued to recruit all available practitioners on the assumption that the demand would equal, if not exceed, the supply. The progressive depletion of the civilian medical services by recruitment in previous years, and by death and retirement, made it more than ever difficult in 1945 to obtain recruits in any considerable numbers from sources other than the 'Young Practitioner' pool.

The number of practitioners supplied to the Services between January 1 and August 31, 1945, was 792. At the latter date the total number supplied by the committee since the beginning of the war was 15,445. By the end of 1945 this figure had risen to 15,701. The total number of specialists recruited during 1945 was 80. Of these, 37 were of full specialist status and 43 were graded specialists.

The task given to the Central Medical War Committee to perform was one of immense importance and great difficulty. In taking up its work at the outbreak of war the committee had the advantage of plans carefully prepared beforehand, largely based on the experience of its predecessor in the War of 1914–18. But it was realised that the official medical field was wider now than then, for not only had the needs of the Armed Forces to be met overseas, but a hospital service was to be provided at home on a scale sufficient for returning battle casualties, for the great civilian army of war workers and for the vast numbers of air raid victims which were expected to require hospital treatment. Nor could the committee overlook the continuing needs of the ordinary civilian sick. To make a right allocation of available resources at the outbreak of war and to vary distribution with changing circumstances as the struggle proceeded, with varying fortunes, to its victorious end, required wise appreciation of the many factors involved, and demanded of the chairman, members and officers of the committee, and of its various sub-committees, sacrifice of time and thought that was always freely offered. The heaviest burden undoubtedly fell upon the Services Sub-committee, under the leadership of a succession of able chairmen, viz:

Mr. H. S. Souttar, C.B.E., D.M., M.Ch., F.R.C.S. (afterwards Sir Henry Souttar).
Sir Alfred Webb-Johnson, Bt., K.C.V.O., C.B.E., D.S.O., T.D., F.R.C.S. (afterwards Lord Webb-Johnson).
Sir Girling Ball, F.R.C.S.
Dr. Peter Macdonald, M.A., M.D.,

Throughout the war Mr. Souttar served with distinction as chairman of the Central Medical War Committee, of which Dr. G. C. Anderson, C.B.E., LL.D., was secretary until his death on January 1, 1944, when he was succeeded by Dr. Charles Hill.

After the end of the war with Germany, the following letter was received by the Secretary of the Central Medical War Committee from the Minister of Health:

'Now that the war in Europe has ended I feel I must convey to the Central Medical War Committee my warm thanks for their valuable help and co-operation during the last six years. The task which the committee readily undertook at the outbreak of war assumes a magnitude and complexity greater than could have been foreseen, but they have faced its problems and shouldered the great volume of work with a determination and efficiency which is very highly appreciated.

'Their first duty was to provide the practitioners necessary for the medical needs of the Armed Forces and I well know how successfully this was achieved. It was, indeed, a positive contribution to victory. I know, too, what difficulties were entailed in meeting the demands of the Services—how the committee had, throughout, to weigh the counter-claims of civilian needs in general practice, hospitals, public services, teaching, research and other fields. As the war lengthened and civilian medical resources were progressively depleted it could almost be said that each individual case became a problem, but the committee could always be relied upon for a sound and fair-minded judgment in striking the balance between civil and military needs.

'This was the committee's main task, but they have also devoted much careful consideration to safeguarding the interests of serving practitioners and have had before them the claims of civilian services overseas, relief and missionary work, problems affecting aliens and a wide range of other matters. The same care has been evident in the committee's handling of all of them.

'The success of their work in meeting the demands of the Services has inevitably placed a heavy strain upon general practitioners, hospital staffs and others remaining in civilian life. Many of them have carried on under conditions of great difficulty and almost intolerable strain. I cannot allow this opportunity to pass without expressing the Government's thanks to all those practitioners for the manner in which their burdens have been borne.

'The committee's work is not yet finished and what remains will present many new problems, but I am confident that they will meet the calls upon them with the same success as have attended their efforts in the past.

'I would also ask you in your capacity as Liaison Officer to convey to members of the Committee of Reference my sincere thanks for the valuable work they have done within their special field of reviewing the hospital staffs of Greater London.

'Finally, I should be glad if you would let members and secretaries of Local Medical War Committees know how deeply I appreciate their contribution to this work, to which they have given voluntarily and without stint so much of their time and energies throughout the years of war.'

In acknowledging this letter the Services Committee took the opportunity of expressing gratitude for the invaluable assistance given to the Central Medical War Committee by officials of the Ministry of Health and other Government departments. The letter from the Minister was communicated to the Local Medical War Committees and to the medical press.

The Central Medical War Committee continued to discharge its functions as a recruiting agency for the Services after the end of hostilities. They also dealt with many matters concerning the demobilisation of doctors from the Services and their replacement by an adequate number of suitable recruits in order to facilitate the release of all classes of practitioners, including those whose services were urgently required to meet the needs of the civilian population. This latter class entailed a large amount of work, no less than 431 applications for special release being received during 1944, and 1,186 during 1945.

As the committee were under the obligation to recruit a substitute for every officer released in this class the greatest discrimination had to be exercised, particularly in regard to specialist officers. The great majority of these applications had therefore to be rejected in fairness to those whose normal release with their age groups might be retarded.

The work of the Central Medical War Committee in this connexion is dealt with under the Demobilisation section in Chapter 6 of this volume, and in the Service Volumes of this History.

THE EMPLOYMENT OF ALIEN MEDICAL PRACTITIONERS

INTRODUCTION

The immigration of alien medical practitioners as a result of racial discrimination and political oppression in certain European countries during the years immediately preceding the war created a situation of some difficulty for the medical profession in Britain. It was unthinkable that the profession should decline to contribute to the solution of the refugee problem by welcoming a proportion of the exiles into its ranks, but as these ranks were at that time in no particular need of recruits it was clearly desirable to consider the possibility of their becoming inconveniently congested. The position was radically changed by the outbreak of war; it was then no longer a question of finding room for large numbers of foreign doctors as permanent residents in Britain, but rather a question of making appropriate use of their services in the national interest.

The influx of medical refugees began in the year 1933, when a considerable number of Jewish practitioners, fugitives from Nazi oppression, arrived from Germany. These refugees could not immediately undertake medical work in Britain since the professional employment of aliens was controlled by the Aliens Order, 1920, and German medical qualifications did not entitle the holder to registration in the Foreign List of the Medical Register of the United Kingdom. It was necessary for the refugees, having obtained sanction from the Home Office, to undertake a course of study with a view to acquiring a registrable diploma. The Home Office had decided to limit strictly the number of refugees permitted to settle in medical practice after acquiring a registrable qualification, and between 1933 and 1935 approximately 180 German doctors were granted this privilege. Thereafter, permission to study for a British medical diploma was given with rare exceptions only on the understanding that the candidate would leave the country after qualification.

In 1938, as a result of the annexation of Austria, many doctors in that country sought permission to settle in Britain, and in July of that year, the Home Secretary, with the concurrence of the leading medical organisations, decided to grant this privilege to fifty Austrian refugees. These were required by the Home Office to undertake a course of study of not less than two years' duration before qualifying, in order that they might have time to become well acquainted with British medical methods and traditions.

When Czechoslovakia was invaded in 1939, the Home Secretary, again after consultation with the medical profession, decided to admit a quota of fifty medical refugees from that country under the same conditions. This quota, which was finally completed early in 1940, contained a somewhat larger proportion of specialists than did the similar quota of medical refugees from Austria.

Thus before the war arrangements had been made for some 300 medical refugees to settle in Britain on the understanding that they would be permitted to establish themselves in independent practice after admission to the Medical Register. In addition, the Home Office, apparently regarding psychological medicine as extending beyond the province of the registered medical practitioner, had allowed a small number of refugee doctors to practise psychotherapy without first acquiring a registrable qualification, and some fifty medically qualified research workers had been permitted to pursue research but not engage in practice. There remained some hundreds of foreign medical practitioners, of various nationalities, who had been permitted to land in Britain (including a number with prospects of admission later to America) but had not found an opportunity of resuming their professional activities in this country.

THE EARLY WAR PERIOD

When war came, the foreign doctors who had found permanent homes or temporary shelter in Britain were not slow to offer their services as medical officers in the Forces. Like many of the British volunteers, they had to be informed that there was no immediate opportunity for them, but some of the refugees who had acquired British qualifications were able to obtain permits from the Aliens War Service Department for employment in emergency hospitals.

After the fall of France in 1940, the lot of the medical refugees in Britain was not a happy one. Many were interned in this country and some were sent for internment to Australia or Canada. On June 10, 1940, the Ministry of Health, at the request of the Aliens War Service Department, issued instructions[9] that the services of all Germans, Austrians and Czechs working in any capacity in hospitals providing treatment for members of H.M. Forces must be dispensed with forthwith. On June 18, these instructions were applied also to persons of Italian nationality. On July 3, the restrictions were modified, and emergency hospitals were permitted to retain the services of Czechs, subject to the approval of the Aliens War Service Department. Hospitals and other institutions not treating members of the Forces could continue to employ Germans, Austrians and Italians on condition that they would be dismissed immediately on the admission of Service cases for treatment.[10] As the result of these regulations a considerable number of alien doctors, even if they escaped internment, were obliged to give up their hospital work and join the ranks of their unemployed compatriots.

In August 1940, when the Government was reconsidering its internment policy, the Home Office Medical Advisory Committee recommended that the restrictions on the employment of 'enemy' aliens should be relaxed and that those aliens who were considered suitable to be exempted or freed from internment should be allowed to undertake the work for which they had previously been granted permits. On November 4, 1940, the Ministry of Health issued a Circular[11] which allowed doctors of enemy alien nationality, if approved by the Aliens War Service Department, to be employed in emergency hospitals under certain conditions. In particular, it was laid down that not more than ten per cent. of the total medical staff (20 per cent. in hospitals of less than 100 beds) might be enemy aliens, and that such aliens must not be employed in wards set apart for Service patients.

During 1940, the many alien doctors not in possession of British diplomas remained without opportunity of professional service. The number of these doctors was increased during the year by the arrival of additional refugees from the Continent after the fall of France. Towards the end of the year, however, when the recruitment of British doctors for service in the Forces was beginning to create a shortage of candidates for resident hospital posts, the position of the unregistered alien practitioners was reviewed by the Home Office and the Ministry of Health and eventually arrangements were made for the services of these practitioners to be available for hospital work by a provision which enabled the General Medical Council to admit them temporarily to the Foreign List of the Medical Register after they had been selected for approved appointments.

TEMPORARY MEDICAL REGISTRATION

By an Order in Council, dated July 24, 1940[12] a new Regulation, numbered 32B, was added to the Defence (General) Regulations, 1939. The effect of this Regulation was to empower the General Medical Council to register in the Medical Register any person by law entitled to practise medicine, surgery and midwifery in any territory outside the United Kingdom to which the Regulation was applied, provided that it was shown to the satisfaction of the General Medical Council that the applicant for registration fulfilled such conditions as to nationality, character, professional qualifications and otherwise, as might be prescribed by the Order. It was laid down that persons registered by virtue of the Regulation should cease to be registered when the Regulation expired or was revoked.

The Regulation was made to facilitate the temporary employment, if found to be desirable in the national interest, not only of refugee doctors from the Continent but also of medical volunteers from North America whose diplomas were not registrable in the ordinary way in the United Kingdom, and in 1941 was extended to the following groups of territories : (1) Australia, Burma, Canada, India, Newfoundland, New Zealand and South Africa; (2) His Majesty's Colonies, Protectorates and Mandated Territories; (3) Belgium, Czechoslovakia, France,

Greece, Holland, Norway and Poland; and (4) Germany and Italy. The extending Order[13] embraced also 'any oversea territory or possession' of these countries, and it was interpreted as including Austria. Under this Order registration in the Medical Register could be effected only after the applicant had been selected for an appointment, and only if the appointment for which he had been selected was certified by the appointing authority to be of an approved kind. The work approved for the purposes of the Order included both medical service in the Armed Forces and civilian medical employment. Private medical practice was excluded, for it was considered that there was as yet no need to call on foreign and other oversea practitioners for assistance in this field.

On January 15, 1941, the Ministry of Health issued to local authorities and to voluntary hospitals a circular[14] which explained the general effect of the temporary registration orders and defined the hospitals and services which the Minister, in pursuance of his powers under the 1941 Order, had approved for the purposes of that Order. These were: (1) hospitals provided by local authorities; (2) other hospitals included in the Emergency Hospital Scheme; and (3) service at or in connexion with any first-aid post provided under the Civil Defence Acts. The circular added that the Minister would be prepared to consider applications for his approval to any further hospital, institution or service under the Order. A similar circular was issued to the appropriate authorities in Scotland at the direction of the Secretary of State.

The Central Medical War Committee accepted an invitation to act as a clearing house in connexion with the employment and temporary registration of alien and other overseas practitioners under the Order of 1941.

DEVELOPMENTS IN 1941

Although the Temporary Registration Orders brought hope to many refugee doctors who had been anxious to play their part in the national effort, the dearth of British candidates for hospital posts was not yet such as to provide opportunities for a large proportion of the available aliens. Even those who were immediately selected for appointment were kept waiting for some weeks before they could begin work, but by June 1941, approximately 300 practitioners had been selected for approved civilian employment, of whom 240 were already registered in the Medical Register, and by the end of 1941, approximately 600 practitioners had obtained appointments.

In certain of the Allied Forces in Britain there were medical officers who were supernumerary to the establishment or had been removed from the active list because of age or physical disability; and from this source also a number of practitioners were made available for civil employment. Some hundreds of applications for temporary registration from medical officers continuing to serve in Allied or Associated Forces were transmitted to the General Medical Council. Registration in these cases of course did not add to the number of practitioners actively engaged in medical work.

Early in 1941, the regulations prohibiting the entry of aliens to Aliens Protected Areas were modified to enable alien doctors to accept work in emergency hospitals in these areas. Certain modifications were made also in the restrictions imposed on the employment of doctors of enemy alien nationality in emergency hospitals generally. A circular issued by the Ministry of Health on March 17, 1941, gave permission for such doctors to be employed in separate wards set apart for Service patients, although it stated that, wherever practicable, they should work only in wards where British doctors and nurses were also engaged.[15] A later circular permitted the employment of one doctor of enemy alien nationality, provided that the resident staff included two British doctors, even though the total medical staff, resident and visiting, might be less than five (in a hospital with less than 100 beds) or ten (in a hospital with 100 beds or over).[16]

At first the appointments secured by temporarily registered practitioners were, almost without exception, hospital appointments of the house officer type, but the Order had not been long in operation before applications were received for approval of appointments of other kinds.

By July 1941, the increasing shortage of British candidates for appointments in general practice had made it necessary to consider the advisability of permitting temporarily registered practitioners to undertake this work. An inter-departmental conference was held at the Ministry of Health and it was decided to recommend that the Temporary Registration Order should be so amended as to permit of the appointment of temporarily registered doctors as assistants to private practitioners. The British Medical Association, which was represented at the conference, concurred in this recommendation on the understanding that individual appointments of this kind would be subject to the approval of the Central Medical War Committee. In addition, approval was given to alien doctors serving in British ships and in the public health, school and child welfare services of local authorities.

In July 1941, the Home Office, after consultation with the Ministry of Health, suggested that the Medical Advisory Committee, consisting of the medical members of the committee constituted in 1938 for selecting medical refugees to be admitted from Austria, should be dissolved and replaced by a sub-committee of the Central Medical War Committee. Accordingly, the Central Medical War Committee appointed an Aliens Committee with the following terms of reference: 'To advise the Home Office and the Ministry of Health upon questions relating to the employment of alien practitioners'.

PROGRESS IN 1942

During 1942, the absorption of foreign medical practitioners by the medical services of the country continued but at a distinctly slower pace. An obstacle in the way of finding work for the practitioners who remained unemployed lay in the fact that many of them were elderly specialists. It was not that these men were inclined to stand on their dignity, for the majority were ready to accept any employment, however humble; but for obvious reasons they were not regarded by hospitals as the most appropriate candidates for junior posts. On the other hand, the decision to allow temporarily registered practitioners to act as assistants in general practice resulted in a limited but gradually increasing demand for their services in this sphere; and recruitment in the field of public health also increased owing to the withdrawal of British doctors for service with the Forces.

The Ministry of Health in February 1942, issued a further circular permitting the employment of an enemy alien practitioner even if there were only one British resident in addition, and promising special consideration of applications for permission to appoint an alien in hospitals where only one resident was employed. The circular also relaxed to some extent the previous regulations regarding the proportion of enemy aliens permitted in the larger hospitals.[17]

Although newcomers from abroad were extremely rare, the pool of available foreign practitioners was slightly augmented during 1942 from various sources. For example, additional medical officers of certain of the Allied Forces in Britain became available for civil employment. Again, a number of aliens, including a small group of Egyptians, who had begun medical study in Britain before the war, completed their training and obtained registrable diplomas. These practitioners, having been allowed to land for the purpose of study only, were restricted to work approved for the purposes of the Temporary Registration Order, although registered in the ordinary way.

A notable event of 1942 was a special qualifying examination held by the English Conjoint Examining Board, at the request of the Czech Government, for a group of Czech medical students who had not completed their studies before leaving their own country. The diploma awarded to these students did not admit them to the Medical Register except under the Temporary Registration Order, but it entitled them to practise in Czechoslovakia after the war. The majority of the students had served in the ranks of the Czech Army. Having passed the special examination, they became eligible for employment as medical officers in their own national Forces or, possibly, in the Royal Army Medical Corps. Earlier, even more notable arrangements to enable Polish students to complete their medical education had been made at the University of Edinburgh, where a Polish Medical School was established, staffed by Polish professors and lecturers. As a result of this outstanding example of international co-operation in the academic sphere, a number of young Polish graduates became available for employment in civil hospitals under the Temporary Registration Order.

The Allied Powers (War Service) Act, 1942, provided that, after the Act had been applied by Order in Council to a particular Allied Power, subjects of that Power who were of military age would become liable in certain circumstances to conscription into the British Forces if they had not joined their own national Forces. It was agreed that there should be a close liaison between the British and Allied authorities and that arrangements for the recruitment of doctors of Allied nationality under the Act should be arranged through the machinery of the Central Medical War Committee.

In December 1942, an analysis was made of the employment of alien practitioners in civilian work under the Temporary Registration Order, the results of which are given below. The 'miscellaneous' category includes practitioners engaged in a variety of situations—for example, as ship surgeons, factory medical officers, psychiatrists in child guidance clinics, and medical officers serving on the staff of Allied Ministries or in special clinics of various kinds, including clinics in London for impecunious refugees and clinics at the ports for Allied seamen. In addition to those represented in the list, fifteen alien practitioners, including eleven Czechs, obtained temporary registration after applying successfully, through the Central Medical War Committee, for medical commissions in H.M. Forces. A number of others were granted commissions after direct application to the Service departments.

Temporary Registration Order

1. Numbers of alien practitioners who obtained civilian medical employment:

(a) Germans and Austrians	459
(b) Czechs	239
(c) Poles	63
(d) Other nationalities	90
Total	851

2. Numbers of alien practitioners in various types of employment:

(a) Hospital appointments	530
(b) General practice	164
(c) Public Health appointments	28
(d) Dental appointments	34
(e) Miscellaneous	95
Total	851

3. Numbers of alien practitioners known to be available and still unemployed:

(a) Germans and Austrians	155
(b) Czechs	30
(c) Poles	11
(d) Other nationalities	17
Total	213

THE PERIOD 1943-5

Apart from discussions of policy and consultations with Government departments, the Central Medical War Committee continued to undertake a large volume of office work in connexion with the employment of alien practitioners. There was continual correspondence with employing bodies who sought information as to names and qualifications of available candidates, and with organisations and individuals interested in the prospects of employment for particular alien doctors. When aliens had completed hospital or other appointments and had not themselves written about their future plans, they were 'followed up' in order that the record of their activities might be kept up to date and any possible help given in securing fresh employment. Much of the daily correspondence originated from the foreign doctors themselves, and many of them called at the office of the committee and were granted repeated interviews. They were given friendly advice and assistance in difficulties of many kinds. When work had been obtained and permits were delayed, appeals were made on their behalf to the security departments. When local police authorities obstructed them in their professional activities through misunderstanding of what was permitted under the Order, prompt remedies were effected. When doubts arose on ethical matters, advice was given regarding the professional standards and customs of the country. In short, the office of the Central Medical War Committee was not merely a clearing house for forms, but a source of guidance and practical help, both to the refugees themselves and to those in need of their services.

During the last three years of the war there were no major changes of policy in regard to the employment of alien doctors. The progressive depletion of the ranks of their British colleagues as a result of recruitment to the Forces created more numerous opportunities of employment for the aliens, both in general practice and in hospital appointments.

In 1944 the Aliens Committee, thinking it unreasonable that refugee alien doctors should be debarred from undertaking medical relief work abroad, entered into correspondence with the United Nations Relief and Rehabilitation Administration regarding the possibility of employing Austrian doctors who wished to find opportunities of this kind.

The first response was not favourable, but eventually, in 1945, it was decided by U.N.R.R.A. that the services of Austrian doctors could be accepted, provided they were refugees resident in the United Kingdom, and that individual clearance certificates for their employment could be obtained from the military authorities.

Early in 1945, a number of Czechoslovakian doctors were released from medical employment in Britain, after consultation with the Central Medical War Committee, and returned to Czechoslovakia to assist in the rehabilitation of that country. A number of Austrian doctors also were able to go back to their own country after the end of the war in Europe. On the other hand, a number of aliens released from military service became available for civilian medical work in Britain.

THE END OF TEMPORARY REGISTRATION

As early as 1944, many refugee alien doctors in Britain were becoming anxious as to their fate at the end of the national emergency, when the Temporary Registration Order would be revoked. The Aliens Committee felt some anxiety also regarding the prospect that British doctors, on return from the Forces, might find themselves in competition with aliens for civilian employment. Early in 1945, it brought this potential problem to the notice of the Central Medical War Committee, but the latter committee took the view that discussion of the matter at that time would be premature.

At its next meeting, in January 1946, it was reported to the Central Medical War Committee that, in the Emergency Laws (Transitional Provisions) Bill it was proposed that the Temporary Medical Register should remain in being until December 31, 1947, but that no new admissions to the Temporary Register should be made after February 24, 1946. The committee decided to watch medical man-power carefully with a view to recommending an earlier termination of the Temporary Registration Order should this seem desirable in the interests of British doctors.

The total number of alien practitioners admitted to the Temporary Register during the war was:

        (a) For civilian employment .   1,185
        (b) For the Forces   .   .   1,986

Of the latter the largest number serving in the British Forces was about 200, the rest were serving in the various Allied Forces in the United Kingdom.

These figures do not include doctors from the United States serving either in civil posts or in the Forces.

The Aliens Committee ceased to function after February 1949.

APPENDIX I

THE AMERICAN HOSPITAL IN BRITAIN, 1940-2

A UNIT OF VOLUNTEER AMERICAN SURGEONS

by

JOHN MARQUIS CONVERSE
M.D.

The Hospital for Special Surgery, New York

THE American Hospital in Britain was born from the desire of a group of American surgeons to give assistance to the British people in their hour of danger. It constituted the vanguard of the numerous members of the American medical profession who were later to come to Great Britain with the United States Army.

In 1939, Dr. Philip D. Wilson, Surgeon in Chief of the Hospital for Special Surgery (Hospital for the Ruptured and Crippled), New York City, was present at the meeting of the British Orthopaedic Association. He expressed to his British colleagues his desire, should hostilities be declared, to bring over to Great Britain a number of volunteer surgeons to assist in the treatment of the war casualties.

Early in 1940, after an exchange of correspondence with Professor Harry Platt of Manchester, who served as an intermediary with the Ministry of Health, the unit was formed. The unit was named 'The American Hospital in Britain' and was financially supported by the British War Relief Society from funds donated by American friends of Great Britain.

On August 24, 1940, the first group of the unit, under the leadership of Dr. Philip D. Wilson, left New York on the ill-fated *Western Prince* which was torpedoed on her next voyage to England.

On September 9, 1940, the unit arrived in London, where its members were entertained as guests of the Government. The German air raids on London had started on September 7, and the members of the unit were able to act as close observers of the Emergency Medical Service as it functioned in the treatment of the casualties from air raids.

From October 1, 1940, until December 31, 1941, the American Hospital in Britain carried out its medical activities in orthopaedic surgery and plastic surgery at Park Prewett Emergency Hospital, Basingstoke. The American section of Park Prewett Hospital was designated as a Regional Orthopaedic Centre. The equipment was brought over from the United States, and an operating theatre and a clinical laboratory were organised.

During the first year of service in England, the American Hospital in Britain consisted of the Orthopaedic Centre, comprising 300 beds at Park Prewett Hospital and of two detached units, one under the direction of Dr. John M. Converse, at the Plastic Surgery Centre at Rooksdown House, Park Prewett Hospital, and the other under the direction of Dr. Henry Heyl in the Neurosurgical Centre of the Queen Elizabeth Hospital, Birmingham. When Dr. Heyl returned to the United States, in August, 1941, he was succeeded by Dr. William Sweet who remained in charge of the neurosurgical centre (at Birmingham) throughout the war.

During this period the unit was under the leadership of Dr. Philip D. Wilson (until January 1941); of Dr. Wallace Cole of Minneapolis, Minnesota (until August 1941); and of Dr. Charles Bradford, of Boston (until January 1942).

During its first year of service in Britain, the Hospital provided surgical care to over 2,500 orthopaedic patients, to 200 patients treated in the plastic surgery centre, and approximately the same number treated at the Neurosurgical Centre at Birmingham.

On January 1, 1942, the Hospital took over the administration of the Churchill Hospital of the Emergency Medical Service in Oxford. The Churchill Hospital rapidly developed into a much bigger organisation than that at Basingstoke. More personnel, including both doctors and nurses, arrived from the United States. The medical staff of the hospital increased to eleven doctors and the hospital was equipped with X-ray machines, laboratories and almost every type of equipment usually found in a hospital in the United States. Nurses were sent over from the United States and worked under the direction of Miss Lorraine Setzler, who became Superintendent of Nursing.

The Churchill Hospital was officially opened by Her Royal Highness the Duchess of Kent, on January 27, 1942, in the presence of Mr. Ernest Brown, the Minister of Health, Vice-Admiral Robert Ghormley, U.S.N., representing the United States Ambassador, Mr. Winant, and Professor (afterwards Sir Francis) Fraser, Director-General of the Emergency Medical Services.

In January 1942, Dr. Philip D. Wilson returned to England to assume once more the leadership of the unit at Oxford and remained until April 1942. He was succeeded by his brother, Dr. Harlan Wilson.

It became evident after the entrance of the United States into the war, that there was no longer a place for a volunteer civilian organisation and that the United States Army would be in need of all the hospital accommodation it could obtain. On July 15, 1942, the transfer of the Churchill Hospital to the United States Army took place. The hospital was occupied by the Second General Hospital organised from the staff of the Presbyterian Hospital of New York City.

During the twenty-one and one-half months that the American Hospital in Britain worked in England, 3,634 patients came under its care and 2,858 operations were performed by its surgeons, in addition to many other minor surgical procedures. During this period, the organisation sent over from the United States 23 doctors, 40 nurses and 14 technicians and secretaries. In addition, nurses and physiotherapists were engaged in England. It sent over from the United States 357 cases of equipment including surgical instruments, laboratory apparatus, gloves, medical supplies and surgical dressings.

From the beginning until August 1, 1942, it paid out for salaries, travelling expenses and purchase of equipment the sum of $295,000, all but about $20,000 of which was given it by the British War Relief Society, Inc.

APPENDIX II

THE AMERICAN RED CROSS—HARVARD FIELD HOSPITAL UNIT

Based on a contribution from
PROFESSOR JOHN E. GORDON
M.D.
Professor of Preventive Medicine at Harvard University

ON the initiative of Dr. Conant, President of Harvard University, Dr. C. Sidney Burwell, M.D., Dean of the Harvard University Medical School, in June 1940, communicated with Professor F. R. Fraser and expressed the desire of the Harvard University Authorities to assist the medical profession in the United Kingdom in their war effort, as it was expected that a heavy strain would be thrown on our medical organisation owing to the fall of France, the threat of invasion and the possibility of an increase in the incidence of infectious disease. He therefore intimated that Professor R. P. Linstead, F.R.S., late Professor of Chemistry at Cambridge University, and then working in the same capacity at Harvard, was leaving for England to discuss with the Chief Medical Officer, Ministry of Health, Sir Arthur MacNalty and Professor Fraser proposals of assistance consistent with the United States Neutrality Act. The Harvard University considered that a group of experts in bacteriology, epidemiology, nutrition, sanitary engineering, medicine and surgery might be able to render valuable assistance to the Ministry of Health. President Conant broadcast a speech on the subject in the United States.

In July, the Ministry of Health expressed the opinion that it would be difficult to fit American experts into its organisation on account of their lack of knowledge of local conditions and English Public Health administration, and suggested that Harvard should send a complete infectious diseases unit, consisting of a hutted hospital, with full staff and equipment. After discussing these proposals with Professor Linstead, this plan was agreed to and it was also decided that Professor Gordon, the Professor of Preventive Medicine at Harvard, should be in charge of the unit.

As an exception to the general rule in England, it was also agreed that this hospital should form an integral part of the Emergency Hospital Scheme.

Professor Linstead proposed that the hospital should have about 100 beds to start with, a fully-equipped laboratory to rank as an emergency public health laboratory under the M.R.C., and a fully-equipped field unit to undertake investigations in the field in connexion with infectious diseases in all parts of the country. After further discussions with Professor Gordon and Dr. Mote of Harvard University, who had also come to England, it was finally agreed, and published in America and in England, that this unit would be despatched under the auspices of the American Red Cross Society, which would avoid breach of the neutrality regulations.

Professor Gordon returned to America in September to take charge of the preliminary arrangements and the mobilising of the necessary personnel. As was to be expected, considerable difficulties had to be overcome, e.g. the U.S.A. State Department insisted that the personnel must sail in neutral ships, which involved the expenditure of dollars which it was the policy of the British Treasury to avoid, if at all possible. The material for the hospital, however, such as prefabricated huts and equipment could be sent in belligerent ships without breach of neutrality regulations. The shipping of the latter commenced from New York in March 1941, and at the same time the staff, which consisted of 10 medical officers, 65 nurses and 10 technical assistants, were being found passages in neutral ships.

Dr. J. R. Hutchinson of the Ministry of Health was deputed to assist Professor Gordon in choosing a suitable site for the erection of the hospital and one was eventually found at Combe Road on the borders of the City of Salisbury. Many difficulties supervened in arranging for the unloading of the material at ports as it arrived and assembling it on the site, owing to the lack of suitable storage accommodation and of labour. These difficulties, however, were eventually overcome and the construction of the hospital began.

The arrangement with the American authorities was that Harvard University and the American Red Cross would provide the funds for the prefabricated buildings, the equipment of the hospital and laboratory, and would pay the salaries of the American personnel, while the Ministry of Health would provide the site and finance the necessary services, such as drainage, water supply, electric supply, etc., and would be responsible for the running expenses of the hospital, which was expected to be ready to go into operation on September 22, 1941. The first wards opened in September and the hospital gradually filled up, so that when it was handed over to the U.S.A. authorities in July 1942, it was fully occupied. During the short period in which it functioned as an Emergency Service hospital it admitted 918 cases, of which 734 were

Service cases, there being a serious shortage of beds in the Southern Command for this purpose. The remaining 184 civilian cases accounted for 2,334 'patient days', or an approximate average of thirteen days each. The laboratory was fully occupied and the mobile teams made about 40 field investigations between January 1941, and July 1942, including one visit to Northern Ireland.

The hospital, as above mentioned, was handed over in July 1942, to the U.S.A. authorities at the request of General P. R. Hawley, Chief Surgeon, European Theatre of Operations, U.S.A., as an urgent need for this kind of unit was felt by the U.S. military medical authorities. It was, however, agreed that the hospital would still admit civilians when necessary, that the mobile unit would still continue to make investigations into the outbreak of infectious diseases in any part of the country, and that Professor Gordon (later Colonel Gordon, M.C., U.S.A.) would remain in England to act as liaison officer between the U.S.A. military authorities and the Ministry of Health.

It was also decided, by the desire of the Harvard University Authorities and the American Red Cross, that as soon as possible after the cessation of hostilities, the whole of the hospital buildings and equipment should be handed over to the Ministry of Health as a free gift from Harvard University. This munificent gift was suitably acknowledged by the Ministry of Health who at the same time expressed their high appreciation of the very valuable work done by the Harvard Unit during the short period that it had been functioning under their auspices. The Chief Medical Officer, Sir Wilson Jameson, suggested that this unit, being the first of its kind in the United Kingdom, might be the prototype of similar units to be established in the United Kingdom as a part of the ordinary health organisation of the country.

REFERENCES

[1] Min. of Labour and National Service Press Notice, April 9, 1940; Min. of Health Circulars 2014 and 2015, May 11, 1940; Emergency Medical Services Instruction 148, May 14, 1940.
[2] Emergency Medical Services Instruction 158, May 25, 1940.
[3] Min. of Health Confidential Report of Committee of Inquiry on Medical Personnel, January 1, 1941.
[4] Emergency Medical Services Instruction 285, March 14, 1941.
[5] Min. of Health Circular 2312, March 17, 1941.
[6] *Parliamentary Debates*, 5th Series, Vol. 372. *House of Commons Official Report.* June 19, 1941, Cols. 807-9. (372 H.C. Deb. 807-9).
[7] Min. of Health, First and Second Reports of the Medical Personnel (Priority) Committee, H.M.S.O., 1942.
[8] *Brit. med. J.* Supplement, 1940, 1, 47.
[9] Min. of Health Circular 2045, June 10, 1940.
[10] Min. of Health Circular 2080, July 3, 1940.
[11] Min. of Health Circular 2193, November 4, 1940.
[12] *Statutory Rules and Orders*, 1940, No. 1328.
[13] *Statutory Rules and Orders*, 1941, No. 24.
[14] Min. of Health Circular 2264, January 15, 1941.
[15] Min. of Health Circular 2312, March 17, 1941.
[16] Min. of Health Circular 2405, June 14, 1941.
[17] Min. of Health Circular 2569, February 10, 1942.

CHAPTER 15

THE CIVIL NURSING SERVICES IN WAR-TIME

by

DAME KATHERINE WATT
D.B.E., R.R.C.

Chief Nursing Officer and Principal Matron, Ministry of Health

THE SHORTAGE OF NURSES

IN the years immediately before the war it had become evident that recruitment to the nursing services was insufficient to meet the needs of the rapidly expanding health services. The shortage was more marked in some parts of the country than in others; more popular areas were better nursed than the less popular. It was evident that in the event of war a large increase in nursing personnel would be required to meet the nursing needs of hospitals and other emergency services which would be provided under an Emergency Medical Scheme.

The question of providing reserves of nurses for the Defence Services in time of war had already been considered by a sub-committee of the Committee of Imperial Defence in 1927 and again by a sub-committee in 1936.

THE 'ATHLONE' COMMITTEE

In 1937 an inter-departmental committee known as the 'Athlone' Committee had been appointed to advise how recruitment could be improved. As a result the Sub-committee on Supply of Nurses in War was reconstituted in October of that year under the chairmanship of Sir Arthur MacNalty, Chief Medical Officer of the Ministry of Health, with the following terms of reference:

(*a*) To attempt to secure for the trained nurses, the establishment of an emergency committee to work on the lines parallel to those of the Emergency Committee of the British Medical Association.

(*b*) To concert with the Order of St. John and the British Red Cross Society (who already had certain commitments for the provision of staff in an emergency) and other suitable organisations, arrangements for the supply of auxiliary and unqualified nursing staff.

This committee found that in March 1938, there were 89,254 trained nurses on the register, but that there was no information available as to how many unregistered trained nurses were in existence. They advised that the Royal College of Nursing should be asked to compile a register of all nurses and assistant nurses, and that the British Red

Cross Society and the Order of St. John be asked to compile one for auxiliary nurses who were prepared to offer their services. It was suggested that use be made of appropriate organisations, including the Women's Voluntary Services, in dealing with the supply of all hospital auxiliaries other than nurses. It appeared to be a vital necessity to appoint a co-ordinating body for the nursing profession. They therefore recommended in their report in September 1938, that a Central Emergency Committee for the nursing profession, similar to the Central Medical War Committee for the medical profession, should be set up.

ORGANISATION OF THE CIVIL NURSING RESERVE

Part VII of the Civil Defence Act required the Minister of Health to make arrangements for the training in advance, in nursing, of persons willing to offer their services in the event of war. The services for which they were specially wanted were new or enlarged hospitals for the treatment of casualties, first-aid posts, and for district nursing in the reception areas, where the health services had to be expanded on account of the Government evacuation scheme.

THE CENTRAL NURSING EMERGENCY COMMITTEE

A Central Emergency Committee was set up early in December 1938, under the chairmanship of Sir Malcolm Delevingne; Miss Z. L. Puxley, O.B.E., of the Ministry of Health, was appointed secretary to the committee. Members of the committee included representatives from the General Nursing Council, the Royal College of Nursing, the Women's Voluntary Services, the Matrons-in-Chief of the Navy, Army and Air Force, and representatives from the County Councils Associations, the Association of Municipal Corporations and the London County Council. The functions of the Central Emergency Committee were to ascertain what nursing personnel was available in the employment of hospitals and institutions, and to compile a register of all other nurses and assistant nurses, and a register of nursing auxiliaries. The members of this register became known as the Civil Nursing Reserve. The three categories of trained nurses, assistant nurses and nursing auxiliaries were sub-divided into (*a*) mobile members prepared to serve anywhere in England and Wales; (*b*) immobile whole-time members prepared to serve locally only (including as a special class those who volunteered to serve in specified districts); and (*c*) immobile part-time members. The Central Emergency Committee approved a distinctive badge in silver and blue for issue to all members of the Civil Nursing Reserve. It also approved indoor uniform for the three grades of nursing members enrolled in the Reserve. Standard rates of pay and conditions of service were drawn up, and it was made clear that authorities who wished to use the services of members of the Reserve must observe these rates and conditions.

Many retired trained nurses and assistant nurses, married and unmarried, came forward for enrolment, and many V.A.D.s of the War of 1914–18 again offered their services, which were gladly accepted. Arrangements were made to train as nursing auxiliaries, women without previous nursing experience who wished to join the Reserve.

There were also available for services at first-aid posts women trained in first-aid only, who were registered by the local authorities and were not included in the Civil Nursing Reserve. Those, however, who desired, could qualify for membership of the Civil Nursing Reserve by undertaking the course of instruction and practical work in hospital which formed the second part of the training of the nursing auxiliary.

As the Civil Nursing Reserve was formed to supplement existing services, and as it was desired to prevent those already engaged in essential nursing duties from giving up their appointments to join the Reserve, certain conditions of enrolment were imposed. Trained nurses in a hospital of any kind or in any other form of public health service, in district nursing, or in industrial nursing, were ineligible, as were also assistant nurses employed in public institutions.

By the end of June 1939, some 7,500 trained nurses and 2,900 assistant nurses had been enrolled, and 45,000 women had applied for training as nursing auxiliaries. In addition, about 24,000 immobile nursing members of Voluntary Aid Detachments were released from their Service obligations so that they might become available as nursing auxiliaries.

The local work of the Reserve, in connection with recruiting, training and registration, was assigned to Local Emergency Organisations which were set up in each county and county borough, with the medical officer of health in charge, and which worked under the direction of the Central Emergency Committee in London. In London and elsewhere the Women's Voluntary Services undertook, on behalf of the Local Emergency Organisation, the arrangements for the selection and preliminary training of those nursing auxiliary applicants who did not join the British Red Cross Society or St. John Ambulance Brigade, and for their subsequent hospital experience.

It was intended that the Civil Nursing Reserve in any county or county borough should be organised in teams or units, and allocated in advance to the particular sphere of work in which they would be called upon to serve in an emergency. Thus organised, the members of a unit would, when emergency arose, know in advance where and for what duty they were required.

Local Emergency Organisations were advised to set up small advisory committees to assist with the local work of administering the Reserve, and it was suggested that the composition of these committees should include representatives of the hospitals and the medical professions, the local branch of the Royal College of Nursing, and members of the

Women's Voluntary Services, British Red Cross Society and St. John Ambulance Brigade. Where these advisory committees were set up, they assisted the Local Emergency Organisation with the work of selecting and training nursing auxiliaries, scrutinising application forms, interviewing candidates and assessing their suitability for nursing. The main points for consideration were age, health, physique and intelligence. Offers of part-time as well as full-time service were welcomed.

These committees started to function early in 1939 and gave valuable advice and assistance to Local Emergency Organisations.

THE TRAINING OF NURSING AUXILIARIES

Training was in two parts and was given free. The first part comprised two courses of instruction, one in first aid and one in home nursing, on the same lines as the training in those subjects given to persons joining the St. John or Red Cross organisations. Red Cross and St. John members who joined the Civil Nursing Reserve and had already taken either or both these courses were excused from taking them again.

The second part was a course of instruction and practical work in hospital, common to all candidates, including members of the St. John and Red Cross organisations. This instruction was given as far as possible at recognised training schools for nurses. In order to qualify in this part of the training, candidates were required to attend the hospital for at least fifty hours within a period of six months, but it was recommended that where possible, attendances should cover ninety-six hours, and that the minimum period of continuous attendance should be two hours. Where a candidate was able to give a longer continuous period of attendance, and so complete the course in a shorter period of time, this was encouraged. Overalls and caps were provided. At the end of the course of instruction the matron of the hospital was asked to report on the attendances and work of the candidate. On receiving a satisfactory report from the matron, the Local Emergency Organisation informed the Central Emergency Committee that the candidate had qualified for enrolment as a nursing auxiliary and entered her name in the appropriate section of the local register; and a certificate of enrolment and badge were issued to the candidate by the Central Emergency Committee.

The object of the hospital experience given to each nursing auxiliary was to fit her to assist the trained nursing staff in carrying out routine ward duties, and thereby to release as many of the trained staff as possible for staffing other expanded or new hospitals, and to free those remaining for supervising nursing activities in the ward. It was realised that only by this dilution of existing staff could the necessary numbers of nursing personnel be secured for the working of the Emergency Hospital Scheme.

The position of the nursing auxiliary was clearly defined as being that of an emergency aid to a nursing staff in time of war, and as such she was distinct from the student nurse in training and the ward domestic staff. The course of instruction in simple nursing procedure and ward routine was drawn up with a view to making her familiar with hospital atmosphere and enabling her to cultivate a quiet assurance and the ability to carry out instructions deftly and correctly with an understanding of their purpose and importance. Hospital authorities co-operated willingly in this scheme and, at the outbreak of war, there was already a considerable reserve of nursing auxiliaries trained to undertake hospital and other duties.

At a later date, during the course of the war, it was found convenient to organise, in place of the two-part courses, combined intensive courses in hospital. The courses lasted a fortnight. The syllabus covered was generally the same as in the two-part courses.

THE OUTBREAK OF WAR

The Sector Matrons and Distribution of Nursing Staff. With the declaration of war the Emergency Hospital Scheme came into operation, the evacuation of some hospitals, the opening up or expansion of others, and distribution of staff and equipment, followed according to pre-arranged plans. To assist the Group Officers at Sector headquarters in the area of their Groups, matrons had been appointed, called, on the analogy of the special Emergency Hospital arrangements in the London Region, *Sector Matrons*. They were, in general, the matrons of large voluntary training schools. There were ten Sector Matrons for the London Sectors; six Sector Matrons were subsequently—in August, 1939—appointed in the Provinces, namely—Birmingham, Liverpool, Manchester, Leeds, Bristol and Newcastle. The function of the Sector Matrons was to arrange the distribution of nursing staff between hospitals and generally to supervise all matters affecting nurses, the controlling authority of each hospital remaining responsible for internal administration. They helped in planning the distribution of nurses and the general arrangements in the short time available before war broke out. Their work was co-ordinated by the Principal Matron of the Civil Nursing Reserve, Miss K. C. Watt, C.B.E., R.R.C. (afterwards D.B.E.), who was appointed in June 1939, to the Ministry of Health. In the London Sectors, each Sector Matron had working with her a matron from the L.C.C. nursing staff, who acted as a channel of communication between the Sector Matron and the local authority hospitals on nursing matters, and acted with the Sector Matron in maintaining a proper distribution of nursing personnel throughout the Sector. Despite the many initial difficulties, arrangements proceeded more or less satisfactorily when the emergency came, and the spirit of co-operation and willingness to help did much to pave the way for smooth functioning. Great adjustments of nursing staff had to be made in the London Sectors. Base hospitals and advanced base hospitals had to be staffed by nurses from the inner hospitals supplemented by members of the Civil Nursing Reserve. With the reduction of hospital beds in London and the opening up of large numbers of additional beds in hospitals in the outer zones of the Sectors, trained and student nurses were transferred from their accustomed surroundings to strange hospitals whose administration was often very different from that of their parent hospital.

THE CONTINUATION OF TRAINING

The question of continuation of training had received considerable thought, and it was recognised that training should be continued unless the intensity of war conditions made it impossible to do so. When, therefore, the expected aerial bombardment of London did not come immediately arrangements were made to preserve continuity of training for those student nurses who had been evacuated to other hospitals. Many of these receiving hospitals had not previously been recognised as training schools and consequently had neither accommodation nor facilities for teaching student nurses. Sister tutors had to be distributed to the best advantage and teaching equipment transferred or borrowed. Considering all these difficulties it is interesting to note that it was necessary to postpone only one State Examination—that scheduled to take place in November 1939. Since that date State Examinations continued to take place regularly, although they were reduced in number each year.

THE STAFFING OF THE HOSPITALS

On the outbreak of war, members of the Civil Nursing Reserve were called up by the Sector Matrons in the London Region, and by the local emergency organisations in the provinces, and were distributed to the hospitals and other services to which they had received prior notice of allocation. In general, the members responded well to the call for service, although some dropped out owing to home and other circumstances. The twenty casualty evacuation trains stationed round London, and three in the provinces, had to be brought into commission immediately. The staff for each of these trains had been previously fixed as three trained nurses, ten nursing auxiliaries and eight male orderlies. No nursing auxiliaries were at that time available for these posts and the Joint War Organisation of the British Red Cross Society and the St. John Ambulance Association on appeal furnished all the nursing auxiliaries for staffing the trains. For hospital service the response from trained nurses, assistant nurses and others with nursing experience, was magnificent. The letters received from members anxious to give their services numbered about 2,000 a day. Telephone calls were extremely numerous and there was a continuous stream of callers at the Ministry of Health and at the Headquarters of the Civil Nursing Reserve of people who wished to be mobilised for nursing service. Many of the offers of service were of no great value, but it showed an excellent spirit in people who wanted to serve in hospitals.

There were many difficulties in fitting square pegs into round holes during the uncertain course of the war, with its change of plans and the long periods of relative inactivity. The task of fitting in staff who were members of the Civil Nursing Reserve was no easy matter. Many trained nurses sent to the hospitals were recruited from the ranks of retired nurses, and without their help the hospitals could not have carried on so well in the early days of the war, and during the rush that followed the evacuation from Dunkirk and the severe air raids of the year 1940–1. Accommodation for the nurses was not always adequate, particularly as a result of the upgrading of hospitals and the consequent increase in the number of beds and of nursing staff required in these hospitals. This meant problems arising out of the blackout, crowded dormitories and dining rooms, lack of facilities for recreation, and difficulties in transport, intensified by war conditions. Nurses faced these conditions well, and a special word of praise is due to all members of hospital staffs, trained nurses and nurses in training, who were transferred from their parent hospital to other hospitals, and who had to adapt themselves to the different conditions of work and living and fit into new surroundings.

One of the greatest difficulties in connexion with the Civil Nursing Reserve was to secure an even distribution of personnel. Attempts to secure a more even distribution were often frustrated by the fact that so many members were not able or not willing to serve outside their home districts. Figures available at the end of June 1941, showed a total of 48,627 whole-time Civil Nursing Reserve members, of whom 12,139 were mobile and 36,488 immobile.

SUBSEQUENT DEVELOPMENTS

The Civil Nursing Reserve Advisory Council. In January 1940, the Central Emergency Committee completed its initial task of organisation of the Civil Nursing Reserve, and was dissolved. Its executive functions were transferred to the Ministry of Health and its advisory functions entrusted to a new body—the Civil Nursing Reserve Advisory Council, under the chairmanship of Miss Florence Horsbrugh, C.B.E., M.P., Parliamentary Secretary to the Ministry. Meetings of the Council took place every three months. When the Central Emergency Committee was dissolved, the local emergency organisations, which had been set up to administer the Reserve in each county and county borough, remained in being.

THE REGIONAL NURSING OFFICERS

In order to co-ordinate the work in Regions it was considered essential to strengthen the organisation by appointing Regional Nursing Officers at the Ministry of Health Regional Offices. These Regional Nursing Officers were appointed in January 1940. Their main duties were to supervise the local working of the Civil Nursing Reserve, to assist hospitals that met special nursing difficulties, to promote recruitment of nurses within the Region, to maintain a proper balance of staff between the different hospitals, and generally to promote the efficiency of the nursing services, visit hospitals and keep in touch with the medical officers of health and organisations such as the Red Cross and Order of St. John and the Women's Voluntary Services. They took over the work of allocating mobile members of the Reserve. Local emergency organisations continued to allocate the immobile members, as well as doing the general work connected with the enrolment of members and the training of nursing auxiliaries.

The work of the Regional Nursing Officers continued to increase, particularly from the time of the Dunkirk crisis when staff had to be transferred rapidly from one hospital to another and from Region to Region. It was necessary therefore to appoint Deputy Regional Nursing Officers in addition.

PROGRESS OF RECRUITMENT

At the time of the Dunkirk crisis, Miss Horsbrugh made a broadcast appeal for more volunteers for the Civil Nursing Reserve, particularly trained nurses. A good response followed the appeal from trained nurses and assistant nurses, and during the quarter ended June 30, 1940, over 2,000 new members of these two grades were enrolled in the Reserve. This was the largest number of either grade recruited in any quarter since the initial rush of volunteers.

In January 1941, it was decided to issue to nursing auxiliaries a red star to be worn on the uniform, indicating completion of one year's satisfactory service in the Reserve. In March 1942, further arrangements were made by which a nursing auxiliary could, in addition, become eligible for a blue star, showing that she had gained special experience by giving a specified amount of service in a sanatorium or tuberculosis hospital, or an infectious diseases hospital. At this time also, it was arranged to extend the awards for satisfactory service to trained and assistant nurses. The former became eligible for a red stripe for each year of satisfactory service and for blue stripes for special experience in the nursing of tuberculous or infectious patients; the latter became eligible in the same way for red and blue stars.

In January 1941, it was necessary to find additional staff for isolation hospitals, tuberculosis hospitals and sanatoria, for expected large seasonal increase in infectious diseases, which gave considerable anxiety as to how patients were to be nursed. The Minister of Health, then Mr. Malcolm MacDonald, broadcast another appeal to nurses, especially those with training and experience in fever and tuberculosis. The response amounted to about 900 trained and assistant nurses and women without any experience offering their services. After enquiries, 400 of these were referred to the local medical officers of health.

In March 1941, generally speaking, there was an adequate nursing staff in the hospitals included in the Emergency Hospital Scheme for the number of beds occupied, and also to meet the first demands that any sudden emergency might make, but the position was less satisfactory in hospitals outside the Scheme, particularly in infectious diseases hospitals, public assistance institutions and sanatoria, although the position had improved after the Minister's broadcast.

On April 3, 1941, the Minister of Health, Mr. Ernest Brown, repeated in the House of Commons that in hospitals for infectious diseases and sanatoria, and in institutions for the old and infirm, the shortage of nurses in some cases was still acute. He announced that he was arranging with the Minister of Labour to secure that the vital importance of the nursing service would be brought to the notice of girls when they registered, and emphasised the importance of securing a larger number of women prepared to take up nursing as a life career.[1]

Registration of girls and women at the Employment Exchanges helped to maintain a steady flow of student nurses and nursing auxiliaries. The number of names on the general and supplementary parts of the State Register increased from 94,200 in April, 1939, to 103,700 in April, 1942, an increase of 9,500. By March 31, 1943, the total number of nurses on the Register had increased to 108,625. Of these 8,928 appeared twice and 53 three times. After allowance was made for names which appeared two or three times, the total number of nurses on the State Register worked out at 99,591.

THE NURSING DIVISION OF THE MINISTRY OF HEALTH

Early in April 1941, a Nursing Division was specially created within the Ministry of Health to deal with general and professional questions affecting nursing and the supply of midwives. A Chief Nursing Officer was appointed, Miss K. C. Watt, C.B.E., R.R.C. (who was already Principal Matron of the Civil Nursing Reserve), and two Deputy Chief Nursing Officers were added to the Division.

PAY OF THE NURSING SERVICES

The Minister announced in the House of Commons certain changes relating to increases in the rates of pay for Civil Nursing Reserve members, and also a scheme whereby women who were registering and wished to become student nurses would be sent to hospitals paying at least £40 a year with an increase of £5 a year, with free board and lodging, laundry and uniform. He asked hospital authorities throughout the country to review the rates of pay for their nursing staffs in the light of these increases. The Minister also announced that he intended to give effect to one of the most important recommendations of the Athlone Committee by setting up a committee to draw up national salary scales.[1]

THE RUSHCLIFFE COMMITTEE

After consultation with the various organisations interested, this committee was appointed in November 1941, under the chairmanship of Lord Rushcliffe. It consisted of two panels, each with twenty members, representing employers and nurses respectively, and its terms of reference were originally to draw up agreed scales of salary and emoluments for State Registered Nurses in England and Wales in hospitals and in the Public Health services, including the service of district nursing, and for student nurses in hospitals approved as training schools by the General Nursing Council for England and Wales. The Minister agreed that emoluments might be interpreted to include the conditions of service which are closely bound up with salaries, such as hours of work, length of holidays and interchangeability of pensions. Subsequently the terms of reference of the committee were extended to include nurses possessing or studying for the certificate of the Tuberculosis Association, and also assistant nurses. A similar committee, with 24 members, under the same chairman, was set up to draw up agreed scales of salaries and emoluments for midwives, including pupil midwives.

In February 1943, the first report of the Nurses Salaries Committee was issued.[2] It dealt with the salaries and emoluments of female nurses in hospitals. The recommendations of the committee covered salaries, emoluments, certain conditions of service such as hours of duty, annual leave and sick leave. There were also recommendations about the training of sister tutors, training for tuberculosis nursing and the recognition by the General Nursing Council of certificates in different branches of nursing. The committee also considered other classes within its terms of reference—male nurses, public health nurses, district nurses, and trained and assistant nurses in nurseries; a second report from the committee containing their recommendations was issued in December 1943.[3]

THE NURSES ACT, 1943

In March 1943, the Nurses Bill was introduced in the House of Commons after discussions with various nursing and other interested organisations and was passed in April. The Act[4] gave effect to a further series of recommendations of the Athlone Committee. Its main objects were to give a proper status and recognition to the grade of assistant nurses by setting up a Roll under the control of the General Nursing Council, to protect the general public by restricting the use of the title 'nurse' to persons with some nursing qualifications and to bring under control agencies for the supply of nurses. Provision was also made to compile a list of nurses who could have applied for admission to the State Register without examination as existing nurses under the Nurses Registration Act, 1919, but had omitted to apply within the time allowed for the purpose. The restriction on the use of the title 'nurse' was to operate from such date as the Minister directed. This direction was issued in May 1945, with effect from October 15, 1945.[5] After the restriction took effect only State Registered and enrolled assistant nurses were able to use the title 'nurse'; this would enable the public to distinguish between the qualified and unqualified person. An exception was made in the Act in favour of children's nurses, who were allowed to continue to use the title 'nurse' except in circumstances or in a context which would suggest they were something other than children's nurses; the Minister also took power to make other exceptions for the benefit of any particular classes on whom the restriction might operate with undue harshness.

NATIONAL ADVISORY COUNCIL FOR THE RECRUITMENT OF NURSES

Early in 1943, the Minister of Labour and National Service, in consultation with the Minister of Health, set up a National Advisory Council for the recruitment and distribution of nurses and midwives under the chairmanship of Mr. M. S. McCorquodale, M.P., Parliamentary Secretary to the Ministry of Labour and National Service. The object in appointing the council was to consider what measures could be taken to relieve the shortages of nurses and midwives, which had become increasingly acute, largely owing to the demands of other services. Officers of the Ministry of Health attended meetings of the council which included in its membership representatives of nurses, midwives and their employers. The detailed work of the measures decided upon to improve distribution and recruitment was carried out in the Appointments Offices of the Ministry of Labour and National Service, and local Advisory Committees assisted them. The Regional Officers of the Ministry of Health attended the local committees to give help and advice.

On April 10, 1943, on the advice of the National Advisory Council, a national registration of nurses and midwives was carried out. An intensive publicity campaign was also undertaken to improve recruitment.

PROGRESS OF THE CIVIL NURSING RESERVE

The Civil Nursing Reserve on February 1, 1943, was supplying to hospitals 3,297 trained nurses, 2,814 assistant nurses and 12,843 nursing auxiliaries. During 1942, 8,000 women were under review for training as nursing auxiliaries. Other members were employed in first-aid posts, casualty evacuation trains, nurseries, emergency maternity homes and hostels, or were assisting in district nursing and in other health services. Thus, it will be seen that the Civil Nursing Reserve has played a most important part in helping to staff emergency services.

Many shortcomings came to light, but taking into consideration the short time in which the Reserve was brought into existence and the sources from which recruitment was originally made, namely, retired nurses, private nurses, assistant nurses and women without any experience in nursing who had to be instructed, the result was on the whole fairly satisfactory. Had there been more time for planning a civilian Reserve to augment the permanent nursing staffs of hospitals and public health services, and had the expected need not been so large, more time could have been devoted to closer scrutiny of application forms, obtaining references and medical examination of candidates. Such procedure would have eliminated many undesirable candidates who, in a rush of enthusiasm, offered their services for nursing but, from one cause or another, were unsuitable; it was in fact gradually adopted during the progress of the war, and latterly all candidates were most carefully scrutinised.

Early in 1944, preparations were being considered for the landing of troops in France and the inevitable influx of casualties which would result. Schemes were drawn up to send nurses from hospitals in London and elsewhere to the units on the South Coast, and to the reception hospitals at the ports to which the casualties would come—also to the hospitals marked as 'transit hospitals' throughout the South of England. Some 800 civilian nurses were moved, the transfer being carried out in complete secrecy. Nurses, including the Civil Nursing Reserve, prepared for the move without demur, even although it meant a good deal of uprooting and, in some cases, discontinuance of their studies. Throughout the months that followed nurses worked where they were asked to work. Hospitals took in convoys morning, noon and night. As the Minister of Health said in the House of Commons, 'the whole scheme worked most smoothly'. Between D-day and VE-day some 160,000 casualties from North-West Europe passed through E.M.S. hospitals, in addition to more than 20,000 flying bomb casualties in Southern England.[6]

It should be noted that in addition to the reception of British casualties, large numbers of wounded German prisoners-of-war were admitted. The nurses attended these patients most efficiently, and made no distinction between British and enemy casualties.

During the latter part of 1944, the position of the Reserve on the termination of hostilities in Europe was considered. The Civil Nursing

Reserve Advisory Council were consulted and expressed the opinion that, as there was likely to be an acute shortage of nurses after hostilities in Europe ceased, the Reserve should remain in being and recruitment of all grades should continue. This advice was accepted.

The distribution of the Reserve then altered in character owing to the shortage of all types of hospital other than those in the Emergency Hospital Scheme, including sanatoria, public assistance institutions and maternity hospitals. Members of the Civil Nursing Reserve, when they could be spared, were sent to these hospitals.

NURSES FROM CANADA

An offer from Canada of trained nursing personnel was made and accepted. The stipulation made by the Canadian authorities, however, was that trained nurses coming to Britain to join the British Civil Nursing Reserve should be those who were ineligible to join the Canadian Army Nursing Service. Fifty-two trained nurses came. They joined the British Civil Nursing Reserve on the same terms and conditions as members recruited in this country, and gave good service. Most of them were married or were, for other reasons, ineligible for service with the Canadian Army Nursing Service.

A further offer of V.A.D. members was made by the St. John Ambulance Brigade and Red Cross Society in Canada, and was gratefully accepted by the Ministry of Health. These members joined the Reserve on the same conditions as nursing auxiliary members, most of them guaranteeing to serve for one year, and many giving more than a year's guarantee. In September 1946, all the St. John members and all but five of the Red Cross members returned to Canada, the latter intending to stay until January 1947.

During 1945, the shortage of nurses and midwives continued, and the vacancies at one time reached the figure of 32,000 nurses.

General and special hospitals suffered badly through lack of nursing staff, and also acutely through lack of domestic staff. Nurses in many cases had to do much more domestic work than was desirable. Matrons and nurses in the hospitals gave most efficient service, and rose to every occasion, but despite their efforts beds had to be closed.

DISTRIBUTION OF AVAILABLE NURSING PERSONNEL THROUGHOUT THE WAR

The following tables give some information as to the distribution of the available nursing personnel to meet the demands of the civil population, the civil hospitals and the Services during the period of the war. Mental and maternity nurses are excluded from these figures:

CIVIL NURSING SERVICES IN WAR-TIME

PRE-WAR DISTRIBUTION

TABLE I

Numbers of Beds and Nursing Staff Employed in the Civil Hospitals in England and Wales on January 1, 1939

Total number of beds	Approx. number of occupied beds	Nursing staff employed			
		Trained nurses	Assistant nurses	Student nurses	Total
270,587	216,700	25,036	15,879	30,602	71,517

The estimated numbers of trained and untrained nurses employed in industrial and private nursing were, in each case 4,000 and 6,000 respectively. Exact figures are not available.

The approximate maximum number of trained and untrained nurses potentially available from which to meet the requirements of a war was therefore 51,000 trained and assistant nurses and 40,000 untrained nurses of all categories, plus an unknown number of retired nurses from which recruits might be obtained.

DISTRIBUTION DURING THE WAR

TABLE II

Civil Hospitals: Numbers of Beds and Nursing Staff Trained and Untrained Employed in the Civil Hospitals in England and Wales at Various Dates during the War:

Date	Total no. of beds	Total no. of beds occupied	Nursing staff employed					
			Trained nurses	Assistant nurses	Student nurses	Other trainees	Nursing auxiliaries	Totals
March 1, 1942	408,864	240,582	28,573	15,868	30,903	3,649	11,316	90,309
February 1, 1943	401,901	243,372	27,215	14,266	33,518	3,670	12,843	91,512
February 1, 1944	393,166	248,628	26,687	15,302	38,343	3,513	12,545	96,390
February 1, 1945	393,255	259,158	27,278	15,281	36,861	3,400	11,882	94,702
August 1, 1945	363,925	242,599	26,977	15,767	35,522	3,010	8,871	90,147
November 1, 1945	350,708	240,127	25,685	15,731	36,212	3,054	6,753	87,435

From these tables it will be seen that the number of trained nurses employed in the civil hospitals was considerably higher than in the pre-war period, assistant nurses remained about the same, student nurses increased in numbers, and auxiliary help was available in the shape of over 15,000 others. Bed occupancy was increased by an average of about 30,000 beds, mainly due to the admissions of civil and military war casualties.

CIVIL DEFENCE SERVICES

TABLE III

Numbers of Trained Nurses, Whole-time and Part-time Employed in the First-aid Posts—Fixed or Mobile—and the Ambulance Services at Various Dates during the War

	Trained nurses			
	Whole-time		Part-time	
	C. N. R. Mobile and immobile	Others	C. N. R.	Others
March 31, 1940	951	455	624	1,817
March 31, 1941	1,224	408	668	1,766
March 31, 1942	1,184	228	598	1,200
March 31, 1943	961	278	507	1,092
September 30, 1944	727	234	416	936
March 31, 1945	337 (Mobile under 5 per cent. of total)	129	204	359

This table shows that before the reduction of the establishment of the Civil Defence Services began in 1942, the numbers of whole-time nurses employed averaged about 1,500 and part-time nurses 2,300, after which the numbers in both categories gradually diminished with the cessation of widespread enemy attacks. These nurses were almost wholly recruited from retired nurses with domestic ties, which accounts for the large proportion who were only able to serve near their homes.

TABLE IV

Numbers of Auxiliary Nurses Employed in the Civil Defence Services during the War at Various Times:

	Auxiliary nurses			
	Whole-time		Part-time	
	C. N. R. Mobile and immobile	Others	C. N. R.	Others
March 31, 1940	2,768	12,899	7,376	69,134
March 31, 1941	6,394	11,694	11,433	62,465
March 31, 1942	6,742	9,890	10,855	48,629
March 31, 1943	3,944	5,678	9,783	63,507
September 30, 1944	2,889	4,938	7,926	58,734
March 31, 1945	963 (Mobile under 5 per cent. of total)	1,798	3,868	31,556

Here again the figures show that the great majority could only do local duties, and that of these only a small proportion were available for whole-time service.

AUXILIARY HOSPITALS

In addition to the above, 1,581 trained nurses and about 8,000 V.A.D.s were recruited during the war for duty with the 240-odd auxiliary hospitals brought into being and staffed by the Joint War Organisation of the British Red Cross Society and St. John Ambulance Association. Of these the maximum numbers employed at any one time were about 500 trained nurses and 3,500 V.A.D.s. It would appear therefore that on the average over 5,000 more trained nurses were employed in the hospitals and first-aid posts than those serving in the civil hospitals before the war.

TABLE V

The Nursing Services of the Navy, Army and Royal Air Force Annual Strengths 1939–1945

	Royal Navy		Army		Royal Air Force	
	Q.A. R.N.N.S. and reserve (fully trained)	V.A.D.*	Nursing officers (fully trained)	V.A.D.	P.M. R.A.F. N.S. (fully trained)	V.A.D.
Pre-war establishment	87	—	629	—	227	—
At December 31, 1939	312	241	2,390	3,238	249	117
At December 31, 1940	380	497	3,708	2,733	450	157
At December 31, 1941	457	763	4,853	3,682	607	260
At December 31, 1942	658	1,564	6,800	4,456	783	255
At December 31, 1943	892	2,735	8,650	4,548	989	253
At December 31, 1944	1,095	3,824	10,315	4,051	1,215	205
At December 31, 1945	981	3,527	9,340†	3,564†	995	82

* Approximate.
† Number serving at August 31, 1945.

At the peak period at the end of 1944 the Services were employing 12,625 fully trained nurses as compared with 27,278 in the civil hospitals, but the latter, of course, were also employing large numbers of assistant nurses and much larger numbers of auxiliaries and student nurses, without whose services the civil hospitals could not adequately have met the needs of the civil population and of Service patients in the E.M.S. hospitals. The maximum number of trained nurses employed in all Services, at the end of 1944, whole or part-time, was 42,216.

DEMOBILISATION

With the general demobilisation of women from the Forces, it was decided in 1946 to release members of the Civil Nursing Reserve in accordance with a scheme of release from the Reserve which had been drawn up and announced at the end of 1945, the date of release depending on the length of service given, and whether this was mobile or immobile.[7] Members were allowed to take their release, although their attention was drawn to the serious shortage of nurses, and every encouragement was given to them to remain in the Reserve.

At June 30, 1946, the numbers in the Reserve were 1,824 trained nurses, 2,540 assistant nurses, and 6,291 nursing auxiliaries.

The Civil Nursing Reserve remained in being, but it was decided that in addition a National Reserve of Nurses should be set up to deal with emergencies arising in peace-time. The composition of this new Reserve would be the same as that of the Civil Nursing Reserve, namely, trained nurses, assistant nurses and nursing auxiliaries. These would be drawn from nurses who have retired from the nursing profession and from those who could serve in an emergency. No trained nurse or assistant nurse serving in a hospital or health service would be eligible for enrolment.

A great tribute must be paid to members of the permanent staffs of hospitals, members of the Civil Nursing Reserve, and to all nurses and midwives who served both in hospitals in the Emergency Scheme and in other spheres, including those in the Public Health Services, in district work in maternity hospitals and special hospitals, for the valuable contribution they made during the war years, for their unselfish devotion to duty and the work they carried out under most difficult conditions.

Members of the nursing and midwifery professions gave little heed to themselves, but at all times put the welfare of their patients before all else.

Tribute should also be paid to all Matrons and to Sector Matrons, for their unselfish and devoted service.

REFERENCES

[1] *Parliamentary Debates*, 5th Series, Vol. 370, *House of Commons Official Report*, April 3, 1941, Col. 1169. (370 H.C. Deb. Col. 1169).
[2] *First Report of the Nurses Salaries Committee.* Cmd. 6424. H.M.S.O., February, 1943.
[3] *Second Report of the Nurses Salaries Committee.* Cmd. 6487. H.M.S.O., December, 1943.
[4] The Nurses Act, 1943. (6 and 7 Geo. 6. c. 17).
[5] *Statutory Rules and Orders*, 1945, No. 637, May 31, 1945.
[6] *Parliamentary Debates*, 5th Series, Vol. 411, *House of Commons Official Report*, June 12, 1945, Col. 1525. (411 H.C. Deb. Col. 1525).
[7] Min. of Health Circular 229/45, December 31, 1945.

INDEX

Airborne casualties, reception and distribution, 157, 289
Aircraft, crashed, training in rescue of crews from, 257
Air raid casualties, civilian, in U.S. military hospitals, 189
    in London, recording and notification of, 88
    total, in United Kingdom, 180
    injuries, atlas of, 265
Air Raid Precautions:
    Act, 1937, 8, 223
    Department, 7
    Handbook, 230, 265
    Official Publications on, 206
    organisation of, 223
    services (*see also* Casualty Services), 223
        Assistant Hospital Officers appointed to, 241
        change of title of, 247
        co-ordination of industrial A.R.P. schemes with, 248
        provision of uniforms for, 229
        transfer of direction of technical training in, 239
Air raids on England, first, 242
    in July 1941—December 1942, 143
    during 1943, 145
    during 1944-5, 169, 264
    daylight, on ports and aerodromes, 113
    experiences and lessons of, 117
    lessons learned from, in Civil Defence, 250, 260, 268
    night, on industrial centres, 114
Alien doctors, 65
    employment of, 424
Ambulance(s), 52
    adaptation of stretcher fitments for, 247
    American (Plate XXXV), 302
    river, 307
    Services (Plates XXIX–XXXV), 276–308
        authorised unit establishment of, 248
        local, separation from Fire Service control, 249
Ambulance trains (Plates XXIX–XXXIII), 276
    description of (Plates XXX–XXXIII), 279
    detraining from, 163
    disbandment of, 290
    equipment and food supplies, 281
    in evacuation of hospital patients, 277
    maintenance and control, 280
    numbers and location of, 278
    number of patients carried, 290
    operations, 282
    personnel, 280
    preparations for D-day, 285
    in transport of casualties, 277
    types of cases carried, 285
    transport, British assistance to U.S. military personnel in, 189
    inter-hospital (Plate XXXIV), 290
American Ambulance (Plate XXXV), 302
    Hospital in Britain, 433
    Red Cross–Harvard Field Hospital Unit, 435
Anti-coagulants, 342
Anti-gas precautions, 244
Army Educational personnel, 138
    physical training coaches, 385
Artificial limbs, supply of, 127
'Athlone' committee, 438
Auxiliary hospitals, nurses in, 453

Battle of Britain (Plates VII–IX), 113
Bedstate returns, 1940, 113
Belgium, Medical Services of, in Great Britain, 190
Blind, treatment of, 73
Blood group determination, 343
Blood Transfusion Service:
    civilian (Figs. 6–10), 334–355
    general commentary, 355
    London, 334
        administration of, 335
        apparatus of (Figs. 6–10), 338
        development of depots, 344
        donors of, 336, 353
        recipients of, 337
        records of, 336
        research by depots, 344
        staffing depots of, 335
    pre-war organisations, 334
    provision of, 42
    Regional, 113, 347
        apparatus, 352
        progress of scheme, 349
        work of centres, 351
'Bomb alley', 175
Britain, period of active operations in, May 1940—July 1941 (Plates V–IX), 96–124
British Expeditionary Force, evacuation from France (Plates V, VI), 100
Buildings, protection of, 43
Burns, first-aid treatment of, 266

Cambridge Infiltration and Drying Plant, work of, 354
Canada, nurses from, 450
Casualties (see also Air Raid Casualties; Civilian Casualties)
    accommodation for, July 1941, 122
    admission to port hospital, 161
    airborne, reception and distribution, 157

INDEX

Casualties among Civil Defence Casualty Service units, 273
   documentation of, on ambulance trains, 288
   labelling of, 258
   plan for reception of, from invasion of continent, 151, 156
      for transport of, by train (Plate XXIX), 277
   recording, 86
   seaborne, 152
   total, in United Kingdom, 180
   treated by Civil Defence Casualty Services, 249, 257, 260, 272
Casualty beds, 90
   variations in numbers available, 91, 93
   Bureaux, 51
   Evacuation trains (see Ambulance Trains)
   Hospital Scheme, London (Fig. 4), 44
   organisation, early steps to create, 7–28
Casualty Services, Civil Defence:
   (See also Air Raid Precautions Services, 51 (Plates XVI–XXVII), 221–275)
   awards to, 274
   casualties among, 273
      treated by, 249, 257, 260, 272
   changes in organisation of, 253
   consolidation and training of, 240
   consultant adviser to, 242
   co-ordination of, with Home Guard medical organisation, 248
   direction of new part-time entrants into, 254
   early organisation and policy, 1925–39, 221
   enrolment of personnel for, 225
   first years of active warfare, 1940–41, 240
   formation of headquarters staff of, 246
   issue of metal stretchers to, 229
   local authorities and (Fig. 5), 223
   middle years, 1942–43, 253
   Ministry of Health and, 225
   mobile units of, 228
   at outbreak of war, 230
   personnel, discipline among, 263
      and vehicles, standards of accommodation, 261
      reduction of whole-time, 255
      training of, 256
   preparedness of, prior to outbreak of war, 229
   reduction in, 266
   renewed heavy raids, flying bombs and rockets, 264
   requirements for London, 221
   service badges and markings of, 247
   strength of, at close of enemy attacks, 273
   work of, 1940–41, 250
      1942, 260
      1944–45, 268
Central Medical War Committee, 404
   Nursing Emergency Committee, 439
Children's hospitals, 92

Civil Defence Act, 1939, 53
   Casualty Services (see Casualty Services)
   Rescue School, 266
   Reserve, 249, 255
   Services, demobilisation in, 196
      nurses in, 452
      reorganisation of, 144
      rôle of, during invasion, 129
   Nursing Reserve, 439
      progress of, 448
      of recruitment, 445
      services in war-time, 438–454
Civilian admissions to hospital, 1944, 1945, 183, 185
   E.M.S., 144, 146
   Blood Transfusion Service (Figs. 6–10), 334–355
   casualties, recording, 86
      treatment of, 71
   evacuation trains, 65
   sick, reflux of, 68
   relaxation of restrictions on admissions of, 166
   transferred, 70
   treatment of, 67
Coastal and transit hospitals, 153
Conscription of practitioners, 112, 389, 410
Consultant Advisers at E.M.S. Headquarters, 207
   in port hospital, 162
Convalescent depots, 84
Convoy hospitals, expansion of, 83
Cross-channel shelling, 180, 264
Crushing or crush injury, 259

D-day, preparations of ambulance trains for, 285
   radiological, 364
Daylight raids on ports and aerodromes, 113
Decentralisation, 105
Decontamination, rescue and first-aid parties, interchangeability of, 244
   units, 52, 136
Demobilisation, 195
   of nurses, 454
Dental Committees, Central, 22
   treatment, 74
Doctors, demobilisation of, 196
   incident, 245
Domiciliary medical attendance, 72
Drugs, national reserve of, 321

Electro-diagnosis, 379
Emergency Hospitals Commission, 103
   Pathological Services, 326–333
   Service (see Hospital Service)
      quantities of supplies obtained under lend-lease for, 324
Emergency Medical Services:
   administrative changes, 1941, 125
   administration and personnel, 109
   civilian transferred patients, 209
   classes of patients, 210
      in hospital, 216

INDEX

Emergency Medical Services :
  expansion of (Figs. 1–4), 29–60
  further expansion and organisation, 61–95
  July 1941, 122
  May 1, 1940, 94
  medical personnel of, 55, 62
  at outbreak of war, 58
  period of active operations (Plates XVII–XXVI), 149, 218
    consolidation and improvement, July 1941–December 1943, 125–148
  physical medicine in, 367
  quantities of supplies bought centrally for, 323
Evacuation of B.E.F. from France, 100
  of chronic sick, 121
  of hospitals in invasion area, 106
  of patients from transit hospital, 165
  of population in invasion area, 106, 107
  scheme, medical supplies for, 317
  trains, civilian, 65
Eve's 'rocking' method of resuscitation, 259

First-aid equipment for London heavy and light rescue parties, 260
  parties, uniforms for, 244
  party equipment panel, 243
  points, up-grading of, 246
  post and ambulance services, authorised unit establishment of, 248
    male personnel of, 243
    first-aid parties, etc., equipment of, 254
    medical establishment of, 65
    reduction of numbers of fixed, 247
  and Rescue Party Services, amalgamation of, 257
  rescue and decontamination parties, interchangeability of, 244
  training, intensification of, 242
  modifications in, 240
  treatment of burns, 266
  of fractures of spine, 266
  units, light mobile, 247
  mobile, 52
Flying bombs (Plates XI, XVI–XXIV), 170, 264, 298
Fracture clinics, 370
  institution of special centres for treatment of, 126
  of spine, first-aid treatment, 266
France, evacuation of B.E.F. from (Plates V, VI), 100
Francis sub-committee, 222
Free French Naval Forces, 191

Gas casualties, treatment of, 75, 135
Gas-cleansing units, mobile, 246
Gastric cases, military, investigation of, 86
'Goodwin' Committee, 9
'Green belt' scheme, 109
Gymnasia, 370
Gymnastic and games equipment, 379

Health, Ministry of, and casualty services, 225
  Nursing Division of, 446
Home base hospitals, 158
  Guard medical organisation, co-ordination of Civil Defence Casualty Services, 248
  Office, Air Raid Precautions Department of, 7
  Security, formation of, Ministry of, 240
Hospital(s) accommodation, 29
  May 1940–July 1941, 96
  1942, 1943, 145, 147
  1944, 1945, 181, 184
  increase of (Plate I, Figs. 1–3), 32, 104
  American, in Britain, 433
  ancillary services for, 42
  auxiliary, nurses in, 453
  in Battle of Britain (Plates VII–IX), 117
  casualties evacuated from France admitted to, 100
  children's, 92
  clearance, 61
  coastal, 153
  convoy, expansion of, 83
  demobilisation in, 195
  effect of conscription of practitioners on, 389
  of demobilisation of doctors on, 197
  E.M.S., patients admitted to, for disabilities due to enemy action, 218
    not due to enemy action, 217
  rehabilitation policy in, 136
  rôle of, during invasion, 129
  Service, 128
    and civilian admissions to, 144
    treatment of U.S. military personnel in, 188
  equipment, 20
  evacuation of London, 289
  in invasion area, evacuation of, 106
  medical establishment of, 64
  mental, 30
  patients, plans for evacuation of, by train, 277
  pool, 63
  port, 159
  reclassification of, 29
  returns of casualties, 90
  Schemes, London, 19
    Casualty (Fig. 4), 44
    publication of, 44
    Regional, 18
  segregation of service cases in, 84
Hospital Services, 14
  administrative responsibility, June 1918, 16
  advances and improvements in, 149
  Emergency, September 1938, 27
  long-term policy, 29
  short-term policy in provinces, 17
  special centres, additional, 150
  May 1940–July 1941, 96
Hospital(s), staffing of, 443
  Survey, January–May 1938, 14
  suspended or withdrawn, 92

INDEX

Hospital(s) Territorial Army General, 15
    transit (*see* Transit Hospitals)
    with wards for officers, 84
Hutted annexes and hospitals, 91

Imperial Defence, Committee of, 3
Incident control, 259
    doctor, 245
    Inquiry Points, 265
Industrial workers, recuperative treatment for, 149
Inter-hospital ambulance transport (Plate XXXIV), 290
    in action, 293
    during flying bomb attacks, 298
    in 1944, 297
    in 1945, 298
    number of patients carried, 304
    in provinces, 301
Invasion, action to be taken on, 212
    arrangements for ambulance trains in case of, 284
    of continent of Europe, medical arrangements, 151
    co-ordination of civil and military medical services during, 129
    medical arrangements in area considered liable to, 106

Labour and National Service, Ministry of, rehabilitation scheme of, 137
Lectures on special subjects, courses of, 126
Lend-lease, medical supplies obtained under, 324
Lister Institute, work of, 354
London, air raid casualties in, recording and notification of, 88
    Blood Transfusion Scheme, 334
    Casualty Hospital Scheme (Fig. 4), 44
        services requirements for, 221
    heavy and light rescue parties, first-aid equipment for, 260
    hospitals, evacuation of, 289
        hospital scheme for, 19
        inception of Pathological Services scheme in, 326
        inter-hospital ambulance fleet, 291
        organisation changes in, 110
    return of hospital patients to, 290
Long-range rocket (Plates XXV, XXVI), 177, 264
Lung irritant gases, 135

'MacNalty' Committee, 12
Masseurs, 376
Medical arrangements for invasion of continent of Europe, 151
    Boards, 85
    conscription, 112, 389, 410
    establishment of first-aid posts, 65
        of hospitals, 64
    Officers of Health, work of, 274
    personnel, 53, 62
    administrative and clinical establishments, 388
    allocated to invasion area, 106
    (Priority) Committee, 394, 397
    provision of, 21, 388–437
    registration, temporary, 426, 430, 432
    Services of Allied forces in Great Britain, 190
        co-ordination of civil and military during invasion, 129
    students, teaching of, 50
Medical supplies, 309–325
    assistance from America and other sources, 317
    basis of supply, 310
    deterioration problems, 319
    developments in scope of arrangements, 315
    difficulties of, 312
    establishment of central stores, 313
    for evacuation scheme, 317
    headquarters organisation, 310
    method of acquisition of, 312
    policy and organisation, 309
    problems arising through war-time restrictions, 319
    special arrangements, 314
        maintenance arrangements, 315
    stock records, 318
    volume of, 322
Mental hospitals, 30
Mobile, first-aid units, 52
    light, 247
    gas-cleansing units, 246
    surgical teams, 63
Mobilisation, 61
Mortuary service, 238, 256
Munich Agreement, period of crisis leading to, 25

National Advisory Council for recruitment of nurses, 448
    Civil Defence Rescue School, 266
    War formulary, 128
Nurses Act, 1943, 447
    demobilisation of, 454
    from Canada, 450
    recruitment of, 445, 448
    shortage of, 438
Nursing auxiliaries, training of, 441, 443
    Division of Ministry of Health, 446
    personnel, 66
        distribution of, throughout war, 450
        provision of, 22
    Services, civil, in war-time, 438–454
        pay of, 446
Norway, Medical Services of, in Great Britain, 192

Occupational therapy, 384
    quantity of items supplied for, 325
Operational orders for outbreak of war, 57
Optical Committee, Central, 23
Out-patients, 386
Oxygen supplies, 135

INDEX

Park Prewett Hospital, administration arrangement at, while acting as transit hospital, 163
Pathological Services:
  inception of scheme in London area, 326
  lessons learnt from working of scheme, 331
  provision of, 42
  scheme in provincial regions, 329
Pathology, teaching of, 329
Penicillin, 162
Pharmaceutical War Committee, Central, 24
Physical medicine:
  (Plates XXXVI-XLI), 366-387
  advisory committees, 380
  comparative survey, 380
  diploma in, 385
  equipment, 377
  extension of outlook and scope, 383
  lessons for future, 383
  medical personnel, 372
  service, accommodation, 367, 372
    organisation, 367
  specialist advice, 372
  technical personnel, 374
Physical training, 151
  coaches, Army, 385
Physiotherapy (see also Physical Medicine), 74, 151
  hut, standard, 368
  refresher courses, 376
  schools, training in, 384
  training in, 375
Poland, Medical Services of, in Great Britain, 193
Pool hospitals, 63
Port hospital, working of, 159
Practitioners, conscription of, 112, 389, 410
Psychoneurotic and psychotic persons, resettlement of, 150

Radiographers, 363
Radiology, 356-365
  difficulties to be overcome, 360
  general commentary, 365
  supply of apparatus, 356
  types of apparatus supplied, 358
  unforeseen features of, 364
Radiological services, provision of, 42
Radiologists, training of, 362
Radio-therapeutic centres, 143
Radium, protection and treatment (Plates II-IV), 76
Recuperative treatment for industrial workers, 149
Regional Blood Transfusion Service, 113
  boundaries, 42
    alterations in, 112
  Hospital Schemes, 18
  Nursing Officers, 445
Regions, organisation of, 48
  renumbering of, 42

Registration, temporary medical, 426, 430, 432
Rehabilitation, 136, 137, 371
  residential, 386
Remedial exercises, quantity of items supplied for, 325
Rescue, first-aid and decontamination parties, interchangeability of, 244
  Party Services, amalgamation of, 257
  Parties, London heavy and light, first-aid equipment for, 260
    uniforms for, 244
  School, National Civil Defence, 266
  Service, basic and operational training for, 265
Resuscitation, 162
  Eve's 'rocking' method, 259
River ambulances, 307
  Emergency Service, 249
'Robinson' Committee, 390
Rocket, long-range (Plates XXV, XXVI), 177, 264
Rushcliffe Committee, 447

Seaborne casualties, 152
  admissions to E.M.S. hospitals, 144, 146
  casualties admitted to E.M.S. hospitals, 100
  hospitals, E.M.S., 128
  sick and casualties, disposal of, 80, 81
    recording, 88
    treatment of, 80
  special centres for, 85
  transportation of, 85
Services, liaison of E.M.S. with, 110
  need for rapid rehabilitation in, 136
Shelling, cross-Channel, 180, 264
Shipwrecked sailors, treatment of, 73
Southampton, Gosport, Portsmouth transit and coastal hospital scheme, 154
Spine, fractured, first-aid treatment of, 266
Stretcher fitments, adaptation of, for ambulances, 247
  to take Army type of stretchers, 258
  method of securing patient to, 244
Stretchers, issue of all metal, 229
  method of blanketing, 243
Surgical teams, mobile, 63
Swimming baths, 379

Territorial Army General Hospitals, 15
'Tomlinson' Committee, 138
Tourniquets, 241
Trains, ambulance (see Ambulance Trains)
Transit and coastal hospitals, 153
Transit hospitals:
  administrative arrangements at, 163
  closing of, 289
  port cases in, 162
  treatment in, 166
Transportation of military cases, 85

Ultra short-wave therapy, 378
United States, medical supplies received from, 317, 324
    Military Hospital, civilian air raid casualties in, 189
        in United Kingdom, 187
        personnel treated in E.M.S. hospitals, 188

V.1 (Plates XI, XVI–XXIV), 170, 264, 298
V.2 (Plates XXV, XXVI), 177, 264

Vegetable Drugs Committee, 321
Vehicles, Civil Defence, standards of accommodation, 261

War injuries, treatment of civilian, 71
White Paper, 1939, 56
'Willesden trigglift', 243

X-ray departments, staffing of, 362
    work in port hospital, 162
    workers, protection of, 363